NUTRITION AND DIET RESEARCH PROGRESS

FOOD FOR HUNTINGTON'S DISEASE

NUTRITION AND DIET RESEARCH PROGRESS

Additional books in this series can be found on Nova's website under the Series tab.

Additional e-books in this series can be found on Nova's website under the eBooks tab.

NEURODEGENERATIVE DISEASES - LABORATORY AND CLINICAL RESEARCH

Additional books in this series can be found on Nova's website under the Series tab.

Additional e-books in this series can be found on Nova's website under the eBooks tab.

NUTRITION AND DIET RESEARCH PROGRESS

FOOD FOR HUNTINGTON'S DISEASE

**M. MOHAMED ESSA
T. MANIVASAGAM
A. JUSTIN THENMOZHI
AND
QAZI A. HAMID
EDITORS**

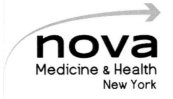

Copyright © 2018 by Nova Science Publishers, Inc.

All rights reserved. No part of this book may be reproduced, stored in a retrieval system or transmitted in any form or by any means: electronic, electrostatic, magnetic, tape, mechanical photocopying, recording or otherwise without the written permission of the Publisher.

We have partnered with Copyright Clearance Center to make it easy for you to obtain permissions to reuse content from this publication. Simply navigate to this publication's page on Nova's website and locate the "Get Permission" button below the title description. This button is linked directly to the title's permission page on copyright.com. Alternatively, you can visit copyright.com and search by title, ISBN, or ISSN.

For further questions about using the service on copyright.com, please contact:
Copyright Clearance Center
Phone: +1-(978) 750-8400   Fax: +1-(978) 750-4470   E-mail: info@copyright.com.

NOTICE TO THE READER

The Publisher has taken reasonable care in the preparation of this book, but makes no expressed or implied warranty of any kind and assumes no responsibility for any errors or omissions. No liability is assumed for incidental or consequential damages in connection with or arising out of information contained in this book. The Publisher shall not be liable for any special, consequential, or exemplary damages resulting, in whole or in part, from the readers' use of, or reliance upon, this material. Any parts of this book based on government reports are so indicated and copyright is claimed for those parts to the extent applicable to compilations of such works.

Independent verification should be sought for any data, advice or recommendations contained in this book. In addition, no responsibility is assumed by the publisher for any injury and/or damage to persons or property arising from any methods, products, instructions, ideas or otherwise contained in this publication.

This publication is designed to provide accurate and authoritative information with regard to the subject matter covered herein. It is sold with the clear understanding that the Publisher is not engaged in rendering legal or any other professional services. If legal or any other expert assistance is required, the services of a competent person should be sought. FROM A DECLARATION OF PARTICIPANTS JOINTLY ADOPTED BY A COMMITTEE OF THE AMERICAN BAR ASSOCIATION AND A COMMITTEE OF PUBLISHERS.

Additional color graphics may be available in the e-book version of this book.

Library of Congress Cataloging-in-Publication Data

ISBN: 978-1-53613-854-2
Library of Congress Control Number: 2018946805

Published by Nova Science Publishers, Inc. † New York

Contents

Preface		ix
Acknowledgments		xi
Chapter 1	The Beneficial Effects of Natural Dietary Products on Neuroprotection *S. Lakshmi, A. Kurian, P. Prakash, A. Firdous and E. Preetham*	1
Chapter 2	Polyphenols and Huntington's Disease *T. Manivasagam, A. Justin Thenmozhi, M. Dhivya Bharathi, T. Sumathi, C. Saravanababu, A. Borah and M. Mohamed Essa*	39
Chapter 3	The Role of Natural Flavonoids in Huntington's Disease *T. Sumathi, A. Justin Thenmozhi and T. Manivasagam*	63
Chapter 4	Spices and Huntington's Disease *R. Balakrishnan, T. Manivasagam, A. Justin Thenmozhi, M. Mohamed Essa and N. Elangovan*	87

Chapter 5	Probiotics, Prebiotics, and Synbiotics on Neurological Disorders: Relevance to Huntington's Disease C. Saravana Babu, N. Chethan, B. Srinivasa Rao, A. Bhat, R. Bipul, A. H. Tousif, M. Mahadevan, S. Sathiya, T. Manivasagam, A. Justin Thenmozhi, M. Mohamed Essa and K.S. Meena	105
Chapter 6	Nutraceuticals: A Novel Neuroprotective Approach against Huntington's Disorder N. J. Dar and R. S. Yadav	141
Chapter 7	Management of Huntington's Disease: Perspectives from the Siddha System of Medicine C. Saravana Babu, M. Mahadevan, B. Srinivasa Rao, V. Ranji, R. Bipul, A. Bhat, N. Chethan, A. H. Tousif, T. Manivasagam, A. Justin Thenmozhi and M. Mohamed Essa	159
Chapter 8	Ascdians as Bioactive Sources for Huntington Disease V. Manigandan, J. Nataraj, V. Arumugam, S. Srivarshini, K. Ramachandran, S. Aruna Devi, S. Umamaheshwari, T. Manivasagam, A. Justin Thenmozhi, and R. Saravanan	181
Chapter 9	Terpenoids and Huntington's Disease R. Balakrishnan, K. Tamilselvam, T. Manivasagam, A. Justin Thenmozhi, M. Mohamed Essa and N. Elangovan	215
Chapter 10	Therapeutic Options for Huntington's Disease: Ayurvedic Medicinal Plants J. Nataraj, T. Manivasagam, A. Justin Thenmozhi, C. Saravana Babu and M. Mohamed Essa	239

Chapter 11	Beneficial Roles of Curcumin, the Curry Spice, in Huntington's Disease *C. Saravana Babu, A. Bhat, R. Bipul,* *N. Chethan, A. H. Tousif,* *A. M. Mahalakshmi, T. Manivasagam,* *A. Justin Thenmozhi and M. Mohamed Essa*	**251**

About the Editors   **269**

Index   **273**

PREFACE

Food for Huntington's Disease focuses on the substitute healing approach for managing Huntington's disease. The curative properties of natural ingredients and bioactive compounds, such as nutraceuticals, from natural products including food, herbs, spices or plant extracts per se have been presented. For example, consuming foods from natural sources that are rich in amino acids, antioxidants, vitamins and alkaloids may reduce the chances of onset for Parkinson's disease and suggests that nutrition and diet have an impact on disease management. In addition, epigenetic modifications in conjunction with Huntington's disease have also been discussed in this book.

Food for Huntington's Disease is another book in series of books related to the benefits of food on brain function. This book designates the possible beneficial effects of edible natural products and their active materials on Huntington's disease. This is a progressive neurodegenerative disease that could cause uncontrolled movements, cognitive difficulties and emotional disturbances. The aim of this book and its series is to create awareness in general audiences about the dietary perception to reduce the occurrence of Huntington's disease. This may enable a better understanding and possibly reduce the cost on medical bills for patients (approximately $4500/year/person) and the insurance companies. Literature revealed that this disturbing neurodegenerative disorder has a higher prevalence in Europe (3-7 in 100,000), North America (4-5 in 100,000), and Australia than in Asian countries.

Studies suggest that mutation in the HD gene and the repeat expansion play an important role in the pathophysiology of this disease. The genetic defect underlying Huntington's disease is unstable, caused by an abnormal CAG expansion within the first exon of the Huntingtin gene (HTT), leading to an expanded polyglutamine (polyQ) track in the HTT protein. This disease is an inherited one. Even though the prevalence rate is moderate, scientists predict that a lot of people possess the possibility of carrying this disease. Mitochondrial dysfunction and oxidative stress could very highly play a role in this disease. In the last decade, the benefits of food on many diseases – including brain diseases – were explored. This book aims to summarize the recent updates on the benefit of natural edible materials and their active principles on the prevention or delaying of the progression or the management of this disease.

The editors feel highly obligated to all the contributors for this initiative. Undeniably, they believe that the information provided in this book would raise the awareness of the readers and could possibly help them to understand the disease process and the benefits of food items on Huntington's' disease management.

M. Mohamed Essa
T. Manivasagam
A. Justin-Thenmozhi
Qazi A. Hamid

ACKNOWLEDGMENTS

We, as editors, thank the almighty for giving support and courage to finish this project successfully.

We are highly thankful to all the authors who contributed for this sequel with effective evidence on the benefit of food on Huntington's disease.

As editors, we thank our family members for their unrestricted support by letting us to devote additional time to complete this book.

Internal grant from CAMS, SQU, Oman (IG/AGR/FOOD/17/02) is highly acknowledged.

We sincerely thank Nova Science Publishers for assisting this edited book to get published.

M. Mohamed Essa
T. Manivasagam
A. Justin-Thenmozhi
Qazi A. Hamid

Chapter 1

THE BENEFICIAL EFFECTS OF NATURAL DIETARY PRODUCTS ON NEUROPROTECTION

S. Lakshmi, A. Kurian, P. Prakash,
A. Firdous and E. Preetham[*]
Department of Biochemistry,
School of Ocean Science and Technology,
Kerala University of Fisheries and Ocean Studies (KUFOS),
Panangad, Kerala, India

ABSTRACT

Lifestyle factors and health beneficiaries are highly emerging co-equal hands in the current world. At a point, therapeutic applications of drugs were found ineffective in reverting or pausing life-threatening diseases like neurodegenerative disorders. Realizing this paucity and hazardous side-effects of drugs on affected individuals, clinicians and scientific researchers step forwarded with low cost and easily accessible lifestyle factors- nutrition and physical activities- as natural treatment remedies. A productive tenure has crossed in successfully underpinning

---

[*] Corresponding Author Email: preetham@kufos.ac.in.

the mechanism of natural products as proud pioneers in health management. Aging is the major predisposing factor in neurodegenerative disorders. As age progresses, apart from the usual entropy factors hailing in the stage, people began to fight with severe cognitive and learning impairments. Brain health is the solid platform for total human health. Owing to the utmost significance in neuroprotection, the chapter summarizes select few herbal and dietary natural products which boons brain health through their individual neuroprotective activities.

Keywords: neurodegeneration, oxidative stress, mitochondrial dysfunction, EGCG

INTRODUCTION

Neurodegenerative diseases represent hereditary and sporadic conditions involving progressive structural and functional loss of neurons or any damage that happens to the brain as well as the spinal cord (Dauer and Przedborski, 2003). Neurodegenerative diseases like Parkinson's disease (PD), Alzheimer's disease (AD), Huntington's disease (HD), and Amylotrophic lateral Sclerosis (Mandel et al., 2003) are always life-threatening and economic hurdles. Apart from aging being the prime risk factor, genetic mutation, protein aggregation or misfolding, debilitated ubiquitin-proteasome system, neuroinflammation, exhaustion of endogenous antioxidants, increase in iron, nitric oxide and pro-apoptotic proteins, and the reduced expression of trophic factors play their roles coequally in neurodegenerative diseases (Figure 1) (Riederer et al., 1989; Fahn and Cohen, 1992; Berg, 2001). Degradation of neurons in the brain and spinal cord leads to ataxia (impaired voluntary coordination by the nervous system) or dementia (sensory dysfunction).

Oxidative stress and mitochondrial dysfunctions are listed top among the key players in neurodegeneration (Emerit and Edeas, 2004). Oxidative stress, uniquely termed as an aging contribution factor is a dominating performer in the incidence and onset of neurodegenerative disorders. The main contributors to Oxidative stress are reactive oxygen species (ROS) such as superoxide anions, hydrogen peroxide, hydroxyl radical, among others, as well as reactive nitrogen species (RNS) like nitric oxide, peroxynitrite, and more. Oxidative stress is reduced with effective enzymatic and non-enzymatic defense mechanisms; cells maintain a homeostasis of synthesis and anti-oxidation of ROS and RNS. Catalase, Superoxide dismutase, glutathione reductase, glutathione peroxidase, and thioredoxin/thioredoxin reductase are the important enzymes involved in the retention of homeostasis. Any disturbance in the equilibrium between antioxidant/pro-oxidant homeostasis leads to oxidative stress thus generating excess ROS and free radicals that are harmful to neurons. Both metabolic and anatomic factors contribute to neuronal cell hypersensitivity and oxidative stress. Different glial cells, surrounded by endothelial cells, are present in the brain. These endothelial cells are less permeable, and therefore, have a reduced uptake of molecules and macrophages. Moreover, brain glial cells consume more oxygen and glucose in ATP generation, making them more prone to oxygen overload and thus generating free radicals (Lepoivre et al., 1994) (Oliveira et al., 2014). Mitochondrial dysfunction accompanies oxidative stress, as the mitochondria is central source of cellular oxidants. ROS formed within mitochondria will contrarily affect the different constituents of the Electron Transport Chain (ETC), which in turn causes a dissipation in ATP formation and the subsequent deterioration of mitochondria as well as other cellular organelles (Oliveira GL et al., 2014).

Decades have gone with society battling brain dysfunctions; people with neuro-disorders are multiplying as age and time progress. Treatment strategies like commercial drugs or hormonal therapies have stayed aback due to high costs, adverse side effects, and an inability to completely cure or revert the disease. However, lifestyle factors such as nutritional therapies, diet, and exercise are heading to counteract brain disorders, owing to their cut rates and easy access.

This chapter describes some important nutritional strategies as well as herbal treatments in neuroprotection:

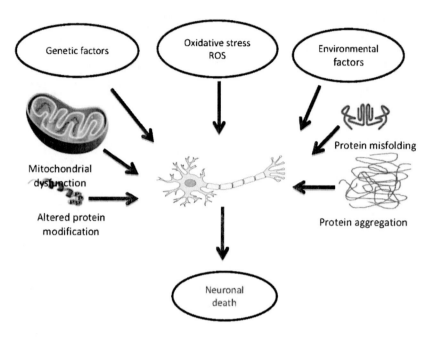

Figure 1. Factors associated with neurodegenerative diseases.

GREEN TEA

Tea is an aromatic beverage consumed all around the world. This popular drink is prepared from the leaves of *Camellia sinensis*, which belongs to Theaceae family. The different forms of tea are black, green and oolong. This classification is based on the refinement process or harvested leaf development. Black tea is completely fermented, green tea is unfermented, and oolong tea is partly fermented. The young tea leaves that undergo withering, pan firing, drying and grading yield green tea. It is estimated that about 20% of world annual tea production is green tea. Around the world, black tea consumption is about 78%, whereas green tea consumption is 20% and oolong is less than 2% (Wu and Wei, 2002). Green tea is widely accepted to possess antioxidants and thus has been well studied for its health benefits (Mukhtar and Ahmad, 2000). Health promoting effects of Green tea, such as anti-inflammatory, anticancer, antiarthritic, antioxidative, and neuroprotective effects have gained interest (Naghma and Hasan, 2007).

Chemical Components of Green Tea

Green tea contains a complex mixture of compounds. It mainly contains polyphenols, majority of which are flavanols that are commonly known as catechins. Catechins come in four different types, epicatechin, epigallocatechin, epicatechin-3-gallate, and epigallocatechin-3-gallate. In addition to catechins, green tea also has gallic acid, caffeine, and amino acids such as theanine, aspartic acid, valine, tryptophan, serine, and lysine; and also carbohydrates like glucose, sucrose, cellulose, fructose, and pectin; as well as minerals like aluminum and manganese, chlorophyll pigment, vitamin B, E, and C, esters, hydrocarbons, aldehydes, and alcohols (Sano et al., 2001).

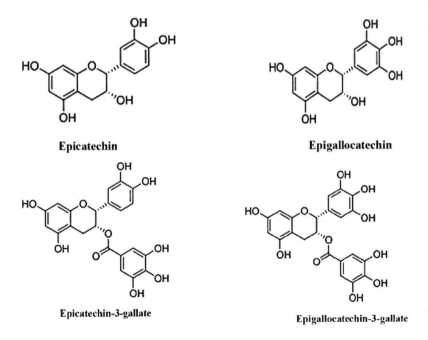

Figure 2. Structure of catechins in green tea.

Green Tea in Neuroprotection

Several studies have proved that green tea extracts can provide neuroprotection. Daily intake of more than 2 cups of tea has shown to reduce the incidence of Parkinson's disease (PD) (Checkoway et al., 2002). Epigallocatechin-3-Gallate (EGCG) and green tea extract have shown to avert striatal dopamine deficiency in mice and dopaminergic neuron loss in *Substantia nigra* through studies using N-methyl-4-phenyl-1,2,3,6-tetrahydropyridine (MPTP) (Levites et al., 2001). The structural resemblance to catechol may contribute to the neuroprotective role of green tea, owing to the presence of potent anti-oxidants in catechol containing compounds (Guo et al., 1996). According to the studies of Pan et al. in 2003 the inhibitory effect of green tea polyphenols in blocking the neurotoxin 1-methyl-4-phenylpyridinium (MPP^+) uptake also accounts for the structural similarity to catechols. This was understood when the inhibitory effect of green tea polyphenol on dopamine (DA) uptake was studied. Levites et al. in 2002, through *in vitro* studies demonstrated that EGCG inhibits MPP and 6-hydroxydopamine (6-OHDA) induced neurotoxicity. *In vitro* studies of Levites et al., in 2003 and Choi et al., in 2001 showed that EGCG could inhibit oxidative stress and neurotoxicity, whereas Ono et al. in 2003 found that epicatechin (EC) reduced the synthesis of neurotoxic amyloid fibril in AD. From the studies of Levites et al., in 2003, it was suggested that the polyphenols in green tea could be utilized as therapeutic agent in PD as well as AD as EGCG was found to be effective in regulating the proteolytic processing of amyloid precursor protein pathway (APP). Among all catechins, EGCG has been found to be a more efficient radical scavenger than epicatechin-3-gallate (ECG), epicatechin (EC), and epigallocatechin (EGC). This may be due to the presence of trihydroxyl group on ring B and gallic acid moiety at the 3' position of Ring C (Nanjo et al., 1996). A study carried out in rat brain tissue by Levites et al., in 2002, disclosed the benefits of the extracts of green tea and black tea in preventing lipid peroxidation due to iron ascorbate in the mitochondrial membranes of brain. Similarly, evidence from the study of Guo et al., in 1996 showed that the major polyphenol catechins in green tea could prevent iron-induced lipid peroxidation.

2002). The antioxidant and anti-inflammatory properties of curcumin are believed to prevent the symptoms of Alzheimer's disease.

The aggregation of small fibers of beta amyloid fibrils, the beta-amyloid plaques are considered to be a major characteristic of Alzheimer's disease. Thus the inhibition of Aβ production, prevention of Aβ fibril formation, and the destabilization of pre-formed Aβ would be an attractive therapeutic strategy for the treatment of Alzheimer's disease (Xu et al., 2005). An animal study based on the treatment with curcumin proved that the levels of beta-amyloid were decreased by around 40%. Surprisingly long term dose of small amounts of curcumin given over longer period were actually more effective than high doses in combating the neurodegenerative process of Alzheimer's disease. This is because, curcumin at higher concentration, binds to Aβ and blocks its self-congregation.

Curcumin modulates the levels of norepinephrine, a neurotransmitter involved in attentiveness, emotions, sleeping, and more; as well as dopamine, which is involved in pleasure, emotion, and regulating locomotion; also serotonin which is involved in appetite, sleep, memory, and learning, among others; and inhibits Mono-Amine Oxidase (MAO)-A and MAO-B enzyme, which disintegrate dopamine and serotonin (Kulkarni et al., 2008).

BRAHMI (*BACOPA MONNIERI*)

Bacopa monnieri, a non-aromatic herb, is a bitter creeper plant found in damp and marshy areas and is commonly used in Ayurvedic medicine as a nerve/cardio tonic, diuretic, and as a therapeutic agent against many of the diseases (H K Singh et al., 1982). It is a popular aquarium plant that can grow in water even in slightly brackish conditions. Stems are used to propagate the plant (Oudhia et al., 2004). *Bacopa monnieri* was initially described around the 6th century A.D. in Charaka Samhita, Atharva-Veda, and Susrut Samhita as a class herb taken for intellectual sharpening and to attenuate mental deficits (medhya rasayana). Traditionally, *Bacopa monnieri* was used to improve memory and cognitive function (Stough et al., 2008). *Bacopa monnieri* extracts have been studied extensively for their neuropharmacological effects and nootropic actions (V R Rammohan et al., 2012)

Major Components of Brahmi

Apart from the major constituents, such as saponins and triterpenoid bacosaponins, substances like alkaloids, sterols, betulic acid, polyphenols, and sulfhydryl compounds that accord antioxidant activity are also components in *Bacopa monnieri*. (Calabrese et al. 2008).

Bacoside-A, a family of compounds extracted from the *Bacopa monniera* plant, is a folk-medicinal substance possessing therapeutic properties, particularly enhancing cognitive functions and improving memory. It has been shown that bacoside-A exerted significant inhibitory effects upon cytotoxicity, fibrillation, and particularly membrane interactions of amyloid-beta, the peptide playing a prominent role in Alzeheimer's disease progression and toxicity (Malishev et al. 2017).

Role in Neuroprotection

B. monnieri extracts studies on animals have reported improved cognition encompassing motor learning and acquisition, consolidation, and retention of memory in rats (H K Sing et al. 1997). *Bacopa monnieri* is also known as a cognitive enhancer; it can be applied as a novel therapeutic agent for cognitive deficit in schizophrenia by changing cerebral neuronal density (Wetchateng et al. 2015). A study was conducted on oxidized LDL (low density lipoprotein) which is supposed to possess a role in the pathology of AD. The *B. monnieri* extract diminished the neurotoxicity of oxidized LDL in a dose dependent manner, potentially by the suppression of cellular oxidative stress (Panit Yamchuen et al. 2017).

Recently, a placebo-controlled clinical study of Brahmi was conducted by Swinburne University of Technology, Australia. 24 healthy adults were given either a placebo or standardized extracts of *B. monnieri* at two different dosages, 320 or 640 milligrams. The 320 milligram-treated group showed significant increases in cognition and memory over three different intervals of testing (Downey et al. 2013). The Pharmacy college of Thailand's Naresuan University studied human brain cells after treatment with *B. monnieri* by giving special emphasis to the Aβ induced damage of AD (Adams, 2013). *B. monnieri* treated neurons were found to have a low level of reactive oxygen species. *B. monnieri* extract also exhibited both reducing and lipid peroxidation inhibitory activities (Adams 2013).

AMLA (*PHYLLANTHUS EMBLICA*)

Emblica officinalis Gaertn. Phyllanthus emblica Linn comes under the family Phyllanthaceae. It is distributed in tropical and subtropical regions of India, China, Indonesia, and the Malay Peninsula. It is well known for its therapeutic applications in indigenous systems of medicine. It is rich in vitamin C, minerals, amino acids, and a wide variety of phenolic compounds, such as tannins, phyllembelic acid, phyllemblin, rutin, curcuminoides, and emblicol (Kim et al., 2005). From ancient times, the plant has been utilized for treating diabetes, hyperlipidemia, CNS (Central nervous system) disorders, ophthalmic diseases, and a number of life style illnesses. It exhibits pharmacological aspects including antioxidant, anticancer, immune modulator, anti-inflammatory, cyto-protective properties (Khan, 2009; Kumar, 2012; Singh, 2015). The therapeutic efficacy of Amla in treating dyspepsia was evaluated with positive results in humans (Chawla et al., 1982). It exhibits good results in antisecretory and anti-ulcer studies in rats. The three main varieties of amla are Banarasi, Francis, and Chakaiya. Considering limitations of these varieties, the following varieties were identified at Narendra Dev University of Agricuture and Technology, Faizabad and released for commercial cultivation: Kanchan, Krishna, Narendra Aonla-6, Narendra Aonla -7, and Narendra Aonla – 10.

Characteristics of commercially grown amla varieties is shown in Table 3

Table 3. Characteristics of commercially grown amla varieties

Variety	Characteristics
Kanchan(NA-4)	A seedling selection from Chakaiya. Fruit are with higher fibre content, industrially preference for pulp extraction and manufacture of various products.
Krishna (NA-5)	A seedling selection from Banarasi. The fruits are large, triangular, and conical with color varying from whitish green to apricot yellow with a red spot on the exposed portion. Flesh is pinkish green, less fibrous and highly astringent.
Narendra Aonla-6	A selection from Chakaiya cultivar. Fruits are most attractive and shining, medium to large size, flattened and very low fibre content.
Narendra Aonla-7	A seedling selection from Francis. Fruits are of medium to large size with conical apex. Fibre content is comparitively higher than NA-6.
Narendra Aonla-10	Selected from the Banarasi cultivar. Fruits are attractive, medium to large in size, and flattened round in shape. The skin is rough, yellowish green with pink tinge. Flesh is whitish green, with high fibre content.

Constituents of Amla

E. officinalis is a rich source of tannins, mucic acid, aminoacids, alkaloids, flavone glycosides, methyl gallate, phenolic glycosides, flavonolglycosides, phyllanemblinins, phenolic acids, sesquiterpenoids, norsesquiterpenoids, and carbohydrates (Zhang et al., 2000; Zhang et al., 2001; Krishnaiah et al., 2009). The fruit juice of *E. officinalis* is rich with vitamin C (478.56 mg/100 ml) (Jain et al., 2004). Bansal et al., (2014) has quantified various phytoconstituents, such as gallic acid, chloro-genic acid, ellagic acid, and quercetin from the fruit juice of *E. officinalis* and found to have 37.95, 17.43, 71.20, and 2.01 mg/100 ml of fruit juice, respectively. Coumaric acid, myricetin, caffeic acid, and synergic acid are found to present in both pulp and seeds, whereas gallic acid and quercetin are found to be present only in the pulp rather than the seed of *E. officinalis* (Nambiar, et al., 2015). Moreover, it is a good source of omega 3 Fatty acid (48 mg/100g) and omega 6 fatty acid (276 mg/100g). In addition amla contains various minerals, such as Calcium (25 mg/100g), Magnesium (10mg/100g), Phosphorus 27 mg/100g), and Potassium (198 mg/100g).

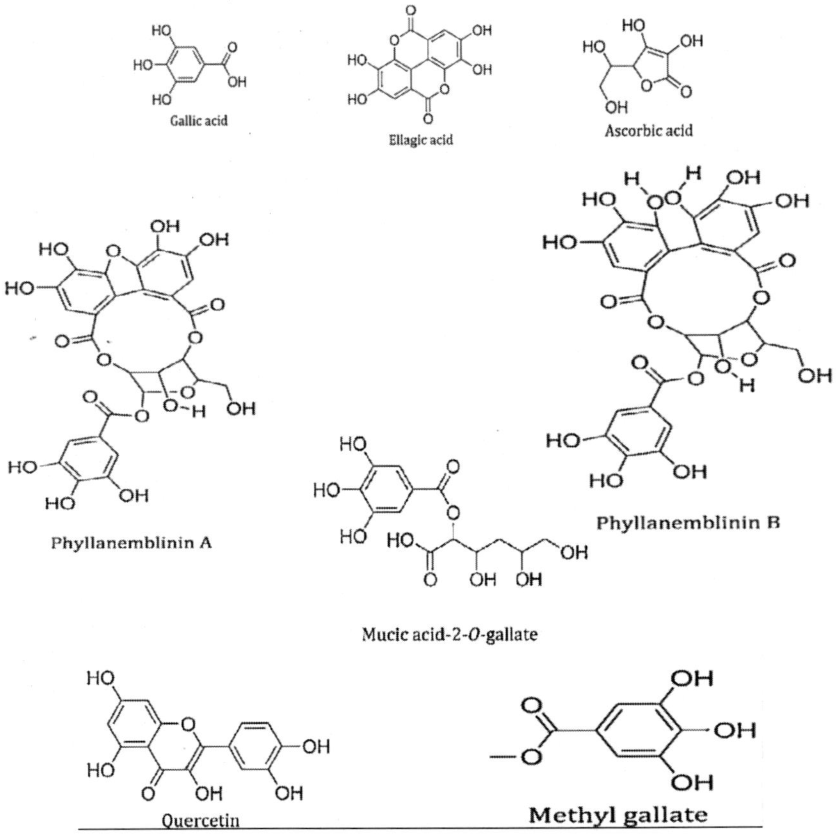

Figure 3. Structure of Major Constituents

Amla in Neuroprotection

Thenmozhy et al., (2016) reported a neuroprotective effect of *E. officinalis* against loss of memory elicited by aluminum chloride ($AlCl_3$)

intoxication. In their study, the co-administration of *E. officinalis* at a dose of 100 mg/kb b.w. reversed neurotoxic effects of $AlCl_3$, including cognitive deficits and apoptosis (Thenmozhi, et al., 2016). *E. officinalis* is supposed to suppress oxidative stress and prevent the hyperphosphorylation via GSK-3b/Akt signaling pathway. Various studies show that *E. officinalis* is a potent candidate against causative factors that are responsible for oxidative stresses by enhancing the antioxidant defense mechanism. *E. officinalis* increases the levels of antioxidant enzymes like catalase, superoxide dismutase, GSH reductase, GSH peroxidase, and GSH S-transferase (Shukla et al., 2009). Anilakumar et al., (2004) suggested that amla may detoxify the dimethyl dydrazine (DMH) partly by enhancing the multi-component antioxidant system in the rat. Linder et al. (1985) revealed that the feeding of amla and the co-administration with DMH significantly reduced the cytotoxic compounds like malondialdehyde MDA and conjugated dienes. They also found that amla increased the hepatic GSH content (Linder et al., 1985). Bhattacharya and Ghosal et al., (1999) investigated the effect of amla on the rat brain frontal cortical and striatal oxidative free radical scavenging enzyme levels. They reported that the antioxidant activity of *E. officinalis* may be due to tannoids, emblicanin A, emblicanin B, punigluconin, and pedunculagin, which possess ascorbic acid like properties (Bhattacharya, et al., 1999). Reddy et al., (2010) and Andican et al., (2005) investigated the ameliorative effect of *E. officinalis* fruit extract against alcohol-induced oxidative stress and established the favorable role of polyphenols such as flavonoids, tannins, and other compounds in mitigating oxidative stress. These polyphenols are mainly present in *E. officinalis* fruit extract and protect against alcohol-induced oxidative stress owing to scavenging effect on NOx which behaves as an antioxidant and pro-oxidant simultaneously (Reddy, et al., 2010; Andican et al., 2005). Similar antioxidant properties of *E. Officinalis* were reported by Shivananjapaa and Joshi (2012) in cellular oxidative stress using a hepatocyte cell line (HepG2). An aqueous extract from fruits of *E. officinalis* significantly improved the antioxidant capacity by increasing the levels of GSH, superoxide dismutase, catalase, GSH peroxidase, GSH reductase, and GSH S-transferase. Stress related oxidative burden is a prime contributing factor in the development of various ailments as well as the process of aging. It has been found that Amlaki Rasayana (AR) promotes long life with enhanced physical and mental strength so that age-related disorders are minimized (Singh et al., 2009; Sarkar and Chaudhary, 2010). The aging-associated DNA damage in neurons and astrocytes has been shown to be reduced in rats supplemented with AR (Swain et al., 2012). Dwivedi et al., (2012) revealed that the dietary supplementation of AR improves the life span and stress tolerance in Drosophila fly models. Studies have proved that amla churna produced a dose-dependent betterment in the memories of young and aged rats. It also reversed the amnesia induced by scopolamine and diazepam. Amla churna may prove to be a useful remedy for the management of Alzheimer's disease due to its multifarious beneficial effects attributed to managemement of memory problems (Vasudevan and Parle, 2007). Bargale and his colleagues carried out a study and found out that amalaki rasayana along with milk has shown a highly significant affect in treating insomnia, constipation, digestive weakness, and hemoglobin percentage, and hence is very effective in treating ageing ailments (Bargale, et al., 2014).

Recently, Guruprasad, et al., (2017) conducted a study on the telomerase activity and telomere length in the peripheral blood mononuclear cells of aged individuals administered with *Amalaki Rasayana* (AR) by administrating AR to healthy, aged (45–60 years) volunteers for 45 days after *koshta shuddhi* procedure. The telomerase activity and telomere length were analyzed on the 0, 45th, and 90th days of administration in peripheral blood mononuclear cells from these individuals and compared with age-matched placebo group and young volunteers (22–30 years) with one comparison made between the groups. Interestingly they found that there was an increase in telomerase activity with no discernible change in telomere length in the *Amalaki* administered participants. The comparison between young and aged participants revealed higher telomerase activity in young participants with no significant differences in telomere length (Guruprasad, et al., 2017).

SPINACH (*SPINACIAO LERACEA* L.)

Spinach (*Spinaciao leracea* L.), is a dark green leafy vegetable, belonging to the family Amaranthaceae (Morelock et al., 2008). Spinach is high in vitamin C. The 3 types of Spinach are:

(i) 'Savoy' - 'Bloomsdale', 'Merlo Nero' and 'Viroflay' are three varieties of Savoy.
(ii) Flat- or smooth-leaf spinach with broad, smooth leaves, often grown for canned and frozen spinach, as well as soups, baby foods, and processed foods. Eg: 'Giant Noble'
(iii) Semi-savoy is a hybrid variety. 'Tyee Hybrid' is a common semi-savoy.

About 90% of the world spinach production is by China (Food and Agriculture Organization of the United Nations). Spinach contains an antioxidant, α-lipoic acid, responsible for reducing glucose levels, increasing insulin sensitivity, lowering the risk of cancer and asthma, and preventing oxidative stress-induced changes in patients with diabetes. It contains almost 17 distinct flavonoid derivatives of patuletin, spinacetin, spinatoside, jaceidin, and flavones (Koh, E. et al., 2012). Accordng to previous studies, α-lipoic acid also decreases peripheral neuropathy and autonomic neuropathy in diabetics. All the functional properties such as, antioxidant, anti-inflammatory, antiproliferative, anti-obesity, hypoglycemic, and lipid-lowering activities of spinach leaves and spinach-derived extracts are considered to be noteworthy.

Constituents of Spinach

Spinach is low in calories, high in complex carbohydrates (3.6%), it has a lower amount of protein (2.9%), contains no cholesterol, has almost no fat (0.4%), and is a good source of fibre (2.2g/100g). Spinach is a rich source of folic acids, oxalic acids, lutein and zeaxanthin, and also contains high amounts of lipophilic antioxidants such as carotenoids (mainly β-carotene and violaxanthin) and β- and β tocopherol involved in the prevention of age-related macular degeneration and cataracts (Moeller, et al., 2000; Olmedilla, et al., 2003; Bunea , et al., 2008). 100 g of fresh spinach contains of ascorbic acid (13–53 mg), β-carotene (5626 µg), carotenoids (17.8 mg), flavonoids (1 – 4 mg), folate (194 µg), folic acid (194 µg), nitrate (31 – 117 mg), oxalate (400 mg), vitamin A (9377 IU), and minerals such as calcium (99 mg), magnesium (79 mg), and potassium (558 mg) (Koh, 2012). It is also has a high concentration of vitamin E, K, and C (Shohag, 2011). It is again another rich source of Glutathione, α-Lipoic acid, D-Glucaric acid, and Coenzyme Q10 (Joseph et al., 2002; Pompella et al. 2003).

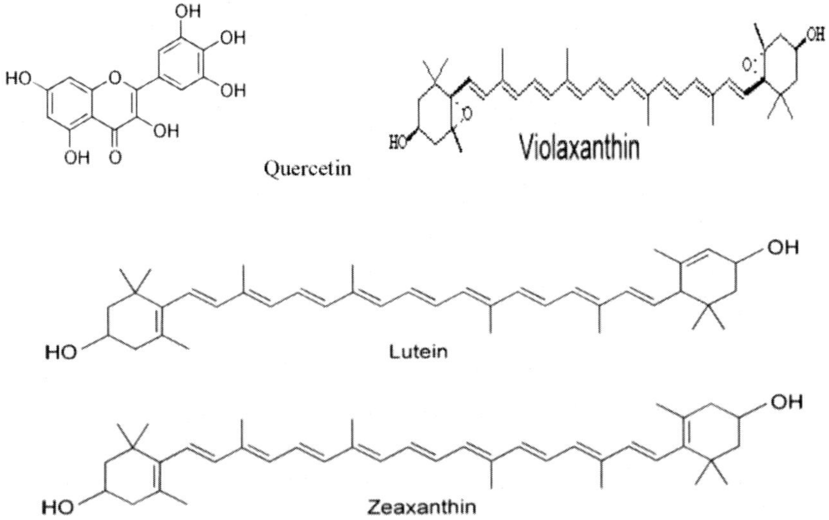

Figure 4. Structure of Major Constituents

Spinach in Neuroprotection

Various studies have already revealed that oxidative stress is a major factor involved in CNS functional anomalies in aging and age-related neurodegenerative diseases and antioxidants may ameliorate or prevent age-associated cognitive declines (Halliwell, 1989; Jenner, 2003; Fahn, and Cohen, 1992; Markesbery, 1997). Endogenous antioxidants like glutathione (Ohkuwa et al., 1997) and glutamine synthetase (Carney et al., 1994), decrease in aging with increases in lipid peroxidation (Migheli et al., 1994; Yu, 1994). Joseph et al. (1998) revealed that phytochemicals present in spinach may be beneficial in retarding functional age-related CNS and cognitive behavioural deficits. Wang et al. (2009) found that spinach protects brain function from premature ageing and reduces the extent of post-ischaemic stroke damage to the brain (Hedges and Lister, 2007; Christen et al., 2000; Morris, 2006). Kang et al. (2005) conducted a study on "Fruit and Vegetable Consumption and Cognitive Decline in Aging Women" and found that increased dietary intake of green leafy vegetables (spinach and romaine lettuce) and cruciferous vegetables (broccoli and cauliflower) revealed less cognitive decline among older women. Their study concluded that spinach had the strongest effect in improving cognitive health (Kang et al., 2005). As oxidative stress has been shown to underlie neuropathological aspects of Alzheimer's disease (AD) and 4-Hydroxy-2-nonenal (HNE) is a highly reactive product of lipid peroxidation of unsaturated lipids, hence HNE-induced oxidative toxicity is a well-described model of oxidative stress-induced neurodegeneration. Abdul and Butterfield (2007) revealed that pre-treatment of neurons with acetyl-L-carnitine (ALCAR) and α-lipoic acid (LA) leads to the activation of phosphoinositol-3 kinase (PI3K), PKG, and ERK1/2 pathways, which play critical roles in neuronal cell survival. This evidence supports the pharmacological potential of co-treatment of ALCAR and LA (which is abundantly present in spinach) in the management of neurodegenerative disorders associated with HNE-induced oxidative stress and neurotoxicity, including AD (Abdul and Butterfield, 2007). Sang-Heui Ko et al. (2014) carried out a study to analyse *in vitro* antioxidant effects of spinach followed by the advantages of spinach supplementation in hyperlipidemicrats. Administration of 5% spinach could give beneficial effects in high fat-cholesterol diet (HFCD) rats, as indicated by decreased liver thiobarbituric acid reactive Substances (TBARS) level, DNA damage in leukocyte, increased plasma conjugated dienes, and manganese superoxide dismutase (Mn-SOD) activity. Thus, the antioxidant property of spinach proves to be an effective way to ameliorate high fat and cholesterol diet-induced oxidative stress (Ko, et al., 2014).

SAFFRON

Crocus sativus or saffron belongs to the family Iridaceae, contains α-crocetin, carotenoids, glycoside crocin, picrocrocin, safranal, lycopene, zeaxanthin, and vitamin B2 (Vijaya Bhargava, 2011). The constituents in saffron namely crocin and safranal have exhibited the ability to act as strong oxygen radical scavengers. In Asian countries, saffron has been used traditionally as an aphrodisiac, antispasmodic, expectorant, sedative, diaphoretic, stomachic, anticatarrhal, and eupeptic (Farahmand et al., 2013). Several studies have proved the multiple effects of saffron extracts in animal models. Ethanolic and aqueous extracts of *C. sativus* petals have helped reduce blood pressure (Fatehi et al., 2003). Xuan (1999) found that crocin analogs were suitable for treating ischemic retinopathy and age related macular degeneration. Papandreou et al., 2011) suggested that treating normal and aged mice with saffron for one week could improve learning and memory.

Saffron Constituents

Around 150 compounds were identified in the stigma of *C. sativus*. Crocetin constitutes 0.3% of the total weight of stigma is contributing the red colour of saffron. Crocetin exists mostly as a trans-isomer in saffron and has a carboxyl group at each end of the polyene chain. Crocin obtained from the dried stigma imparts the red colour to saffron. 80% of pigment content in saffron is crocin and can be directly crystallized. Before or during intestinal absorption, crocin gets hydrolyzed to crocetin and form mono and diglucuronide conjugates. 6 - 16% of saffron is constituted by crocin. The most commonly found crocin in saffron is α –crocin which can be easily dissolved in water (Melnyk et al., 2010). Picrocrocin and saffranal are responsible for the bitterness of saffron. Other constituents seen in saffron are amino acids, starch, lycopene, resins, trace amounts of riboflavin, thiamine, and kaempferol in the alcoholic extracts (Gregory et al., 2005).

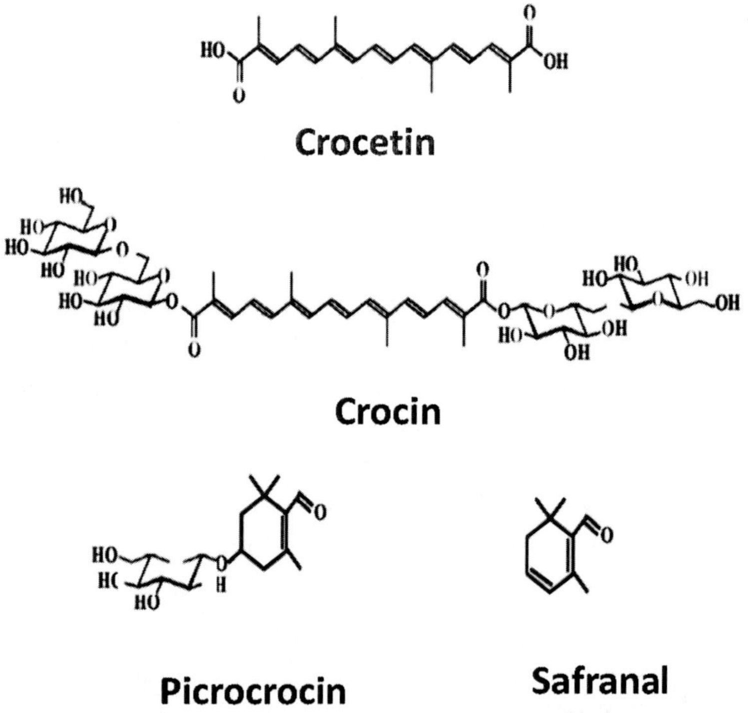

Figure 3. Structure of *C. sativus* constituents.

Saffron in Neuroprotection

Deposition of Aβ fibrils in AD was found to be inhibited in the presence of aqueous-ethanolic extract of saffron, which was mainly due to the carotenoid constituent, trans-crocin-4 (Papandreou et al., 2006). In rats intracerebroventricular (ICV) injection of streptozotocin (STZ) causes cognitive deficits. Treating such animal models of sporadic AD with saffron extract for 3 weeks could improve the condition (Khalili et al., 2010). The study of Geromichalos et al., (2012) suggested that saffron extract could inhibit the breaking down of acetylcholine. Crocin could be effective than safranal in inhibiting the fibrillation of apoalpha-lactalbumin under amyloidogenic condition (Ebrahim-Habibi et al., 2010). Ahmad et al., (2005) reported the neuroprotective effects of crocetin at 25, 50 and 75 μg/kg body weight in 6-hydroxydopamine induced Parkinson's disease in rats, which was suggested to have happened due to the reduction in utilizing dopamine by tissues. Another study concluded that pre-treatment of 1-methyl-4-phenyl-1, 2,3,6-tetrahydropyridine (MPTP) induced Parkinson's disease in rat model with saffron could save dopaminergic cells in the *Substantia nigra* pars compacta (SNc) and retina. They observed 30 - 35% reduction in the number of tyrosine hydroxylase (TH+) cells when compared to control treated with saline in SNc and retina. SNc and retinal TH+ cell count increased by 25 - 35% in MPTP injected mice that were pre-treated with saffron (Purushothuman et al., 2013). Inducing cerebral ischemia in rats by middle cerebral artery occlusion suggested that administration of stigma extract of *C. sativus* at 100 mg/kg for a week could reduce catalase, SOD, K-ATPase, aspartate, and glutamate concentrations (Saleem et al. 2006). A study showed that treatment with 10 and 50 μM crocin and 5 and 25 mg/ml saffron extract diminished the neurotoxic effect caused by glucose in PC12 cells (Mousavi et al., 2010). Mice treated with saffron extract at 200 mg/kg dose administered along with 500 mg/kg of honey syrup for 45 days reduce the aluminium chloride induced neurotoxicity (Shati et al., 2011). Safranal has been proved to provide protective effects in ischemic rats against oxidative damage in the hippocampal tissues (Hosseinzadeh and Sadeghnia, 2005). It also reduced the concentration of aspartate and glutamate following kainic acid administration in the hippocampus of rats (Hosseinzadeh et al. 2008b). In the rat model of ischemic stroke, it was found that crocin reduced the malondialdehyde (MDA) level and increased glutathione peroxidase and SOD activity (Vakili et al., 2013). When saffron was administered along with aluminium it could reverse the alterations in monoamine oxidase activity and lipid peroxidation levels in the cerebellum and brain (Linardaki et al., 2013). It has been suggested that crocetin can increase the antioxidant ability in brain and also can protect against 6-OHDA induced neurotoxicity whereas crocin can improve learning, memory and can also prevent the oxidative stress in hippocampus (Ghadrdoost et al., 2011). Another study revealed that diazinon-induced oxidative stress and inflammation could be prevented by aqueous extracts of saffron at 50, 100 and 200 mg/kg (Moallem et al., 2014).

Conclusion

Dementia and cognitive dysfunctions as close accompaniments of neurodegenerative disorders provides a tiresome period of living for affected people. The increase in the rate of neurodisorders and their treatment have been rising tremendously in the past few years. Natural plant sources is gaining attention in conferring health benefits. The neuroprotective properties of Green tea, amla, saffron, spinach, turmeric, and Brahmi offer natural treatments for neurodegenerative ailments through the contributions of their diverse constituents. Natural bioactive compounds in brain health management will lead to more productive outcomes in the future leading to healthy brain function that can ultimately coordinate learning and memory.

Acknowledgments

We gratefully thank the support of the Center of Excellence in Food Processing Technology, KUFOS for their help in data acquisition. The authors deeply acknowledge the Department of Health Research, ICMR, New Delhi, for their encouragement and financial assistance (No.R. 12013/04/2017-HR) towards the HRD fellowship-Women Scientist with break in career to SL.

REFERENCES

Abdul, HM; Butterfield, DA. Involvement of PI3K/PKG/ERK1/2 Signaling Pathways in Cortical Neurons to Trigger Protection by Cotreatment of Acetyl-L-Carnitine and A-Lipoic Acid Against HNE-Mediated Oxidative Stress And Neurotoxicity: Implications for Alzheimer's Disease. *Free Radical Biology and Medicine*, 2007, 42(3), 371-384.

Ahmad, AS; Ansari, MA; Ahmad, M; Saleem, S; Yousuf, S; Hoda, MN; Islam, F. Neuroprotection by Crocetin in a Hemi-Parkinsonian Rat Model. *Pharmacol Biochem Behav.*, 2005, 81, 805–813.

Ambegaokar, SS; Wu, L; Alamshahi, K; Lau, J; Jazayeri, L; Chan, S; et al. Curcumin Inhibits Dose-Dependently and Time-Dependently Neuroglial Proliferation And Growth. *Neuro Endocrinol Lett.*, 2003, 24, 469–73.

Andican, G; Gelisgen, R; Unal, E; Tortum, OB; Dervisoglu, S; Karahasanoglu, T; Burçak, G. Oxidative Stress and Nitric Oxide in Rats with Alcohol-Induced Acute Pancreatitis. *World Journal of Gastro-enterology: WJG*, 2005, 11(15), 2340.

Anilakumar, KR; Nagaraj, NS; Santhanam, K. Protective Effects of Amla on Oxidative Stress and Toxicity in Rats Challenged with Dimethyl Hydrazine. *Nutrition research*, 2004, 24(4), 313-319.

Arab, H; Mahjoub, S; Hajian-Tilaki, K; Moghadasi, M. The Effect of Green Tea Consumption on Oxidative Stress Markers and Cognitive Function in Patients with Alzheimer's Disease: A Prospective Intervention Study. *Caspian Journal of Internal Medicine.*, 2016, 7(3), 188-194.

Bansal, V; Sharma, A; Ghanshyam, C; Singla, ML. Coupling of Chromatographic Analyses with Pretreatment for the Determination of Bioactive Compounds in *Emblica Officinalis* Juice. *Analytical Methods*, 2014, 6(2), 410-418.

Bargale, SS; Shashirekha, HK; Baragi, UC. Anti-Aging Effect of *Amalaki Rasayana* in Healthy Elderly Subjects. *Journal of Ayurveda and Holistic Medicine (JAHM)*, 2014, 2(1), 10-18.

Berg, D; Gerlach, M; Youdim, MBH; Double, KL; Zecca, L; Riederer, P; Becker, G. Brain Iron Pathways and Their Relevance to Parkinson's Disease. *J Neurochem.*, 2001, 79, 225–36.

Bhargava, V. Medicinal Uses and Pharmacological Properties of *Crocus sativus* Linn (Saffron) *Int J Pharmacy Pharmaceutical Science.*, 2011, 3, 22–26.

Bhattacharya, A; Chatterjee, A; Ghosal, S; Bhattacharya, SK. *Antioxidant Activity of Active Tannoid Principles of Emblica Officinalis (Amla).* 1999.

Bunea, A; Andjelkovic, M; Socaciu, C; Bobis, O; Neacsu, M; Verhé, R; Van Camp, J. Total and Individual Carotenoids and Phenolic Acids Content in Fresh, Refrigerated and Processed Spinach (*Spinacia oleracea* L.). *Food Chemistry*, 2008, 108(2), 649-656.

Chawla, YK; Dubey, P; Singh, R; Nundy, S; Tandon, BN. Treatment of Dyspepsia with Amalaki (*Emblica officinalis* Linn.)--an Ayurvedic Drug. *The Indian Journal of Medical Research*, 1982, 76, 95.

Checkoway, H; Powers, K; Smith-Weller, T; Franklin, GM; Longstreth, WT; Jr. Swanson, PD. Parkinson's Disease Risks Associated with Cigarette Smoking, Alcohol Consumption, and Caffeine Intake. *Am J Epidemiol*, 2002, 155, 732–8.

Choi, YT; Jung, CH; Lee, SR; Bae, JH; Baek, WK; Suh, MH; Park, J; Park, CW; Suh, SI. The Green Tea Polyphenol (-)-Epigallocatechin Gallate Attenuates Beta- Amyloid-Induced Neurotoxicity in Cultured Hippocampal Neurons. *Life Sci*, 2001, 70, 603–14.

Christen, WG; Gaziano, JM; Hennekens, CH; Physicians, FTSCO; Study II, HEALTH. Design of Physicians' Health Study II—A Randomized Trial of Beta-Carotene, Vitamins E And C, and Multivitamins, in Prevention of Cancer, Cardiovascular Disease, and Eye Disease, and Review of Results of Completed Trials. *Annals of epidemiology*, 2000, 10(2), 125-134.

Daily, JW; Yang, M; Park, S. Efficacy of Turmeric Extracts and Curcumin for Alleviating the Symptoms of Joint Arthritis: A Systematic Review and Meta-Analysis of Randomized Clinical Trials. *Journal of Medicinal Food.*, 2016, 19 (8), 717–29.

Daniel, M. *Medicinal Plants: Chemistry and Properties.* Science Publishers. 2005, p. 225.

Dauer, W; Przedborski, S. Parkinson's Disease: Mechanisms and Models. *Neuron.*, 2003, 39, 889–909.

Dwivedi, V; Anandan, EM; Mony, RS; Muraleedharan, TS; Valiathan, MS; Mutsuddi, M; Lakhotia, SC. *In Vivo* Effects of Traditional Ayurvedic Formulations in Drosophila Melanogaster Model Relate with Therapeutic Applications. *PLoS One*, 2012, 7(5), e37113.

Ebrahim-Habibi, MB; Amininasab, M; Ebrahim-Habibi, A; Sabbaghian, M; Nemat-Gorgani, M. Fibrillation of Alpha-Lactalbumin: Effect of Crocin and Safranal, Two Natural Small Molecules From *Crocus Sativus. Biopolymers.*, 2010, 93, 854–865.

Emerit, J; Edeas, MFB. Neurodegenerative Diseases and Oxidative Stress. *Biomed. Pharmacother.*, 2004, 58, 39–46.

Fahn, S; Cohen, G. The Oxidant Stress Hypothesis in Parkinson's Disease: Evidence Supporting It. *Ann Neurol.*, 1992, 32, 804–12.

Fahn, S; Cohen, G. The Oxidant Stress Hypothesis in Parkinson's Disease: Evidence Supporting It. *Annals of Neurology*, 1992, 32(6), 804-812.

Farahmand, SK; Samini, F; Samini, M; Samarghandian, S. Safranal Ameliorates Antioxidant Enzymes and Suppresses Lipid Peroxidation and Nitric Oxide Formation in Aged Male Rat Liver. *Biogerontology.*, 2013, 14, 63–71.

Fatehi, M; Rashidabady, T; Fatehi-Hassanabad, Z. Effects of *Crocus Sativus* Petals' Extract on Rat Blood Pressure and on Responses Induced by Electrical Field Stimulation in the Rat Isolated Vas Deferens and Guinea-Pig Ileum. *J Ethnopharmacology.*, 2003, 84, 199–203.

Finch, CE; Cohen, DM. Aging, Metabolism, and Alzheimer Disease: Review and Hypotheses. *Experimental Neurology*, 1997, 143(1), 82-102.

Food Standards Agency, UK Government. *Producing and Distributing Food – Guidance: Chemicals in Food: Safety Controls; Sudan Dyes and Industrial Dyes Not Permitted in Food.* gov.uk. , 2015.

Frautschy, SA; Hu, W. Phenolic Anti-Inflammatory Antioxidant Reversal of B-Induced Cognitive Deficits and Neuropathology. *Neurobiol Aging.*, 2001, 22, 993–1005.

Garcia-Alloza, M; Borrelli, LA; Rozkalne, A; Hyman, BT; Bacskai, BJ. Curcumin Labels Amyloid Pathology *In Vivo*, Disrupts Existing Plaques and Partially Restores Distorted Neurites in an Alzheimer Mouse Model. *J Neurochem.*, 2007, 102, 1095–104.

Geromichalos, GD; Lamari, FN; Papandreou, MA; Trafalis, DT; Margarity, M; Papageorgiou, A; Sinakos, Z. Saffron as a Source of Novel Acetylcholinesterase Inhibitors: Molecular Docking and *In Vitro* Enzymatic Studies. *J Agric Food Chem.*, 2012, 60, 6131–6138.

Giri, RK; Rajagopal, V; Kalra, VK. Curcumin, the Active Constituent of Turmeric, Inhibits Amyloid Peptide-Induced Cytochemokine Gene Expression and CCR5-Mediated Chemotaxis of THP-1 Monocytes by Modulating Early Growth Response-1 Transcription Factor. *J Neurochem.*, 2004, 91, 1199–210.

Gregory, MJ; Menary, RC; Davies, NW. Effect of Drying Temperature and Air Flow on the Production and Retention of Secondary Metabolites in Saffron. *J Agric Food Chem.*, 2005, 53, 5969–5975.

Guo, Q; Zhao, B; Li, M; Shen, S; Xin, W. Studies on Protective Mechanisms of Four Components of Green Tea Polyphenols Against Lipid Peroxidation in Synaptosomes. *Biochim Biophys Acta*, 1996, 1304, 210–22.

Guo, Q; Zhao, B; Li, M; Shen, S; Xin, W. Studies on Protective Mechanisms of Four Components of Green Tea Polyphenols Against Lipid Peroxidation in Synaptosomes. *Biochim Biophys Acta*, 1996, 1304, 210–22.

Guruprasad, KP; Dash, S; Shivakumar, MB; Shetty, PR; Raghu, KS; Shamprasad, BR; Mana, AE. Influence of *Amalaki Rasayana* on Telomerase Activity and Telomere Length in Human Blood Mononuclear Cells. *Journal of Ayurveda and Integrative Medicine.*, 2017.

Halliwell, B. Oxidants and the Central Nervous System: Some Fundamental Questions. Is Oxidant Damage Relevant to Parkinson's

Disease, Alzheimer's Disease, Traumatic Injury or Stroke? *Acta Neurologica Scandinavica*, 1989, 80(s126), 23-33.

Jenner, P. Oxidative Stress in Parkinson's disease. *Annals of Neurology*, 2003, 53(S3).

Hedges, LJ; Lister, CE. Nutritional Attributes of Spinach, Silver Beet and Eggplant. *Crop Food Res Confidential Rep*, 2007, 1928.

Hosseinzadeh, H; Sadeghnia, HR; Rahimi, A. Effect of Safranal on Extracellular Hippocampal Levels of Glutamate and Aspartate During Kainic Acid Treatment in Anesthetized Rats. *Planta Med.*, 2008b, 74, 1441–1445.

Hosseinzadeh, H; Talebzadeh, F. Anticonvulsant Evaluation of Safranal and Crocin from *Crocus Sativus* in Mice. *Fitoterapia.*, 2005, 76, 722–724. http://www.greenmedinfo.com/blog/ayurvedic-herb-improves-memory-cognition-and-alzheimers.

Jain, SK; Khurdiya, DS. Vitamin C Enrichment of Fruit Juice Based Ready-To-Serve Beverages Through Blending of Indian Gooseberry (*Emblica officinalis* Gaertn.) Juice. *Plant Foods for Human Nutrition (Formerly Qualitas Plantarum)*, 2004, 59(2), 63-66.

Jenner, P; Olanow, CW. Oxidative Stress and the Pathogenesis of Parkinson's Disease. *Neurology*, 1996, 47, (6 suppl3), 161S-170S.

Joseph, JA; Erat, S; Denisova, N; Villalobos-Molina, R. Receptor-and Age-Selective Effects of Dopamine Oxidation on Receptor–G Protein Interactions in the Striatum. *Free Radical Biology and Medicine*, 1998, 24(5), 827-834.

Joseph, JA; Villalobos-Molina, R; Denisova, N; Erat, S; Cutler, R; Strain, J. Age Differences in Sensitivity to H2O2-or NO-Induced Reductions in K+-Evoked Dopamine Release From Superfused Striatal Slices: Reversals by PBN or Trolox. *Free Radical Biology and Medicine*, 1996, 20(6), 821-830.

Khan, KH. Roles of *Emblica Officinalis* in Medicine – A Review, *Bot. Res. Int.*, 2, (2009), 218–228.

Kang, JH; Ascherio, A; Grodstein, F. Fruit and Vegetable Consumption and Cognitive Decline in Aging Women. *Annals of Neurology*, 2005, 57(5), 713-720.

Khalili, M; Hamzeh, F. Effects of Active Constituents of *Crocus sativus* L Crocin on Streptozocin-Induced Model of Sporadic Alzheimer's Disease in Male Rats. *Iran Biomed J.*, 2010, 14, 59.

Khan, N; Afaq, F; Mukhtar, H. Cancer Chemoprevention Through Dietary Antioxidants: Progress and Promise. *Antioxid Redox Signal.*, 2008, 10, 475-510.

Khan, N; Mukhtar, H. Multitargeted Therapy of Cancer by Green Tea Polyphenols. *Cancer Lett.*, 2008, 269, 269-80.

Kim, GY; Kim, KH; Lee, SH; Yoon, MS; Lee, HJ; Moon, DO. Curcumin Inhibits Immunostimulatory Function of Dendritic Cells: Mapks and Translocation of NF-B as Potential Targets. *J Immunol.*, 2005, 174, 8116-24.

Kim, HJ; Yokozawa, T; Kim, HY; Tohda, C; Rao, TP; Juneja, LR. Influence of Amla (*Emblica officinalis* Gaertn.) on Hypercholesterol-Emia and Lipid Peroxidation on Cholesterol-Fed Rats. *Journal of Nutritional Science and Vitaminology*, 2005, 51(6), 413-418.

Ko, SH; Park, JH; Kim, SY; Lee, SW; Chun, SS; Park, E. Antioxidant Effects of Spinach (*Spinacia oleracea* L.) Supplementation in Hyper-Lipidemic Rats. *Preventive Nutrition and Food Science*, 2014, 19(1), 19.

Koh, E; Charoenprasert, S; Mitchell, AE. Effect of Organic and Conventional Cropping Systems on Ascorbic Acid, Vitamin C, Flavonoids, Nitrate, and Oxalate in 27 Varieties of Spinach (*Spinacia oleracea* L.). *Journal of Agricultural and Food Chemistry*, 2012, 60(12), 3144-3150.

Koh, E; Charoenprasert, S; Mitchell, AE. Effect of Organic and Conventional Cropping Systems on Ascorbic Acid, Vitamin C, Flavonoids, Nitrate, and Oxalate in 27 Varieties of Spinach (*Spinacia oleracea* L.). *Journal of Agricultural and Food Chemistry*, 2012, 60(12), 3144-3150.

Krishnaiah, D; Devi, T; Bono, A; Sarbatly, R. Studies on Phytochemical Constituents of Six Malaysian Medicinal Plants. *Journal of Medicinal Plants Research*, 2009, 3(2), 067-072.

Kulkarni, SK; Bhutani, MK; Bishnoi, M. Antidepressant Activity of Curcumin: Involvement of Serotonin and Dopamine System. *Psychopharmacology (Berl)*, 2008, 201, 435–42.

Kumar, K; Bhowmik, D; Dutta, A; Pd Yadav, A; Paswan, S; Srivastava, S; Deb, L. Recent Trends in Potential Traditional Indian Herbs *Emblica Oficinalis* and Its Medicinal Importance. *Journal of Pharmacognosy and Phytochemistry*, 2012, 1(1).

Lepoivre, M; Flaman, JM; Bobé, P; Lemaire, G; Henry, Y. Quenching of the Tyrosyl Free Radical of Ribonucleotide Reductase by Nitric Oxide. *J. Bio. Chem.*, 1994, 269, 21891–97.

Levites, Y; Amit, T; Mandel, S; Youdim, MBH. Neuroprotection and Neurorescue against Amyloid Beta Toxicity and PKC-Dependent Release of Non-Amyloidogenic Soluble Precursor Protein by Green Tea Polyphenol (-)-Epigallocatechin-3-Gallate. *FASEB J*, 2003, 17, 952–4.

Levites, Y; Amit, T; Youdim, MBH; Mandel, S. Involvement of Protein Kinase C Activation and Cell Survival/Cell Cycle Genes in Green Tea Polyphenol (-)-Epigallocatechin-3-Gallate Neuroprotective Action. *J Biol Chem*, 2002, 277, 30574–8.

Levites, Y; Weinreb, O; Maor, G; Youdim, MBH; Mandel, S. Green Tea Polyphenol (-)-Epigallocatechin-3-Gallate Prevents N-Methyl-4- Phenyl-1,2,3,6-Tetrahydropyridine-Induced Dopaminergic Neuro-Degeneration. *J Neurochem*, 2001, 78, 1073–82.

Levites, Y; Youdim, MBH; Maor, G; Mandel, S. Attenuation of 6-Hydroxydopamine (6-OHDA)-Induced Nuclear Factor-Kappa B (Nfkappab) Activation and Cell Death by Tea Extracts in Neuronal Cultures. *Biochem Pharmacol*, 2002, 63, 21–9.

Linardaki, ZI; Orkoula, MG; Kokkosis, AG; Lamari, FN; Margarity, M. Investigation of the Neuroprotective Action of Saffron (*Crocus Sativus* L) in Aluminum Exposed Adult Mice Through Behavioral and Neurobiochemical Assessment. *Food Chem Toxicol.*, 2013, 52, 163–170.

Linder, MC. Nutrition and cancer prevention. In: Linder, M. C., editor. *Nutritional Biochemistry and Metabolism with Chemical Applications.* New York: Elsevier, 1985, p. 347–68.

Luke, A Downey; James, Kaen; Fiona, Nemeh; Angela, Lau; Alex, Poll; Rebeca, Gregory. An Acute Double Blind Placebo Controlled Cross Over Study of 320mg and 640mg Doses of a Special Extract of *Bacopa monnieri* on Sustained Cognitive Performance. *Phytotherapy Research.*, 2013, 27, 1407-1413.

Mandel, S; Grunblatt, E; Riederer, P; Gerlach, M; Levites, Y; Youdim, MBH. Neuroprotective Strategies in Parkinson's Disease: An Update On Progress. *CNS Drugs.*, 2003, 17, 729–62.

Markesbery, WR. Oxidative Stress Hypothesis in Alzheimer's Disease. *Free Radical Biology and Medicine*, 1997, 23(1), 134-147.

Melnyk, JP; Wang, S; Marcone, MF. Chemical and Biological Properties of the World's Most Expensive Spice: Saffron. *Food Res Int.*, 2010, 43, 1981–1989.

Moallem, SA; Hariri, AT; Mahmoudi, M; Hosseinzadeh, H. Effect of Aqueous Extract of *Crocus Sativus* L (Saffron) Stigma Against Subacute Effect of Diazinon on Specific Biomarkers in Rats. *Toxicol Ind Health.*, 2014, 30, 141–6.

Moeller, SM; Jacques, PF; Blumberg, JB. The Potential Role of Dietary Xanthophylls in Cataract and Age-Related Macular Degeneration. *Journal of the American College of Nutrition*, 2000, 19(sup5), 522S-527S.

Morelock, TE; Correll, JC. *Vegetables: Handbook of Plant Breeding*, eds. J. Prohens-Tomas and F. Nuez, Springer, New York, 2008, vol. 1, pp. 189-218.

Morris, MC; Evans, DA; Tangney, CC; Bienias, JL; Wilson, RS. Associations of Vegetable and Fruit Consumption with Age-Related Cognitive Change. *Neurology*, 2006, 67(8), 1370-1376.

Mukhtar, H; Ahmad, N. Tea Polyphenols: Prevention of Cancer and Optimizing Health. *Am J Clin Nutr.*, 2000, 71, 1698S–702S.

Naghma, K; Hasan, M. Tea Polyphenols for Health Promotion. *Life Sciences.*, 2007, 81, 519–533. doi: 10.1016/j.lfs.2007.06.011.

Nambiar, SS; Paramesha, M; Shetty, NP. Comparative Analysis of Phytochemical Profile, Antioxidant Activities and Foam Prevention Abilities of Whole Fruit, Pulp and Seeds of *Emblica Officinalis*. *Journal of Food Science and Technology*, 2015, 52(11), 7254-7262.

Nanjo, F; Goto, K; Seto, R; Suzuki, M; Sakai, M; Hara, Y. Scavenging Effects of Tea Catechins and Their Derivatives on 1,1-Diphenyl-2-Picrylhydrazyl Radical. *Free Radic Biol Med*, 1996, 21, 895–902.

Ng, TP; Chiam, PC; Lee, T; Chua, HC; Lim, L; Kua, EH. Curry Consumption and Cognitive Function in the Elderly. *Am J Epidemiol.*, 2006, 164, 898–906.

NIIR Board of Consultants & Engineers. *Complete Book on Spices & Condiments: (With Cultivation, Processing & Uses)*. Delhi: Asia Pacific Business Press., 2006, pp. 188–191.

Ortiz-López, L; Márquez-Valadez, B; Gómez-Sánchez, A; Silva-Lucero, MDC; Torres-Pérez, M; Téllez-Ballesteros, RI; Ichwan, M; Meraz-Ríos, MA; Kempermann, G; Ramírez-Rodríguez, GB. Green Tea Compound Epigallo-Catechin-3-Gallate (EGCG) Increases Neuronal Survival in Adult Hippocampal Neurogenesis *In Vivo* And *In Vitro*, *Neuroscience*, Volume 322, 2016, Pages 208-220, ISSN 0306-4522, Https://doi.org/10.1016/j.neuroscience.2016.02.040.

Oliveira, GL; et al. Potential Involvement of Oxidative Stress in the Induction of Neurodegenerative Diseases: Actions, Mechanisms and Neuro-Therapeutic Potential of Natural Antioxidants. *Afr J Pharm.*, 2014, 8, 685–700.

Olmedilla, B; Granado, F; Blanco, I; Vaquero, M. Lutein, but not α-Tocopherol, Supplementation Improves Visual Function in Patients with Age-Related Cataracts: A 2-Y Double-Blind, Placebo-Controlled Pilot Study. *Nutrition*, 2003, 19(1), 21-24.

Ono, K; Yoshiike, Y; Takashima, A; Hasegawa, K; Naiki, H; Yamada, M. Potent Anti-Amyloidogenic and Fibril-Destabilizing Effects of Polyphenols *In Vitro*: Implications for the Prevention and Therapeutics of Alzheimer's Disease. *J Neurochem*, 2003, 87, 172–81.

Oudhia, Pankaj. (2004). *Bramhi (Bacopa Monnieri)*. Society for Parthenium Management (SOPAM). Retrieved July 30, 2017.

Pan, T; Fei, J; Zhou, X; Jankovic, J; Le, W. Effects of Green Tea Polyphenols on Dopamine Uptake and on MPP -Induced Dopamine Neuron Injury. *Life Sci*, 2003, 72, 1073–83.

Pandav, R; Belle, SH; DeKosky, ST. Apolipoprotein E Polymorphism and Alzheimer's Disease: The Indo-US Cross-National Dementia Study. *Arch Neurol.*, 2000, 57, 824–30.

Papandreou, MA; Polissiou, MG; Efthimiopoulos, S; Cordopatis, P; Margarity, M; Lamari, FN. Inhibitory Activity on Amyloid-Beta Aggregation and Antioxidant Properties of *Crocus Sativus* Stigmas Extract and Its Crocin Constituents. *J Agric Food Chem.*, 2006, 54, 8762–8768.

Papandreou, MA; Tsachaki, M; Efthimiopoulos, S; Cordopatis, P; Lamari, FN; Margarity, M. Memory Enhancing Effects of Saffron in Aged Mice are Correlated with Antioxidant Protection. *Behav Brain Res.*, 2011, 219, 197–204.

Park, SY; Kim, DS. Discovery of Natural Products from *Curcuma Longa* That Protect Cells from Beta-Amyloid Insult: A Drug Discovery Effort against Alzheimers Disease. *J Nat Prod.*, 2002, 65, 1227–31.

Pendurthi, UR; Rao, LV. Suppression of Transcription Factor Egr-1 by Curcumin. *Thromb Res.*, 2000, 97, 179–89.

Perluigi, M; Joshi, G; Sultana, R; Calabrese, V; De Marco, C; Coccia, R; Cini, C; Butterfield, DA. *In vivo* Protective Effects of Ferulic Acid Ethyl Ester against Amyloid-Beta Peptide 1-42-Induced Oxidative Stress. *J Neurosci Res.*, 2006, 84, 418–426.

Perry, G; Sayre, LM; Atwood, CS; Castellani, RJ; Cash, AD; Rottkamp, CA; et al. The Role of Iron and Copper in the Aetiology of Neurodegenerative Disorders. *CNS Drugs.*, 2002, 16, 339–52.

Pompella, A; Visvikis, A; Paolicchi, A; De Tata, V; Casini, AF. The Changing Faces of Glutathione, a Cellular Protagonist. *Biochemical Pharmacology*, 2003, 66(8), 1499-1503.

Priyadarsini, KI. The Chemistry of Curcumin: From Extraction to Therapeutic Agent. *Molecules.*, 2014, 19 (12), 20091–112.

Purushothuman, S; Nandasena, C; Peoples, CL; El Massri, N; Johnstone, DM; Mitrofanis, J; Stone, J. Saffron Pre-Treatment Offers

Neuroprotection to Nigral and Retinal Dopaminergic Cells of MPTP-Treated mice. *J Parkinsons Dis.*, 2013, 3, 77–83.

Ravindran, PN. ed. *The Genus Curcuma*. Boca Raton, FL: Taylor & Francis., 2007, p. 244

Reddy, VD; Padmavathi, P; Paramahamsa, M; Varadacharyulu, NC. *Amelioration of Alcohol-Induced Oxidative Stress by Emblica Officinalis (Amla) in Rats*, 2010.

Riederer, P; Sofic, E; Rausch, WD; Schmidt, B; Reynolds, GP; Jellinger, K; Youdim, MBH. Transition Metals, Ferritin, Glutathione, and Ascorbic Acid in Parkinsonian Brains. *J Neurochem.*, 1989, 52, 515–20.

Saleem, S; Ahmad, M; Ahmad, AS; Yousuf, S; Ansari, MA; Khan, MB; Ishrat, T; Islam, F. Effect of Saffron (*Crocus Sativus*) on Neuro-behavioral and Neurochemical Changes in Cerebral Ischemia in Rats. *J Med Food.*, 2006, 9, 246–253.

Sabnis, RW. *Handbook of Acid-Base Indicators*. Boca Raton: CRC Press., 2007, p. 219.

Sano, M; Tabata, M; Suzuki, M; Degawa, M; Miyase, T; Maeda-Yamamoto, M. Simultaneous Determination of Twelve Tea Catechins by High-Performance Liquid Chromatography with Electrochemical Detection. *Analyst.*, 2001, 126, 816–820.

Sarkar, PK; Chaudhary, AK. *Ayurvedic Bhasma: The Most Ancient Application of Nanomedicine*. 2010.

Singh SK, Chaudhary AK, Rai DK and SB Rai. Preparation and Characterization of a Mercury Based Indian Traditional Drug Rassindoor. *Indian J. Tradit. Knowl*, 2010, 8, 346–357.

Shati, AA; Elsaid, FG; Hafez, EE. Biochemical and Molecular Aspects of Aluminum Chloride-Induced Neurotoxicity in Mice and the Protective Role of *Crocus Sativus* L Extraction and Honey Syrup. *Neuroscience*, 2011, 175, 66–74.

Shivananjappa, MM; Joshi, MK. Influence of *Emblica officinalis* Aqueous Extract on Growth and Antioxidant Defense System of Human Hepatoma Cell Line (HepG2). *Pharmaceutical Biology*, 2012, 50(4), 497-505.

Shohag, MJI; Wei, YY; Yu, N; Zhang, J; Wang, K; Patring, J; Yang, XE. Natural Variation of Folate Content and Composition in Spinach (*Spinacia oleracea*) Germplasm. *Journal of Agricultural and Food Chemistry*, 2011, 59(23), 12520-12526.

Shukla, V; Vashistha, M; Singh, SN. Evaluation of Antioxidant Profile and Activity of Amalaki (*Emblica Officinalis*), Spirulina and Wheat Grass. *Indian Journal of Clinical Biochemistry*, 2009, 24(1), 70-75.

Singh, RH; Singh, L. Studies on the Anti-Anxiety Effect of the Medyha Rasayana Drug Brahmi (*Bacopa Monniera* Wettst.) *Res Ayur Siddha.*, 1980, 1, 133–148.

Singh, HK; Dhawan, BN. "Neuropsychopharmacological Effects of the Ayurvedic Nootropic *Bacopa Monniera* Linn. (Brahmi)". *Indian J Pharmacol.*, 1997, 29, 359–365.

Singh, MK; Yadav, SS; Yadav, RS; Chauhan, A; Katiyar, D; Khattri, S. Protective Effect of *Emblica Officinalis* in Arsenic Induced Biochemical Alteration and Inflammation in Mice. *Springer Plus*, 2015, 4(1), 438.

Schmidt, Helen, L.; Alexandre, Garcia; Alexandre, Martins; Pamela, B. Mello-Carpes; Felipe, P. Carpes. Green tea Supplementation Produces Better Neuroprotective Effects than Red and Black Tea in Alzheimer-Like Rat Model, *Food Research International*, Volume 100, Part 1, 2017, Pages 442-448, ISSN 0963-9969, Https:// doi.org/10.1016/ j.foodres. 2017.07.026.

Stough, C; Lloyd, J; Clarke, J; et al. The Chronic Effects of an Extract of *Bacopa Monniera* (Brahmi) on Cognitive Function in Healthy Human Subjects. *Psychopharmacology*, 2001, 156, 481–484.

Sultana, R; Ravagna, A; Mohmmad-Abdul, H; Calabrese, V; Butterfield, DA. Ferulic Acid Ethyl Ester Protects Neurons Against Amyloid Beta-Peptide(1-42)-Induced Oxidative Stress and Neurotoxicity: Relationship to Antioxidant Activity. *J Neurochem.*, 2005, 92, 749–758.

Swain, U; Sindhu, KK; Boda, U; Pothani, S; Giridharan, NV; Raghunath, M; Rao, KS. Studies on the Molecular Correlates of Genomic Stability in Rat Brain Cells Following Amalakirasayana Therapy. *Mechanisms of ageing and development*, 2012, 133(4), 112-117.

Turmeric Processing. Kerala Agricultural University, Kerala, India., 2013. Retrieved 10 October 2015.

Turmeric. Drugs.com., 2009. Retrieved 24 August 2017.

Thenmozhi, AJ; Dhivyabharathi, M; Manivasagam, T; Essa, MM. Tannoid Principles of *Emblica Officinalis* Attenuated Aluminum Chloride Induced Apoptosis by Suppressing Oxidative Stress and Tau Pathology Via Akt/GSK-3β Signaling Pathway. *Journal of Ethnopharmacology*, 2016, 194, 20-29.

Tomren, MA; Másson, M; Loftsson, T; Tønnesen, HH. Studies on Curcumin and Curcuminoids XXXI. Symmetric and Asymmetric Curcuminoids: Stability, Activity and Complexation with Cyclodextrin. *Int J Pharm.*, June 2007, 338 (1–2), 27–34.

UK Food Guide. *E100: Curcumin.* UKfoodguide.net. Retrieved 14 April 2017.

US Food and Drug Administration. *Detention Without Physical Examination of Turmeric Due to Lead Contamination.* FDA.gov, 2015.

Vakili, A; Einali, MR; Bandegi, AR. Protective Effect of Crocin Against Cerebral Ischemia in a Dose- Dependent Manner in a Rat Model of Ischemic Stroke. *J Stroke Cerebrovasc Dis.*, 2013, S1052–3057(12), 00345-X.

Vasudevan, M; Parle, M. Memory Enhancing Activity of *Anwala Churna* (*Emblica Officinalis* Gaertn.): An Ayurvedic Preparation. *Physiology & Behavior*, 2007, 91(1), 46-54.

Vaughn, AR; Branum, A; Sivamani, RK. Effects of Turmeric (*Curcuma Longa*) On Skin Health: A Systematic Review of the Clinical Evidence. *Phytotherapy Research.*, 2016, 30(8), 1243–64.

Wang, Y; Chang, CF; Chou, J; Chen, HL; Deng, X; Harvey, BK; Bickford, PC. Dietary Supplementation with Blueberries, Spinach, or Spirulina Reduces Ischemic Brain Damage. *Experimental Neurology*, 2005, 193(1), 75-84.

Wu, CD; Wei, GX. Tea as a Functional Food for Oral Health. *Nutrition.*, 2002, 18, 443–4.

Xu, Y; Ku, BS; Yao, HY; Lin, YH; Ma, X; Zhang, YH; et al. The Effects of Curcumin on Depressive-Like Behaviors in Mice. *Eur J Pharmacol.*, 2005, 518, 40–6.

Xuan, B; Zhou, YH; Li, N; Min, ZD; Chiou, GC. Effects of Crocin Analogs on Ocular Blood Flow and Retinal Function. *J Ocular Pharmacol Therap.*, 1999, 15, 143–152.

Yang, F; Lim, GP; Begum, AN; Ubeda, OJ; Simmons, MR; Ambegaokar, SS; et al. Curcumin Inhibits Formation of Amyloid Beta Oligomers and Fibrils, Binds Plaques, and Reduces Amyloid *In Vivo*. *J Biol Chem.*, 2005, 280, 5892–901.

Zhang, YJ; Tanaka, T; Iwamoto, Y; Yang, CR; Kouno, I. Novel Norsesquiterpenoids from the Roots of *Phyllanthus Emblica*. *Journal of natural products*, 2000, 63(11), 1507-1510.

Zhang, YJ; Tanaka, T; Iwamoto, Y; Yang, CR; Kouno, I. Novel Sesquiterpenoids from the Roots of *Phyllanthus Emblica*. *Journal of natural products*, 2001, 64(7), 870-87.

In: Food for Huntington's Disease ISBN: 978-1-53613-854-2
Editors: M. Mohamed Essa et al. © 2018 Nova Science Publishers, Inc.

Chapter 2

POLYPHENOLS AND HUNTINGTON'S DISEASE

T. Manivasagam[1], A. Justin Thenmozhi[1,],
M. Dhivya Bharathi[1], T. Sumathi[2],
C. Saravanababu[3], A. Borah[4] and M. Mohamed Essa[5,6,7]*

[1]Department of Biochemistry and Biotechnology, Faculty of Science, Annamalai University, Annamalainagar, Tamil Nadu, India
[2]Department of Medical Biochemistry, University of Madras, Taramani Campus, Chennai, Tamil Nadu, India
[3]Cellular and Molecular Neurobiology Laboratory, Department of Life Science and Bioinformatics, Assam University, Silchar, Assam, India
[4] Department of Pharmacology, JSS College of Pharmacy, JSS Academy of Higher Education and Research, SS Nagar, Mysore, Karnataka, India
[5]Department of Food Science and Nutrition, CAMS, Sultan Qaboos University, Muscat, Oman
[6]Ageing and Dementia Research Group, Sultan Qaboos University, Muscat, Oman
[7]Food and Brain Research Foundation, Chennai, Tamil Nadu, India

---

* Corresponding Author Email: justinthenmozhi@rediffmail.com.

Abstract

Huntington's disease is the most common neurodegenerative disease, characterized by notable cognitive impairment and specific movement disorder. Currently used medications offer symptomatic relief to HD, without preventing the disease progression. Various pre-clinical experiments and clinical trials have shown that the multi-target ability of the traditional herbal medicine and its phytochemicals could offer therapeutic ailment for HD. Plant derived polyphenols are the ubiquitous compound with multiple pharmacological activities including anti-oxidant, anti-inflammatory, mitochondrial protective and anti-apoptotic activities. They can improve cognitive functions and prevent/delay the onset of certain neurodegenerative disease including HD.

Keywords: Huntington's disease, polyphenol, oxidative stress, mitochondrial dysfunction, neuroprotection

Introduction

Huntington's disease (HD) is a progressive, complex, and inherited neurodegenerative disease (roughly 85 to 95% of cases), symptomatic as a triad of movement, cognitive, and psychiatric disorders. HD affects middle-aged people between 30 and 50 years, with an onset from 2 to 85 years, usually leads to death 15 to 20 years after onset. Juvenile cases develop more rapidly and can prove fatal within 7–10 years from the commencement of the disease. Pneumonia is the main cause of death in HD patients. The disease was initially called "chorea" due to the fact that people affected by this disease have a tendency towards erratic movement similar to dancing. Now it is more commonly called Huntington's (or Huntington) Disease. The first occurrence of HD is believed to be in the 1600s, but it was misunderstood as a "dancing disorder" and was viewed as witchcraft (Lee et al., 1842). A disease with symptoms similar to HD had been found in families in colonial New England for generations and was known locally as "magrums" or "megrims". The patients were treated as disgraceful witches and burnt to death openly. In addition it was believed that their families were also to be cursed. Most of the sufferers in the well-known Salem Witch Trials, held in Salem, Massachusetts, USA from 1692 to 1693, were in fact, sufferers of HD.

Charles Waters published his observations on HD patients in Dunglison's "Practice of Medicine" in 1842 and later in "American Medical Times" in 1863.In 1872, Johan Christian Lund found a high incidence of dementia combined with jerky movements in subjects in Norway; due to these symptoms the disease is frequently called "setesdalrykkja" in that country (Stien, 1991). But it was not until 1872, that George Huntington developed a model for the disease's phenotypes and then called it Huntington's chorea. He published a full description of the disease in the scientific document entitled "On Chorea". In 1958 another physician, Americo Negrette, observed the features of HD patients; his findings were presented by his coworker, Ramon Avilla Giron at New York in 1972 when United States of America had been commemorating the centenary year of HD (Bhattacharyya, 2016).

CLINICAL SYMPTOMS

The Motor Symptoms and Signs

Impaired movement is the cardinal symptom of HD; it causes dysfunction in involuntary and voluntary motor functions. Fast-uncontrolled movements of the distal limb muscles and proximal muscles of the trunk characterized the choreatic movements associated with HD. Initially, the movements occur in the fingers, toes, and in the small facial muscles. After which the unwanted movements extend to other muscles in distal to proximal or axial directions. If the patient wants to move their tongue it can become a struggle of uncertainty and difficulty. In the hands, the palmsmoves upward and then back, keeping the hands rolling. Other symptoms include shrugged shoulders, the perpetual motion of feet and legs, turned and averted toes, crossed and sudden movement of feet, and varied, irregular and completely un-describable motions as well as unconceivable attitudes and expressions. Patients show unstable walking with a slightly inebriated look. They also develop akinesia, hypokinesia, and rigidity (symptoms like Parkinson's disease), which result in bradykinesia, a slowness in the movement, and akinesia, an obscurity in starting movements. Furthermore, difficulties in daily activities like taking a bath or shower, dressing, getting out of bed, cleaning the house, using the toilet, cooking, and eating are found.

Behaviour and Psychiatric Symptoms and Signs

Psychiatric symptoms precede the onset of motor symptoms and are present mainly during the early stage of HD. The psychiatric signs in HD patients vary between 33% and 76%, depending on the methods used to evaluate them. Due to the negative impact on everyday activities, these symptoms severely impair a patient's functioning and are also hard on the families of the patients. The behavioral and psychiatric symptoms include depression, weight loss, apathy, inactivity, low self-esteem, and feelings of guilt and anxiety. Early symptomatic individuals and pre-manifest gene carriers commit suicide more frequently. Obsessions and compulsions lead to disturbance in the life of the patient and result in aggression and irritability. Enhanced passive behavior and a loss of interest are also found as a part of the apathy syndrome. Psychosis may appear along with cognitive dysfunction, mainly in the final stages of HD. In the later stages hypo-sexuality can also occur.

Secondary Symptoms and Signs

Unintended weight loss, diminished appetites, slower functioning, difficulty in food intake and swallowing, hypothalamic neuronal loss, disturbances in the circadian rhythm of sleep are the common symptoms. Autonomic disturbances can result in attacks of profuse sweating. Speech impairment with reduced intelligibility, executive dysfunction, such as poor decision-making, as well as irritability and impulsivity are also found in HD patients. Language and visual-spatial deficits such as lowered attention, verbal fluency, and abstract reasoning are also found in the late stage of the disease.

DIAGNOSIS OF HUNTINGTON'S DISEASE

As the clinical symptoms of HD are always typical, the diagnosis is easy for a patient with choreiform movements, a known family history, and cognitive dysfunction. But it is difficult for patients with uncharacteristic presentations or a lack of family history. Sometimes HD maybe confused with chorea gravidarum, vascular hemichorea, hyperthyroid chorea, tardive dyskinesia, unilateral post-infectious (Sydenham's) chorea, and chorea linked to auto-antibodies raised against phospholipids. Compared to HD, the characteristics of these disorders are not familial, have a different time line, do not have impaired saccades, motor impersistence, and cognitive decline. Choreiform movements are unpredictable and irregular, but the movements are stereotyped to involve both the upper and lower limbs. Patients are unaware and do not have any explanation for these unpurposed movements. This gait disorder is always awkward, nonspecific, or tilt on a broad base. During the disease progression, patients may develop postural instability that leads to a "dancing" symptom. The neurologic examinations indicate the presence of gait, rigidity, the loss of saccadic eye movements, and dystonia. They struggle to preserve certain fixed postures.

Genetic testing is normally used to confirm the diagnosis and identify the patients with atypical clinical symptoms. It can be used for patients who don't have the family history of HD or those having negative family history (early parental death, misdiagnosis adoption, or non paternity). Brain imaging techniques have shown atrophy in caudate nuclei, which may be used to diagnosis even before the onset of motor symptoms.

PATHOLOGY OF HD

HD affects both the men and women. The Huntingtin protein (HTT) gene, located in the short arm of chromosome 4 (4p16.3 region), shows an increased number of CAG nucleotide repeats during HD. It encodes to the 350 kDa protein consisting of several sub domains. At the N-terminal, the polyglutamine (polyQ) extension, coded by the CAG repeats, acts as a membrane association signal. The polyQ domain is trailed by a polyproline sequence, which stabilizes the protein conformation in mammals. The amino-terminal of the HTT is followed by three clusters of HEAT repeats, which are needed to bind with the interacting proteins. Both the onset and severity of the disease is directly connected with the number of CAG repeats, but the actual function of this remains elusive. The exon-1 of the HTT gene contains 6 to 35 CAG repeats, but an intermediate number (36–40) will lead to a low progression of the pathology. If the HTT has more than 40 glutamine repeats, then the disease is expressed during the adult stage. If the number of glutamine repeats exceeds 60, then the juvenile form of the HD develops.

NEUROLOGY OF HUNTINGTON'S DISEASE

The mutant Huntingtin protein (mHTT) induces selective neurodegeneration in the striatum and the inner parts of the cortex during the early stages of HD. In the advanced cases the hippocampus, cerebellum, hypothalamus, thalamic nuclei, andamygdale are also affected. Severe atrophy was found in other brain regions like the lateral tuberal nucleus of the hypothalamus. The neurons that are severely affected in HD are the striatal projection neurons, which are linked to the different brain regions through its axons. These neurons are the GABAergic medium-sized spiny neurons (MSNs), and they represent about 95% of the total neurons. The striatum receives glutamatergic input from the cortex and is innervate to the globus pallidus and substantia nigra. The progressive loss of MSN in HD leads to glutamate excitotoxicity. However, there are interneurons that transmit somatostatin NADPH diaphorase, neuropeptide Y, cholinergic interneurons, and a subclass of GABAergic neurons.

MECHANISM OF NEUROGENERATION

The exact molecular mechanism, by which HTT mutation induces the striatal neurodegeneration, is still elusive. This mechanism is multifactorial, complex, and develops a coexistence of both loss and gain of functional effects. The mHTT is reported to negatively affect several different processes includingtranscription, autophagy, ubiquitin-proteasome system, vesicular trafficking, calcium homeostasis, and mitochondrial function. In addition, the mutation may also hamper the HTT protein from exerting its normal activities that are central for the function and viability of striatum neurons.

MITOCHONDRIAL DYSFUNCTION

Numerous experiments have indicated various changes in the structure and functions of the brain mitochondria in HD patients and HD postmortem tissues. These include:

1. A reduction in glucose uptake and an energy depletion in the striatum and cortex.
2. A diminished activity of aconitase (a tricarboxylic acid cycle enzyme) activity with an enhanced ROS synthesis, excitotoxicity, and mitochondrial dysfunction in the striatum and the cerebral cortex.
3. A lowered level of mitochondrial complexes II–III and IV activity in the striatum.
4. Increased lactate levels in the cerebral cortex and the striatum.
5. An enhanced lactate/pyruvate ratio in the cerebrospinal fluid.
6. A reduced phosphocreatine/inorganic phosphate ratio in skeletal muscle.

7. Diminished mitochondrial ATP generation.
8. Morphological changes and diminished mitochondrial membrane potential.
9. A depletion of leukocytic mitochondrial DNA.

OXIDATIVE STRESS IN HD

Oxidative free radicals are highly reactive oxygen derivate, which have an unpaired electron in their outer most shell, and are lethal to cells. If their levels are become enhanced, it leads to a condition called oxidative stress. Various mechanisms lead to the development of oxidative stress in HD including excitotoxicity, nitric oxide dysregulation, cellular energetic defects, inflammatory reactions, and heavy metal toxicity. Mitochondrial respiratory complexes are the main source of ROS; defects in its structure or function leads to the over production of ROS. Inhibition of complex II in experimental models leads to the formation of oxidative stress in HD. Another important mechanism that induces mitochondrial ROS production is the Ca^{2+} dyshomeostasis. Energy depletion or diminished ATP synthesis leads to the partial depolarization of the outer mitochondrial membrane and the release the voltage dependent Mg^{2+} ion. This blocks the Ca^{2+} channel in the NMDA receptor complex. Glutamate removes the inhibition and allows the steady entry of Ca^{2+} into the cell, leading to the excitotoxic events that involve oxidative stress. Sodium ions can enter through the NMDA receptor; under energy-deprived conditions it will be extruded less effectively from the cytoplasm by the ATP dependent Na^+/K^+ATPase. Impaired mitochondrial function affects the intracellular Ca^{2+} concentration, as the normal mitochondrion is involved in Ca^{2+} sequestration. Diminished mitochondrial capability lowers the proton gradient maintenance and a negative potential on the inside of the inner membrane will diminish their capacity to attract Ca^{2+}. Enhanced mitochondrial matrix Ca^{2+} loading induces superoxide production by the mitochondria in HD neurons. This leads to an enhanced mitochondrial DNA damage impeding the mitochondria function. Evidence links the redox-transition metals such as copper and iron as mediators of oxidative stress in neurological diseases. However, the presence of iron in the basal ganglia is a risk factor for developing the disease. Iron has been showed to damage synapses leading to lowered GABA uptake and elevated dopamine uptake. Ceruloplasmin, a protein involved in copper metabolism, is also involved in iron homeostasis. Enhanced levels of ceruloplasmin were described in HD. The susceptible brain regions (caudatenucleus) are mostly associated with neurodegeneration and astrogliosis. 3-Nitro Propionic acid, an inducer of HD in experimental animals caused oxidative stress from an inflammatory response.

EXCITOTOXICITY

Many experiments have demonstrated the link between the intracellular signaling pathways and excitotoxicity during HD. The NMDA receptors along with kainite, c-Jun-N-terminal kinase (JNK), mixed lineage kinase (MLK), and a postsynaptic density protein 95 (PSDP-95) are considered important elements in this cascade. Existing reports indicate that the stimulation of the Glutamate receptor is connected with the activation of MLK-1. Further, the activated JNK pathway is involved in apoptosis. The scaffold protein, PSDP-95 contains guanylate cyclase activity and it is reported to link with many intracellular proteins. In addition it is also binds to NMDA receptor through some small repeat units called PDZ domains, thereby regulating the synaptogenesis and synaptic plasticity. Then, both NMDA and kainate receptors get hyposensitized due to the interference of the mHTT with the PSDP-95, which facilitates the enhanced Ca^{2+} uptake and the stimulation of the MLK-2 activation. This allows the activation of MAP kinase 4 and 7 and the stress signaling kinases (SEK-1), which subsequently enables the JNK-2 activity by phosphorylating the N-terminal fragment of c-Junthatis one half of the transcription factor AP-1. The phosphorylation of the MLK-2 at the C-terminal fragment is caused by JNK-2 activation, which could be one of the significant events in stimulating apoptosis in HD.

INFLAMMATION

In the brain, the non-neuronal glial cells play different roles in neuronal function and tissue homeostasis. Microglia represent≤ 10% of the total cells and are considered as the main inhabitants of the immune cells of the CNS. When the tissues undergo infection and damage, it attains an 'ameboid' appearance, showing enhanced phagocytic activity and initiates an innate immune response by producing several inflammatory molecules such as TNF-αand IL-6. After the removal of the triggered stimuli, the microglia participates in the regeneration of the injured tissue. If the provocative stimuli could not be eliminated, the constant production of IL-6, IL-8, and TNF-α occurs, which can drive chronic inflammation and tissue damage that develops the disease further, thereby implicating various acute and chronic neurological disorders. The mHTT expression in the microglia is adequate to give a cell-autonomous augmentation of proinflammatory gene expression.

In the brain, astrocytes comprises about 90% of cells and are responsible for providing physical support to neurons and microglia, removing toxic materials including extracellular glutamate, providing factors necessary for proper function neurons, microglia, and endothelial cells, helping to maintain the extracellular ion balance, and finally offer nourishment in form of lactate. During the neuronal insult, astrocytes enhance the inflammatory process, which was started by microglia that were involved in repairing the spoiled tissue. Several reports have indicated that the mHTT expressing astrocytes are flawed in carrying out functions that hold up neuronal wellbeing.

APOPTOSIS

Apoptosis is the primary cause of progressive death in HD neurons. Neurons undergo apoptosis through information received from internal or external agents. Internal information is mainly correlated with the cell type, state of maturity and differentiation, and developmental stage whereas external features include the presence and absence of growth factors, hormones, cytokines, and interactions of the cell matrix that affect the cell fate. It is morphologically characterized by the presence of peri-nuclear chromatin condensation, membrane blebbing, the swelling of the intracellular organelles, and DNA fragmentation. The nonrandom pattern of DNA fragmentation produces a ladder formation during agarose gel electrophoresis. Moreover, the mitochondrial function was needed for the occurrence of apoptosis. Mitochondrial functional impairment occurring due to the inhibition of the various respiratory chain complexes can lead to apoptosis. An enhanced stimulation of glutamate receptors ends in Ca^{2+} influx by opening the NMDA channels. More Ca^{2+} gets accumulated in the mitochondria. It results in the mitochondrial inner membrane potential being transiently depolarized and leads to mitochondrial permeability transition. Then internal and external membranes of mitochondrial proteins get fused, leading to the formation of the mitochondrial PT pore complex. The induction of PT pores is triggered by the enhanced synthesis of reactive oxygen species. Due to the inner membrane potential collapse, cytochrome C and the apoptosis inducing factor (AIF) are released from the pores. Thus oxidative stress, excitotoxicity, and partial energy depletion leads to apoptosis in HD.

In HD, about 30% of brain mass gets reduced and a direct correlation was found between brain weight and disease progression. However severe loss is found in the basal ganglia with about a 60% reduction in the putamen, caudate, and globus pallidus mass. Severe neuropathological changes including neuronal loss and astrogliosis were present in the caudate nucleus. The GABA-nergic MSN of the caudate region is also affected. The cholinergic and aspiny interneurons (NADPH-diaphorase) are left relatively spared. The cerebral cortex and putamen are affected less whereas cerebellum get slightly affected.

TREATMENT AND CARE

Treatment with donepezil (a cholinesterase inhibitor) has not been shown to enhance cognition or motor performance in HD. Recent studies have indicated that the administration of vitamin E and omega-3 fatty acid did not offer any beneficial effects, whereas tetrabenazine, an antidopaminergic monoamine depleting agent, is shown to be effective for treating the involuntary movement, but not for depression or cognitive impairment. Small doses of neuroleptics (haloperidol) and atypical neuroleptics (olanzapine) are used for the treatment of psychotic symptoms and to nullify the aggression. Valproic acid is used to treat the hyperkinesias, whereas anti-Parkinsonic drugs improve the hypokinetic and rigidity symptoms. Medication with L-dopa increases the severity of the choreatic movements in HD. Benzodiazepines are used to reduce aggressiveness, irritability, anxiety, and sleep disorders. Neuropsychiatric problems are mainly treated with psychological drugs in the early phase of HD, which offer a greater relief to the patient and their family. If the patient develops hallucinations or delusions, then a consultation with a psychiatrist is desirable, because a more complex neuroleptic treatment is needed. Neuroleptics produce side effects, which reduce the patient's cognition and therefore, will need to be balanced in treatment. Depression can be treated with ant-depressive agents, with psychological therapy (cognitive behavior therapy), or through regular clinical appointments. Antiepileptic treatment is also indicative in juvenile HD. None of the currently list of drugs offer effective treatment to preventing the onset or reduce the progress of HD. The cognitive deficits associated with HD are generally unresponsive to treatment.

NATURAL PRODUCTS AND NEURODEGENERATIVE DISEASES

Natural phytochemicals obtained through one's natural diet exhibit various biological functions including antioxidant, antimutagenic, anticarcinogenic, antiaging, and neuroprotective activities. Experimental, epidemiological, and clinical studies have indicated there is a link between nutrition and cognition, mood decline, and neurodegeneration; they highlight the efficacy of diet in delaying or preventing NDDs. Edible phytochemicals are considered to be good candidates for preventive and/or protective actions in NDDs due to their low side-effects and history of human use. The safety and effectiveness of herbal formulations for treating dementia were explored by comparing the herbal medicine with a placebo and various pharmaceutical agents. All the studies indicated that the herbal medicine attenuated the symptoms with no severe adverse effects. As there is no effective treatment for HD, research has been focused on developing new drugs from dietary sources, which have multifunctional properties. Novel plant extracts and their major components including polyphenols can have antioxidant effects as well as their various modulatory effects on the cholinergic, glutaminergic, GABAergic, catecholaminergic, serotonergic and histaminergic systems in HD have been studied.

POLYPHENOLS

Polyphenols are secondary metabolites, which offer protection to plants from pests, insects, and ultraviolet light. They are ubiquitously present in fruits, seeds, vegetables, cereals, pulses, and oils, among others. Currently, there are known to be more than 8,000 polyphenolic compounds without substantial nutritional value. Recently, there has been an increased interest in exploring their antioxidative function. Polyphenolic compounds offer a therapeutic affect against various diseases including cancer, atherosclerosis, diabetes, cardiovascular, and neurodegenerative diseases.

CLASSIFICATIONS AND DIETARY SOURCES OF POLYPHENOLS

Polyphenols consists of phenolic structure with several hydroxyl groups, but have variation from simple (phenolic acids) to complex (condensed tannins) polymeric molecules.

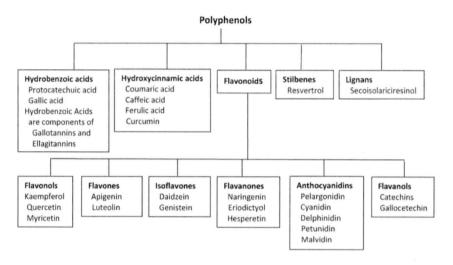

Figure 1. Classification of Polyphenols.

They are classified based on the number of phenolic rings and the structural elements linked to the rings. They include:

(a) **Phenolic acid** (non-flavonoid polyphenols) represent about 1/3 of total polyphenol intake of our diet and further classified into cinnamic acid and benzoic acid derivatives.

(b) **Flavonoids** make up approximately 2/3 of the polyphenolic content in our diet. Their structural backbone contains C6-C3-C6, whose two C6 phenolic rings are named Ring A and Ring B with a linking C3 chromane ring. They are further divided into anthocyanins and anthoxanthins, which are further classified into flavonols, flavones, isoflavones, flavonones, and flavanols.

(c) **Stilbenes** consist of a 1,2-diphenylethylene nucleus with attached hydroxyl groups on the aromatic rings; an example is Trans-resveratrol.
(d) **Tannins** are the water-soluble polyphenols that can be further classified into hydrolysable and condensed tannins.
(e) **Diferuloyl methanes** are characterized by hydroxyls substituting two aromatic rings, linked by an aliphatic chain containing carbonyl groups; an example is Curcumin.

RESVERATROL

Resveratrol is a small polyphenol found in among 70 dissimilar plants such as fruits (plums, grapes, berries, pines, pomegranates, and mulberries), tea, nuts, and some plants sources used in traditional Asian medicine. It exists as two isomers, trans- and cis-resveratrol, in which trans-resveratrol is known to be nontoxic and more potential than cis-resveratrol. After it is administered orally, about 70-75% of resveratrol is taken up quickly and metabolized into glucuronide and sulphate derivatives that are consequently removed from the urine. One published paper about resveratrol safety demonstrated that the utilization of 0.5 - 5.0 g of resveratrol did not cause any serious adverse effects in humans. Resveratrol targets the CNS as it can cross the blood brain barrier (BBB) and it takes on a protective role during various neurodegenerative conditions.

Resveratrol and HD

By targeting several signaling pathways, the resveratrol exhibits its protective role *in vivo*. Resveratrol has been shown to mediate its potential therapeutic action against diseases such as neurodegenerative diseases, diabetes, and inflammatory disorders through the activation of sirtuin-1 (SIRT1). Sirtuin enzymes are important for many cellular processes including cell cycle regulation, fatty acid metabolism, the regulation of p53, gene silencing, and life span extension. Parker et al. (2005) reported that resveratrol prohibited neuronal impairment phenotypes in a transgenic *C. elegans* model, expressing mutant poly-glutamines by enhancing the expression of Sir2.In striatal cultures from the HdhQ111 knock-in mice model of HD, resveratrol offered neuronal protection against the mutant poly-glutamine-mediated cell death (Parker et al., 2005) and HEK293T cells (Li et al., 2007) through the promotion of SIRT1-associated mechanisms. The activation of the tumor suppressor p53 plays a significant role in intervening with the mHTT toxic effects and mediating cytotoxicity in HD cells of the transgenic mouse (Bae et al., 2005). Resveratrol protects cells against the toxic effects of mHTT by inducing SIRT1 activity and inhibiting p53 indirectly as SIRT1 interacts with and deacetylates p53 (Vaziri et al., 2001; Luo et al., 2001). The p53 deacetylation causes the attenuation of its activity and inhibits p53 dependent apoptosis.

The oral administration of resveratrol reverted the impaired cognitive and motor functions as well as the inflammation persuaded 3-nitro-propionic acid (complex II inhibitor of the electron transport chain), which leads to HD symptoms in mice (Kumar et al., 2006). The beneficial properties of resveratrol were shown by Beal and Ferrante (2004) in the N171-82Q transgenic mouse model of HD. In mHTT-expressing nerve cells, the Ras-extracellular signal-regulated kinase (ERK) activation offers neuroprotection, (Apostol et al., 2006), consequently the activation of the Ras-ERK cascade offered neuroprotection against mHTT in the Drosophila model of HD (Maher et al., 2011).

Treatment of SRT501, a proprietary micronized resveratrol formulation in the N171-82Q HD mouse model showed biological effects in the cortex, but did not prevent or improve the HD-type neurotoxicity in the striatum (Ho et al., 2010). As resveratrol can pass through the BBB and mount up in the cerebral cortex after its oral administration, the Ho et al. (2010) indicated that an improved administration or the administration of potent resveratrol analogues or metabolites would be more appropriate for HD. Dopamine induces oxidative stress and triggers apoptosis in dopaminergic neuroblastoma SH-SY5Y cells, hyper-expressing the mutant polyQHTT protein. Resveratrol attenuates the dopamine induced generation of ROS, restores the level of ATG4, allows the processing of autophagosomal-associated isoform (LC3) that plays a fundamental role in facilitating the degradation of polyQ-HTT aggregates, and protects the cells from dopamine toxicity.

CURCUMIN

Curcumin [1, 7-Bis (4-hydroxy-3-methoxyphenyl)-1,6-heptadiene 3,5-dione], from the rhizome of turmeric is one of the most extensively studied naturally derived phytochemicals in recent decades due to its various pharmacological properties. Curcuminoids are the active components attributed to pharmacological properties of turmeric, and they present as a mixture of curcumin (75–80%), demethoxycurcumin (15–20%), and bis demethoxy curcumin (3–5%). A major disadvantage of curcumin is its poor bioavailability due to poor absorption, insolubility in aqueous media, rapid metabolism, and rapid systemic elimination. The administration of curcumin along with piperine/turmeric oil, or in the form of nano-particles, or by complex ationwith phosphatidyl choline and liposome enhanced its bioavailability in tissues. Curcumin has been extensively studied for its therapeutic effects on nervous system, especially the brain, and the diseases related to this vital organ (Table 1).

Table 1. Protective effect of curcumin on neurological diseases

S. No	Protective effect of curcumin on neurological diseases
1.	Parkinson's disease
2.	Alzheimer's disease
3.	Multiple sclerosis
4.	Brain tumor
5.	Traumatic brain injury
6.	Neuroinflammatory diseases
7.	Depression
8.	Ischemia
9.	Encephalopathy (hepatic and/or uremic)

Curcumin and HD

The administration of 3-nitropropionic acid showed body weight loss, diminished motor function, changes in oxidative stress, neuro-inflammatory, and neurochemical variability. Curcumin alone and in combination with piperine showed beneficial effect against 3-NP induced motor deficit, neurochemical, and biochemical abnormalities in rats (Singh et al., 2015). Curcumin encapsulated solid lipid nanoparticles (C-SLNs) and ameliorated the 3-NP-induced diminished mitochondrial complexes, cytochrome levels, glutathione levels, superoxide dismutase activity, nuclear factor-erythroid 2 antioxidant pathway, and neuro motor co-ordination deficits (Sandhir et al. 2014).

(-)-EPIGALLOCATECHINGALLATE (EGCG)

Tea is second most commonly consumed beverage worldwide after water. The consumption of tea is split with ~ 20% green tea, (mainly in China and Japan), ~78 %black tea, (Western countries) and less than 2% is oolong tea (Japan and China).Green tea is unfermented tea and mainly consists of catechins (30-40% of its own dry weight), whereas black tea is fermented and oolong teas are partially fermented; the fermentation process induces the oxidation and polymerization of catechins. Catechins belong to a group of polyphenols that are reported to be responsible for the therapeutic activities of green tea. The catechins flavonoids present in green tea are (+)-catechin, (-)-epicatechin, (+)-catechingallate, (-)-epicatechin allate (ECG), (-)-epigallocatechin, (+)-gallocatechin, (+)-gallocatechin allate, and (-)-epigallocatechin allate (EGCG). EGCG is the most prominent of the catechins in green tea with numerous pharmacological properties (Figure 2).The bioavailability of green tea catechins in humans and animals depends on the route of administration. Orally administered catechins are easily absorbed, get metabolized, and predominantly excreted within 24 h. Abd El Mohsen et al.(2002) stated that the catechin metabolites like epicatechin lucuronide and its methylated derivative were detected in brain after oral ingestion in rats. Recently, catechins, particularly EGCG, have attracted attention as a potential therapeutic agent for neurodegenerative diseases mainly due to their antioxidant, metal chelating, mitochondrial protective, anti-apoptotic, and antiinflammatory properties. It has also been reported to cross the blood–brain barrier and has been demonstrated to be safe though clinical studies.

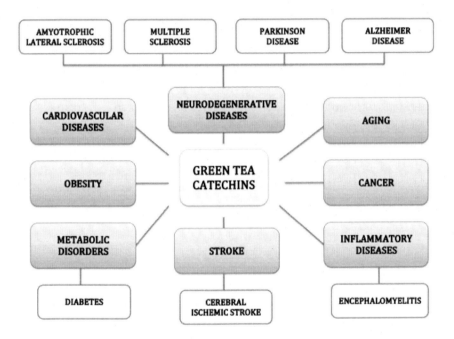

Figure 2. Neuroprotective effect of green tea catechins.

Huntington's Disease and EGCG

Ehrnhoefer et al., (2006) demonstrated that the green tea EGCG potently inhibited the aggregation, misfolding, and oligomerization of mutant HTT exon 1 protein in the yeast model of HD. EGCG administration attenuated photoreceptor degeneration and motor dysfunction in transgenic HD flies over expressing the HTT exon 1 protein.

HD AND GRAPE-DERIVED POLYPHENOLS

Polyphenols from grapes or its derived products are linked with the prevention of cardiovascular disease, cancer, and neurodegenerative disorders. The pharmacological properties of grapes are directly proportional to their polyphenol levels. Resveratrol, anthocyanin and proanthocyanidins are found abundantly in grapes, wines, juice, and grape seed extracts. Due to the popular use of grapes in foods and drinks and the beneficial role of grape-derived polyphenols, scientist focused their research on how they exert their neuroprotective effect. Grape seed polyphenolic extract (GSPE) significantly extended the lifespan of the UAS-Q93 HTTexon1 transgenic drosophila model of HD. It also attenuated HD phenotypes in the R6/2 mouse model of HD through its antioxidant activity and by preventing the abnormal aggregation of mHTT proteins.

CONCLUSION

Even though about 8000 polyphenols have been discovered so far, only very limited research has been carried out on the neuroprotective effects of polyphenols against HD. Better knowledge on the polyphenol bioavailability will facilitate current scientific understanding and offer hope for the prevention of HD.

REFERENCES

Abd El Mohsen, M. M., Kuhnle, G., Rechner, A. R., Schroeter, H., Rose, S., Jenner, P. & Rice-Evans, C. A. (2002). Uptake and Metabolism of

Epicatechin and Its Access to the Brain After Oral Ingestion. *Free Radic Biol Med., 33*, 1693-1702.

Apostol, B. L., Illes, K., Pallos, J., Bodai, L., Wu, J., Strand, A., Schweitzer, E. S., Olson, J. M., Kazantsev, A., Marsh, J. L., et al. (2006). Mutant Huntingtin Alters MAPK Signaling Pathways in PC12 and Striatal Cells: ERK1/2 Protects Against Mutant Huntingtin-Associated Toxicity. *Hum. Mol. Genet., 15*, 273-285.

Ashu Johri, M. Flint Beal. (2012). Antioxidants in Huntington's disease. *Biochimica et Biophysica Acta*, 1822, 664-674.

Bae, B. I., Xu, H., Igarashi, S. et al., (2005). P53 Mediates Cellular Dysfunction and Behavioral Abnormalities in Huntington's Disease, *Neuron, 47*, 29-41.

Beal, M. F. & Ferrante, R. J. (2004). Experimental Therapeutics in Transgenic Mouse Models of Huntington's Disease. *Nature Reviews Neuroscience, 5*, 373-384.

Bhattacharyya, K. B. (2016). The Story of George Huntington and His Disease. *Ann Indian Acad Neurol, 19*, 25-28.

Ehrnhoefer, D. E., Duennwald, M., Markovic, P., Wacker, J. L., Engemann, S., Roark, M., Legleiter, J., Marsh, L., Thompson, L. M., Lindquist, S., Muchowski, P. J. & Wanker, E. E. (2006). Green Tea (2)-Epigallocatechin-Gallate Modulates Early Events in Huntingtin Misfolding and Reduces Toxicity in Huntington's Disease Models. *Human Molecular Genetics, 15*, 2743-2751.

Henning, S. M., Niu, Y., Lee, N. H., Thames, G. D., Minutti, R. R., Wang, H., Go, V. L. & Heber, D. (2004). Bioavailability and Antioxidant Activity of Tea Flavanols After Consumption of Green Tea, Black Tea, or a Green Tea Extract Supplement. *Am. J. Clin. Nutr., 80*, 1558-1564.

Ho, D.J., Calingasan, N. Y., Wille, E., Dumont, M. & Beal, M. F. (2010). Resveratrol Protects Against Peripheral Deficits in a Mouse Model of Huntington's Disease. *Exp. Neurol., 225*, 74-84.

Jun, Wang., Cathie, M. Pfleger., Lauren, Friedman., Roselle, Vittorino., Wei, Zhao., Xianjuan, Qian.,Lindsay, Conley., Lap, Ho. & Giulio, M.

Pasinetti. (2010). Potential Application of Grape Derived Polyphenols in Huntington's Disease. *Translational Neuroscience*, *1*, 95-100.

Kumar, P., Padi, S. S., Naidu, P. S. & Kumar, A. (2006). Effect of Resveratrol on 3- Nitropropionic Acid-Induced Biochemical and Behavioural Changes: Possible Neuroprotective Mechanisms. *Behav. Pharmacol.*, *17*, 485–492.

Lee, J., Hwang, Y. J., Ryu, H., Kowall, N. W. & Ryu, H. (2014). Nucleolar Dysfunction in Huntington's disease. *Biochimica et Biophysica Acta (BBA) - Molecular Basis of Disease*, 1842, 785-790.

Li, Y., Yokota, T., Gama, V., Yoshida, T., Gomez, J. A., Ishikawa, K., Sasaguri, H., Cohen, H. Y., Sinclair, D. A., Mizusawa, H. & Matsuyama, S. (2007). Bax-Inhibiting Peptide Protects Cells from Polyglutamine Toxicity Caused by Ku70 Acetylation. *Cell Death Differ.*, *14*, 2058–2067.

Luo, J., Nikolaev, A. Y., Imai, S. I., et al., Negative Control of p53 by Sir2α Promotes Cell Survival Under Stress, *Cell*, vol. *107*, no. 2, pp. 137–148, 2001.

Maher, P., Dargusch, R., Bodai, L., Gerard, P. E., Purcell, J. M. & Marsh, J. L. (2011). ERK Activation by the Polyphenols Fisetin and Resveratrol Provides Neuroprotection in Multiple Models of Huntington's Disease. *Hum. Mol. Genet.*, *20* (2), 261–270, Jan 15.

Parker, J. A., Arango, M., Abderrahmane, S., Lambert, E., Tourette, C., Catoire, H. & Neri, C. (2005). Resveratrol Rescues Mutant Poly-Glutamine Cytotoxicity in Nematode and Mammalian Neurons. *Nat. Genet.*, *37*, 349–350.

Sandhir, R., Yadav, A., et al. (2014). Curcumin Nanoparticles Attenuate Neurochemical and Neurobehavioral Deficits in Experimental Model of Huntington's Disease. *NeuroMol Med*, *16*(1), 106–118.

Singh, S., Jamwal, S. & Kumar, P. (2015). Piperine Enhances The Protective Effect of Curcumin Against 3-NP Induced Neurotoxicity: Possible Neurotransmitters Modulation Mechanism. *Neurochem Res*, *40*, 1758–1766.

Stien, R. (1991). The History of the Hereditary Progressive Chorea in Norway and Johan Christian Lund and His Contribution to the

Understanding of This Disease. In: Boucher M, Broussole E, editors. *History of Neurology.*, Vol. *1*. Lyon: Foundation Marcel Merieux.

Suganuma, M., Okabe, S., Oniyama, M., Tada, Y., Ito, H. & Fujiki, H. (1998). Wide Distribution of [3H] (-)-Epigallocatechingallate, a Cancer Preventive Tea Polyphenol, in Mouse Tissue. *Carcinogenesis*, *19*, 1771–1776.

Vaziri. H., Dessain, S. K., Eaton, E. N., et al., HSIR2SIRT1 Functions as an NAD-Dependent p53 Deacetylase. *Cell*, vol. *107*, no. 2, pp. 149–159, 2001.

In: Food for Huntington's Disease
Editors: M. Mohamed Essa et al.
ISBN: 978-1-53613-854-2
© 2018 Nova Science Publishers, Inc.

Chapter 3

THE ROLE OF NATURAL FLAVONOIDS IN HUNTINGTON'S DISEASE

T. Sumathi[1,*] *A. Justin Thenmozhi*[2] *and T. Manivasagam*[2]

[1]Department of Medical Biochemistry, University of Madras,
Taramani Campus, Chennai, Tamil Nadu, India
[2]Department of Biochemistry and Biotechnology,
Annamalai University, Annamalainagar, Tamil Nadu, India

ABSTRACT

Huntington's disease (HD) is an inherited disorder damaging nerve cells present in the brain. The brain damage progresses and worsens over time and affects the cognition (awareness, perception, judgement, thinking,) movement and behaviour. The cure for Huntington's disease has not been yet found out, despite, HD gene been discovered many years ago. In recent years, there has been a growing interest in using natural compounds which can be used as a drug for HD and many studies are being carried out in this field. Active compounds from tea, tomatoes, citrus fruits and turmeric has given a positive outcome and have a hope in developing drugs for HD.

Keywords: Huntington's disease, models of HD, flavonoids

---

[*] Corresponding Author Email: sumsthangarajan@gmail.com.

1. INTRODUCTION

1.1. Huntington's Disease

Huntington's Disease (HD) was named after George Huntington who provided a classic account of the disease in 1872. It is a fatal, autosomal dominant neurodegenerative disorder. It is characterized by motor and cognitive impairment, abnormal body movements, chorea and personality changes (Johri and Beal, 2004). The neurodegenerative process primarily degenerates medium spiny striatal neurons and, also cortical neurons, to some extent. The most vulnerable neurons in HD are γ-amino butyric acid (GABA)ergic and enkephalin neurons of the basal ganglia (Smith et al., 2008). Their early dysfunction is responsible for development of chorea. The pathology of HD shows shrinkage of the brain and striking neurodegeneration in the corpus striatum (Imariso et al., 2008). HD is prevalent worldwide at a rate of 5 to 8 per 100,000 people with no gender preponderance. The highest frequencies of HD are found in countries of European origin and Europe. The lowest frequencies are found in China, Africa, Finland and Japan (Kumar et al., 2010).

It is caused by an unstable expansion of a CAG repeat present in the coding region of the IT-15 gene. This gene encodes for a protein called huntingtin (HTT), and the mutation results in elongated stretch of polyglutamine near the N-terminus of the protein (Zuccato et al., 2010). There are 10–29 (median, 18) consecutive repeats of the CAG triplet coding for glutamine, whereas, HD patients have increased numbers of CAG repeats, from 36 to 121 (median, 44). The length of the polyglutamine/ CAG repeat sequence is inversely proportional to the age of the disease onset (Kumar et al., 2010).

Huntingtin (HTT) protein is expressed in all the cell types with highest expression in neurons. Accumulation of proteolytic HTT fragments and their aggregation triggers a cascade leading to increased neuronal dysfunction through oxidative injury, glutamate excitotoxicity, transcriptional dysregulation, mitochondrial dysfunction, apoptotic signals, and energy depletion. These changes comprise of neurochemical alterations, which involve glutamate receptors and other receptors, such as the adenosine receptors and dopamine (DA) having functions in motor coordination (Kumar et al., 2010).

There is no cure for HD till date. Tetrabenazine is the first drug approved by FDA, but it only reduces the chorea symptoms. Many food products containing antioxidants like tea, coffee, turmeric etc. have been shown to have protective effect against various models of HD.

1.2. Models for Huntington's Disease

1.2.1. Chemical Models

1.2.1.1. Quinolinic Acid

Quinolinic acid (QUIN) is an endogenous metabolite which is derived from kynurenine pathway of tryptophan degradation. Quinolinic acid cannot cross blood brain barrier, when it is injected into the brain of rodents. It reproduces same neurodegenerative events in rodents, resembling the one which are observed in the post-mortem brains of HD patients. It causes neurodegeneration by causing excitotoxicity. Quinolinic acid is a glutamatergic agonist which acts on NMDA receptor, preferably in discrete populations of NMDA receptors consisting of NR2A and NR2B subunits. Excitotoxicity is totally dependent on the increase levels of intracellular Ca^{2+} after its influx through NMDA receptor. Calcium activated enzymes like endonucleases, phospholipases and proteases contribute to the cell component degradation and ultimately neuronal death.

1.2.1.2. 3-Nitropropionic Acid

3-nitropropionic acid is a fungal toxin causing neurotoxicity in humans and rodents. It is a reversible inhibitor of complex II of mitochondrial ETC, succinate dehydrogenase. It causes impaired electron transfer in mitochondria which results in an increased generation of reactive oxygen (ROS) and nitrogen (RNS) species, which plays an important role in 3-NP induced pathogenesis (Thangarajan et al., 2016). The 3-NP model is known to cause bilateral striatal lesion that develops spontaneously (Singh et al., 2015).

1.2.2. Genetic Models

HD cell lines are useful as they allow the stable and inducible expression of wild-type and mutant huntingtin protein (mHTT). They have been useful for deciphering the disease mechanisms, and have recently been exploited for the therapeutic screening. A wide range of species like the invertebrate *Drosophila melanogaster* and *Caenorhabditis elegans* non-mammalian species like *Danio rerio* and mammals, such as rat and mouse, have also been genetically engineered to express the HTT mutated gene.

Various genetic mouse lines are divided based on incorporation of the mHTT is into the genome of mouse.

a) Transgenic mice express both alleles of murine wild type HTT and also a fragment of the human HTT gene containing polyglutamine mutations like R6/1 and R6/2.
b) knock- in mice consists of pathogenic CAG repeats which are inserted into the existing CAG expansion of wild type huntingtin.
c) Mice that expresses the full length human HD gene, like mice expressing mutated huntingtin (mHTT) through Bacterial Artificial Chromosome (BAC) or Yeast Artificial Chromosome (YAC).
c) mice in which mHTT can be turned on or turned off at certain stages, mimicking the distinct phases of the Huntington's disease (Sharma et al., 2012).

1.3. Flavonoids

Flavonoids are the plant pigments synthesised from phenylalanine. They display attractive colors known from flower petals, and emit excellent fluorescence when they are placed under UV light, and are ubiquitous to green plant cells. They are well known regulators of plant growth by inhibiting the exocytosis of the auxin indolyl acetic acid, inducing gene expression, and also, they influence other biological cells in various ways and they are less toxic to animal cells (Havsteen, 2002).

Many studies suggest that flavonoids have biological activities like anti-allergic, vasodilation, anti-inflammatory and anti-viral activity. However, antioxidant activity of flavonoids is a field of interest due to their ability to decrease and scavenge free radical formation (Pietta, 2000).

Fruits and vegetables are the main dietary sources of flavonoids for humans, with wine and tea. There is growing interest in the pharmacological potential of natural products and therefore here we have summarized the protective effects of various flavonoids against Huntington's disease.

1.3.1. Tea

Tea is one of the most widely consumed liquid on earth. It is widely consumed socially and habitually since 3000 B.C. It has a pleasing astringent taste which refreshes the person so immensely that its potential medicinal properties and health benefits are not noticed. Recent scientific studies have pointed out certain health benefits which are derived from tea.

The biological name of Tea is *Camellia sinensis L*. It is a cultivated evergreen plant, native to China, which later spread to Japan and India, and then to Russia and Europe, and at last making its presence in the New World in the late 17th century. Green, black and oolong tea are all made from the same plant species, *C. sinensis* L. but they differ in their appearance, chemical content, organoleptic taste and flavour due to the fermentation process they undergo (Sharangi, 2009).

Tea composition varies according to the season, climate, age of the leaf and tea variety, (Uzunalic et al., 2006). The chemical components of tea leaves include alkaloids (caffeine, theobromine, theophylline, etc.), polyphenols (catechins and flavonoids), polysaccharides, inorganic elements (e.g., aluminium, fluorine and manganese), amino acids, volatile oils, vitamins (e.g., vitamin C), lipids, etc (Sharangi, 2009). Figure 1 shows various compounds present in tea.

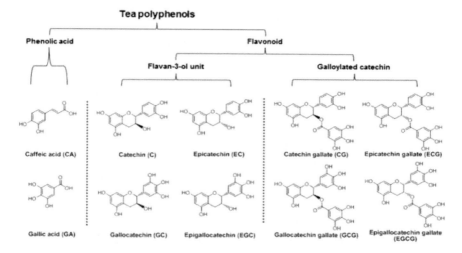

Figure 1. Phenols present in tea (Du G J et al., 2012).

It is well known that consumption of green tea brings relaxation. The chemical substance responsible for the sense of relaxation is theanine. Theanine is a unique amino acid found almost solely in tea plants and is the main component responsible for the exotic taste of 'green' tea (Juneja et al., 1999).

L-theanine increases the synthesis of neurotransmitters and nerve growth factor in infant rats. It exerts neuroprotective activity in a rat model of stroke by preventing glutamate receptor agonist-mediated brain injury (Yamada et al., 2007; Zukhorova, 2013). Others have indicated that L-theanine augments anti-psychotic therapy in schizophrenia and schizo-affective disorder patients (Miodownik C, 2011). More recent studies of psychiatric disorders indicate that L-theanine reduces immobility time in both the forced swim test and tail suspension test in mice (Yin C, 2011) and alters catecholamines in cerebral cortex and hippocampus of mice having chronic restraint stress-induced cognitive impairment (Tian X, 2013).

1.3.2. Hesperidin

Hesperidin is an inexpensive and abundant by-product of Citrus cultivation. It is the major flavonoid in lemons and sweet lime. Hesperidin is commonly used in traditional medicines as a combination product (Garg et al., 2001).

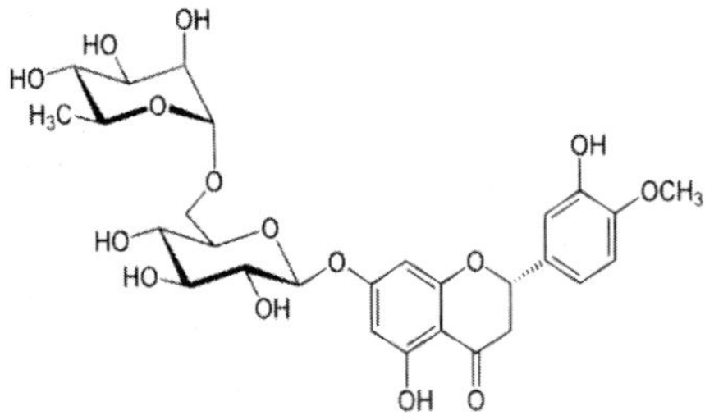

Figure 2. Structure of Hesperidin.

1.3.3. Lycopene

The fat-soluble pigments, carotenoids, are found in tomatoes and their products. Lycopene is an aliphatic hydrocarbon product and is one of the 600 known naturally occurring carotenoids. It is present in high amounts in tomatoes and tomato-based products (Kumar et al., 2009).

1.3.4. Turmeric

Turmeric (*Curcuma longa*) is extensively used as a food preservative, spice and colouring material in South- East Asia, China and India. It is used extensively as a household remedy and in traditional medicine for various diseases. Curcumin (diferuloylmethane) is the main yellow bioactive component of turmeric and is known to have a wide array of biological activities. These include its, antioxidant, anti-inflammatory, antiprotozoal, antimutagenic, anticoagulant, antibacterial, antidiabetic, antifungal, anticarcinogenic, antiviral, antiulcer, antivenom, antifibrotic, hypercholesteraemic and hypotensive activities (Chattopadhyay, 2004).

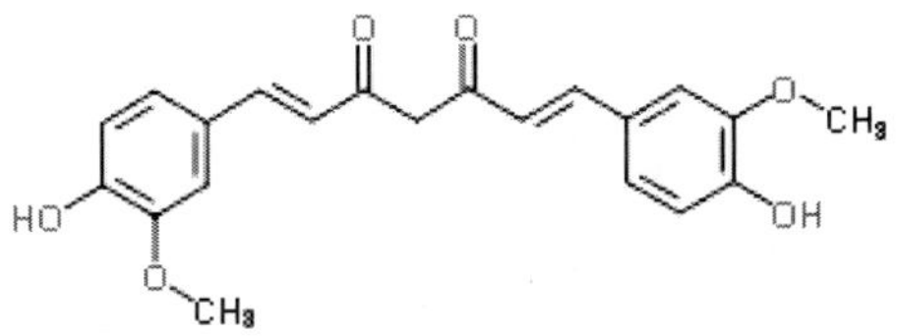

Figure 3. Structure of Curcumin.

2. Effect of Natural Flavonoids in Different Models of Huntington's Disease

2.1. 3-Nitropropionic Acid (3-NP) Induced Huntington's Disease

The effect of epigallocatechin (EGCG) and lycopene was studied on memory impairment as well as disturbed glutathione system against 3-NP administration. Rats were treated with EGCG (10, 20 and 40 mg/kg). Rats showed a reduction in mean transfer latency when treated with EGCG on 11th and 15th day against 3-NP induced rats. EGCG treatment significantly reduced the time spent in the target quadrant on 15th day as compared to the control group.

Chronic EGCG pre-treatment improved memory performance against 3-NP induced rats.

Chronic 3-NP treatment significantly decreased redox ratio (reduced glutathione/oxidized glutathione), glutathione- S-transferase and total glutathione in cortex, striatum, and hippocampus of brain in comparison to the vehicle treated group. Pre-treatments with EGCG restored glutathione levels and redox ratio significantly (Kumar and Kumar, 2009).

Protective effect of L-theanine against 3-Nitropropionic acid induced neurotoxicity in rats was reported by Sumathi et al., in 2014. Rats were treated with L-theanine (100 and 200 mg/kg) orally, 1h prior to 3-NP treatment, once a day. Body weight and behavioral parameters [rotarod activity, Morris water maze test, open field test (OFT) and forced swim test (FST)] were observed on 1st, 5th, 10th and 15th day post-3-NP treatment. Glutathione (GSH), catalase (CAT), Malondialdehyde (MDA) and superoxide dismutase (SOD) levels and levels of mitochondrial enzyme complex II, Succinate dehydrogenase (SDH) were measured on the 15th day in the rat striatum. Systemic 3-NP acid administration caused a significant reduction in the body weight, locomotor activity and oxidative defence of the rats. There was a significant decrease in the mitochondrial activity of 3-NP treated rats. L-theanine (100 and 200 mg/kg b.w.) treatment showed a significant attenuation in the impairment in behavioral, biochemical and mitochondrial enzyme activities as compared to the 3-NP administered group. This study revealed that pre-treatment with L-theanine significantly decreases 3-Nitropropionic acid induced oxidative stress and restored the decreased GSH, SOD, and SDH and CAT activity. L-theanine treatment also decreased the neuronal damage as proved by histopathological analysis of the rat striatum. Thus, above study proved that L-theanine exerts neuroprotective effects against 3-NP induced neurotoxicity (Sumathi et al., 2014).

Jamwal et al., (2016) reported that L-theanine has a neuroprotection action against 3-NP induced toxicity in the striatum by altering Nitric oxide pathway. Rats were administered with 3-Nitropropionic acid for 21 days. L-theanine was administered once a day, 1 hour prior to 3-Nitropropionic acid treatment for 21 days and L-NAME (10 mg/kg,i.p.), a well- known NO inhibitor and L-arginine (50 mg/kg; i.p.). NO precursor was administered 1 hour prior to L-theanine treatment. Body weight and behavioral alterations were assessed on a weekly basis. On the 22nd day, rats were sacrificed, and the striatum were isolated for biochemical (GSH, nitrite and LPO), neurochemical analysis and pro-inflammatory cytokines. Pre-treatment with L-theanine (25 and 50 mg/kg/ day) significantly modified the alteration in body weight in a dose dependent manner as compared to the 3-NP treated group. Systemic administration of 3-NP significantly decreased locomotor activity (day 14th and 21st) and grip strength (on rotarod and grip strength meter) when compared to normal control group and caused the increase in foot errors and latency on narrow beam walk apparatus. All these behavioural alterations were restored by L-theanine treatment.

Pre-treatment with L-theanine significantly decreased the LPO and nitrite levels and increased the GSH levels, thus decreasing oxidative stress. Systemic 3-NP administration significantly increased the pro-inflammatory cytokines levels, i.e., IL-6, IL-1β and TNF-α, levels in the striatum as compared to normal control group. Pre-treatment with L-theanine (25 and 50 mg/kg/day) dose dependently and significantly prevented the increase in levels of IL-6, IL-1β, TNF-α when compared to the 3-NP treated groups (Jamwal et al., 2016).

Neuroprotective effect of lycopene against 3-NP neurotoxicity in rats and the role of nitric oxide mechanism were investigated. Lycopene (2.5, 5 and 10 mg/kg, p.o.) treatment decreased the loss in bodyweight, attenuated the decreased locomotor activity and the decrease in grip strength on rotarod as compared to 3-NP-treated rats. Lycopene (2.5, 5 and 10 mg/kg, p.o.) treatment significantly reduced lipid peroxidation and concentration of nitrite and had also restored the decreasing levels of catalase and superoxide dismutase activities, mitochondrial redox activity and mitochondrial complex activity as compared to the 3-NP-treated animals (Kumar et al., 2009).

Menze and colleagues studied the protective activity of Hesperidin against 3-Nitropropionic acid induced Huntingon's disease. They studied the effect of hesperidin on PPI response locomotor activity, striatal, hippocampal and cortical malondialdehyde levels, electron microscopic examination and immunohistochemistry. Systemic 3-NP administration to rats for 5 days (20 mg/kg) caused 55% deficit of PPI response, reduction of locomotor activity by days 2 and 5, elevation of striatal, hippocampal and cortical malondialdehyde (MDA) levels by 41%, 56% and 63% reduction of respective catalase activity by 50%. Immunohistochemically stained regions of striata, hippocampi and cortex showed presence of iNOS positive cells. Ultrastructural examination by electron microscope showed perivascular edema, mitochondrial swelling and shrunken nerve cells. Pre-treatment with hesperidin (100 mg/kg) before 3-NP administration prevented changes in PPI response or locomotor activity, increased hippocampal, striatal and cortical, MDA levels by 10% and reduced respective catalase activity by 5%, 20% and 22%. Very few iNOS positive cells were seen in sections from rats treated with hesperidin and had also reduced cellular abnormalities due to 3-NP induction. This study proved that hesperidin has a potential neuroprotective role against 3-NP-induced Huntington's disease-like manifestations. This neuroprotection can be referred to its anti-inflammatory and anti-oxidant activities (Menze et al., 2012).

Naringin was also found to have neuroprotective activity against Huntington's disease reported in two different studies. Naringin was given in 6 doses (20, 40, 60, 80, 100 and 120 mg/kg body weight) to study the dose dependent effect of naringin on 3-Nitropropionic acid induced rats. It was seen that of 80 mg/kg b.w dose of naringin modulated the abnormalities of the histopathology of striatum near to normal. At this dose naringin significantly ($p < 0.05$) altered the activities of lactate dehydrogenase (LDH) and alkaline phosphatase (ALP) to normal level. It was also observed that the reduced glutathione and lipid peroxidation levels in the striatum altered to near normal level in 3-NP treated rats after the experimental period. Increasing naringin concentration (100 and 120 mg/kg b.w.) also provides protection to 3-NP-induced rats, but there is no significant difference as compared to 80 mg/kg b.w. then, Naringin at a dose of 80mg/kg was given to animals divided in four groups. The activities of enzymic antioxidants (CAT, GR, SOD and GPx) were also reduced in 3-NP-induced rats as compared to the control animals. Treatment with naringin caused an increase in the levels of non-enzymic antioxidants (Vit E, GSH and vit C) near to the normal levels as compared to 3-NP-induced animals. Naringin treatment ameliorated decreased activities of Ca^{2+}-ATPase, Na+/K+-ATPase and Mg2+- ATPase closer to normal levels as compared with 3-NP-induced animals. There was an increase in the expressions levels of mRNA of Bad and Bax and decrease in the expression of Bcl-2 as compared to control rats. Naringin treatment caused a significant alteration in the expression of these markers near to normal. The release of cytochrome c from mitochondria is an essential step in turning on the apoptosis. Cytosolic and mitochondrial fractions were prepared and used for immunoblotting analysis of cytochrome c. 3-NP-induced rats exhibited an increase in the release of cytochrome c in cytosol from mitochondria with relative decrease in mitochondrial cytochrome c. Following naringin supplementation, the levels of cytochrome c restored to normal. Caspase-3 activation is an important event in apoptosis. Increased expression of cleaved caspase-3 was observed in 3-NP-induced rats. Naringin treatment significantly decreased the cleaved caspase-3 levels in 3-NP induced rats (Kulasekaran et al., 2011).

Treatment with naringin increased the reduced glutathione/ oxidized glutathione ratio by decreasing the levels of hydroperoxide, nitrite and hydroxyl radical in 3-NP-induced rats. Transmission electron microscopic and Nissl staining showed that naringin altered 3-NP induced histological changes. Naringin induces, heme oxygenase-1, NAD(P)H: quinone oxidoreductase-1, P1 and gamma-glutamyl cysteine ligase and glutathione S-transferase, mRNA expressions through the activation of Nrf2 and decreased the expressions of pro-inflammatory mediators like and inducible nitric oxide synthase, cyclooxygenase-2 and tumour necrosis factor-alpha, (Gopinath et al., 2012).

Protective effect of naringin and hesperidin on 3-NP induced rats by was studied by Kumar and Kumar. Protective effect of these two citrus flavonoids was compared with L-NAME and L-Arginine. Naringin (100 mg/kg, p.o.) and hesperidin (100 mg/kg, p.o.) treatment significantly attenuated the decrease in body weight as compared to 3-NP administered group. Naringin (50 and 100 mg/kg, p.o.) and Hesperidin (100 mg/kg, p.o.) pre-treatment significantly improved locomotor activity as compared to 3-NP treated group. Naringin (50 and 100 mg/kg, p.o.) and Hesperidin (100 mg/kg, p.o.) pre-treatment significantly improved muscle grip strength (delayed fall of time) on rotarod, attenuated the increased nitrite concentration, increased lipid peroxidation and restored the decreased levels of catalase and superoxide dismutase enzyme activities as compared to 3-NP treated group. Naringin (100 mg/kg) and Hesperidin (100 mg/kg) treatment significantly restored mitochondrial complex enzyme (I, II and IV) activities as compared to 3-NP-treated group. Naringin (100 mg/kg, p.o.) and Hesperidin (100 mg/kg, p.o) treatment significantly restored the depleting mitochondrial redox activity as compared to 3-NP-treated group.

On intraperitoneal administration of 3-NP (20 mg/kg for 4 days) there was a loss of body weight, poor retention of memory, decline in motor function and changes in oxidative stress (reduced glutathione, nitrite level and lipid peroxidation,) parameters in brain. Continuous pre- treatment with curcumin (10, 20 and 50 mg/kg, p.o.) for a period of 8 days beginning 4 days, once daily, improved the 3-NP-induced cognitive and motor impairment in a dose- dependent manner. Biochemical analyses revealed that curcumin administration significantly attenuated 3-NP induced oxidative stress (reduced glutathione, nitrite activity and lipid peroxidation) in the brains of rats. It also restored the decreased succinate dehydrogenase activity in a significant manner. The results of this study clearly indicated that curcumin through its antioxidant activity showed neuroprotection against 3-NP-induced behavioral and biochemical alterations (Kumar et al., 2007).

2.2. Quinolinic Acid Induced Huntington's Disease

Jamwal et al., (2016) reported the neuroprotective activity of L-theanine against QUIN induced Huntington's like symptoms in rats. Rats were administered with Quinolonic acid (200 nmol/2µl saline) bilaterally on 0 day. L-theanine was administered once a day at dose of 25 & 50 mg/kg orally for 21 days and L-arginine (NOS activator) and L-NAME (NOS inhibitor) were administered 1 hour prior to L-theanine treatment. Behavioral parameters (body weight, grip strength, locomotor activity and narrow beam walk) observations were done on 1st, 7th, 14th, 21st day after QUIN treatment. On 21st day, animals were sacrificed and rat striata isolated for biochemical (nitrite, GSH and LPO), neuroinflammatory markers (IL-6, IL-1β and TNF-α) and neurochemical analysis (glutamate, dopamine, 5-HIAA, DOPAC serotonin, GABA and HVA). QA administration significantly changed body weight, motor coordination, locomotor activity, oxidative defense (increased Nitrite and LPO and decreased GSH), pro-inflammatory levels (IL-1β, TNF-α and Il-6), glutamate, GABA, catecholamines level (serotonin, dopamine and their metabolites). L-theanine treatment (25 & 50 mg/kg/day, p.o.) prevented the alterations significantly. Simultaneous treatment of L-NAME with L-theanine (25 mg/kg/day, p.o.) significantly increased the effect of L-theanine (25 mg/kg/day, p.o.) whereas simultaneous treatment of L-arginine with L-theanine (50 mg/kg/day, p.o.) significantly reduced the protective activity of L-theanine (50 mg/kg/day, p.o.) (Jamwal and Kumar, 2016).

The protective activity of EGCG was studied against QUIN induced toxicity in N18D3 cells, hybrid neuronal cell lines, which are used in the study of sensory neuropathy model. Cells were examined for cell viability after QUIN or EGCG treatment for 24 hrs. Cell viability was measured by MTT assay. EGCG alone (0, 1, 5, 25, 50, and 100 µM) did not decrease cell viability except 50 µM EGCG, which slightly increased the cell viability (104.85 ± 2.19%) as compared with the control. The N18D3 cells were pre-treated with 1, 5, 25, 50, or 100 µM EGCG to investigate the neuroprotective effects of EGCG, and the cells were then exposed to 0 to 50 mM QUIN for 24 h. EGCG pre-treatment for 2 h before 30 mM QA exposure decreased cell death in a dose-dependent manner significantly.

To study the apoptosis-like cell death in N18D3 cells, the cell nuclei were stained with 4′,6-diamidino-2-phenyindole (DAPI). Quinolinic acid (30 mM) induced cell death and showed morphological changes such as DNA fragmentation and nuclear condensation. TUNEL staining also exhibited that QA (30 mM) increased apoptosis in N18D3 cells and pre-treatment with EGCG (100 µM) reduced the number of TUNEL-positive cells.

To investigate the changes in intracellular calcium levels, Fura-2 based calcium imaging experiments were performed in the Quinolinic acid induced excitotoxicity model. N18D3 cells were cultured on coverslips and were pre-incubated with EGCG (5 or 25 µM) for 2 hours prior to treatment with Quinolinic acid (1 mM). Both EGCG and QUIN were present during the calcium imaging procedure. The concentration of calcium was increased rapidly on treating with 1 mM QUIN in the cells, whereas intracellular calcium concentrations were decreased on pretreatment with 5 or 25 µM EGCG for 2 hours.

For testing, the Quinolinic acid induced NO productions, N18D3 cell lines were studied for direct intracellular Nitric oxide (NO) production by using a Nitric Oxide sensitive dye- DAF-2DA. The cells had a fluorescence signal on loading with DAF- 2DA. The QA induced Nitric oxide production in the cells was significantly blocked by pre-treatment with 5 or 25 µM of EGCG.

Further, the neuroprotective action of EGCG, cell survival and apoptosis related gene expression analysis was performed using RT–PCR experiments. By pre-treating with EGCG, anti-apoptotic gene Bcl-XL mRNA levels were increased as compared to that of QUIN. The pro-apoptotic genes such as Caspase-3, and -6, Bax did not show any significant change in expression on treatment with EGCG, QUIN, or the co-treatment. Only the expression levels of capase-9 were increased on stimulation with 30 mM QUIN, which were attenuated by the EGCG pre-treatment. 100 µM EGCG was the most effective concentration when compared with 1 or 10 µM EGCG in showing the anti-apoptotic effects.

EGCG pre- treatment increased the PI-3K activity. However, on addition of LY294002, a PI3K inhibitor, 1 hour before treatment with EGCG, the protective effect of EGCG was inhibited. Quinolinic acid enhanced the immunoreactivity of p-GSK-3β and 100 µM EGCG attenuated the increase remarkably. These results proved that neuroprotective activities of EGCG in proteins were linked to the increasing expression of the p-PI-3K and p-GSK-3β (Jang et al., 2010).

Single intrastriatal administration of quinolinic acid caused a severe reduction in body weight, motor impairment (impaired grip strength in rotarod and decreased total locomotor activity in actophotometer), increase in oxidative stress, impairment in the activities of mitochondrial complexes activities and reduced state 3 respiration (NAD+ /FAD+ -linked) in rats. Caffeine treatment for 21 days attenuated the QA induced behavioural, biochemical and mitochondrial alterations in a significant manner displaying neuroprotective efficacy of Caffeine (Mishra and Kumar, 2014).

Curcumin (CUR) treatment decreased the rotational behavior caused due to QUIN induction and reached to an average of 233 ± 66 ipsilateral turns. Curcumin treatment significantly attenuated this behaviour through a dose of 100 mg/kg (CUR100+QUIN: 155 ± 25 ipsilateral turns). The most prominent protective effect was seen on treatment with 400 mg/kg (CUR400+QUIN: 54 ± 14 ipsilateral turns). The control animals showed a well preserved striatal tissue sections, whereas the surgical administration of Quinolinic acid caused cellular damage as revealed by severe neuronal cell loss in the dorsal striatum, pyknotic cells and shrunken cells, interstitial oedema and retraction of neuropils. All Curcumin doses (100, 200 and 400mg/kg) given were able to prevent histological and morphological alterations provoked by quinolinic acid. Administration of quinolinic acid to rats increased the striatal protein carbonyl content to 157% above the Control group, whereas CUR treatment reduced the protein carbonyl content to normal levels. Animals administered with Curcumin alone did not exhibit any significant change. Quantification of cells positive to Nrf2 showed that QUIN treatment decreased the intranuclear entry of Nrf2 at 62% at 30 min, and 76% at 120 min, while increased its peri- and extra-nuclear localization as compared to Control group. CUR administration prevented this decrease to basal levels. CUR alone significantly increased intra-nuclear Nrf2 localization by 113% at 30 min, and 69% at 120 min, when compared to control group (Ramrez et al., 2013).

In view of emerging role of flavonoids in altering oxidative stress and neuroinflammation, Kumar et al., explored the neuroprotective effect of hesperidin when combined with minocycline (microglial inhibitor), against quinolinic acid (QA) induced Huntington's disease (HD). Intrastriatal administration of Quinolinic acid (300 nmol/4 µl) unilaterally, significantly decreased the body weight, caused an impairment in behavioural activities (beam balance, memory performance and locomotor activity), produced oxidative damage (increased nitrite concentration, lipid peroxidation, reduced glutathione and depleted super oxide dismutase), caused mitochondrial function impairment (decreased Complex I, II, III, and IV activities), enhanced striatal lesions and modulated the levels of caspase-3, TNF-α and BDNF expression, as compared to sham group. Chronic treatment with minocycline (25mg/kg, p.o.) and hesperidin (100mg/kg, p.o.) treatment for 21 days significantly attenuated the behavioral, biochemical and cellular alterations as compared to Quinolinic acid treated (control) animals, whereas hesperidin (50mg/kg, p.o.) treatment was not found to be significant. On treatment of hesperidin (50mg/kg) & minocycline (25mg/kg) combinedly, potentiated the neuroprotective effect of both the compounds which was significant as compared to their effects alone in quinolinic acid induced animals. Thus, the collective results of this study suggested a possible role of microglial modulation and antioxidant effect in neuroprotective potential of hesperidin against Quinolinic acid induced Huntington's Disease like symptoms in rats (Kumar, 2013).

2.3. Transgenic Models for Huntington's Disease

Ehrnhoefer et al., showed that EGCG is effective in preventing the aggregation of mHTT-exon 1 protein in a dose dependent manner. They examined if addition of EGCG to aggregation reactions alters the assembly of such aggregates in-vitro. GST-tagged fusion protein with 53 glutamine residues (GST-HDQ53) was incubated with the site-specific Pre-Scission protease to remove the GST tag and to initiate the aggregation of HDQ53. At 5 hours after GST cleavage, aliquots were analysed by Atomic Force Microscopy for aggregation reactions and the assembly of oligomers. The dominant structure seen was a heterologous proportion of spherical oligomers having a diameter of 0–80 nm. On EGCG administration, the density (particles/field) of these structures was significantly decreased, whereas the number of circular oligomers with a larger diameter (120–200 nm) was enhanced. This indicates that EGCG reduces the aggregation of small HDQ53 oligomers by stimulating the formation of bigger ones. It was also shown that EGCG binds to the unstructured poly glutamine sequence and interferes with the conformational rearrangement presumed to occur just after cleavage.

For testing, whether EGCG affects HTT exon 1 toxicity in-vivo, a yeast model of HD was used. The HTT exon 1 GFP-fusion proteins GFP-HDQ25 and GFP-HDQ72 were over expressed in yeast and cell growth was measured by tracking the optical density at 600 nm. Increased expression of GFP-HDQ25 did not significantly alter yeast cell growth. When GFP-HDQ72 was produced in excessive manner, cell proliferation was completely blocked, which indicated that GFP fused protein with the expanded polyglutamine tract is toxic in yeast. Remarkably, when these cells were treated with 500 mM EGCG, yeast growth significantly improved, which indicated that EGCG can reduce the toxicity of the GFP-HDQ72 protein in-vivo. EGCG treatment did not cause mutations in the yeast genome, which was responsible for the improved growth phenotype.

Fluorescence microscopy proved that EGCG treatment decreases the number of yeast cells containing GFP-HDQ72 protein aggregates. Similarly, when cell extracts were analyzed with the membrane filter retardation assay, a lower amount of SDS-insoluble GFP-HDQ72 aggregates were seen in EGCG-treated cells, which proved that EGCG not only suppresses toxicity but also inhibits aggregation of protein in a yeast model of HD (Ehrnhoefer et al., 2006).

CONCLUSION

The active ingredients of most the medicines are natural products obtained from plants. As seen above, most of the compounds from natural products that are currently in use to be developed as animals are derived from plant sources. Compounds which have been shown to be protective against HD in various models, have been extracted from food sources which are consumed daily all over the world. So the emphasis should be on developing resistance towards HD by encouraging the increased intake of natural fruits, vegetables and beverages.

REFERENCES

Chattopadhyay, Ishita, Biswas, Kausik, Bandyopadhyay, Uday, Banerjee, Ranajit K. 2004. Turmeric and Curcumin: Biological Actions and Medicinal Applications. *Current Science* 87.

Du, Guang-Jian, Zhang, Zhiyu, Wen, Dong-Xiao, Yu, Chunhao, Calway, Tayler, Yuan Chun-Su, and Wang, Chong-Zhi. 2012. Epigallo-Catechin Gallate (EGCG) Is the Most Effective Cancer Chemo-Preventive Polyphenol in Green Tea. *Nutrients* 4(11): 1679–1691.

Ehrnhoefer, Dagmar E., Duennwald, Martinn, Markovic, Phoebe, Wacker, Jeniffer L., Engemann, Sabine, Roark, Margarett, Legleiter, Justin, Marsh, Lawrence J., Thompson, Leslie M, Lindquist, Susan, Muchowshki, Paul J., Wanker, Erich E. 2006. Green tea (2)-Epigallocatechin-Gallate Modulates Early Events in Huntingtin Misfolding and Reduces Toxicity in Huntington's Disease Models. *Human Molecular Genetics* 15 (8): 2743–2751.

Garg A, Garg S, Zaneveld L. J. D, Singla A. K. 2001. Chemistry and Pharmacology of the Citrus Bioflavonoid Hesperidin. *Phytotherapy* 15: 655-669.

Gopinath K and Sudhandiran G. 2012. Naringin Modulates Oxidative Stress and Inflammation in 3-Nitropropionic Acid-Induced Neuro-Degeneration Through the Activation of Nuclear Factor-Erythroid 2-Related Factor-2 Signalling Pathway. *Neuroscience* 227: 134–143.

Harold N. Graham. 1992. Green Tea Composition, Consumption, and Polyphenol Chemistry. *Preventive Medicine* 21(3): 334-350.

Havsteen, Bent H. 2002. The Biochemistry and Medical Significance of the Flavonoids. *Pharmacology and therapeutics* 96 (2-3): 67-202.

Imarisio, Sara, Carmichael, Jenny, Korolchuk Viktor, Chen, Chien W., Saiki, Shinji, Rose, Claudia, Krishna, Gauri, Davies, Janet E, Tofi, Evangelia, Underwood, Benjamin R and Rubinsztein, David C, 2008. Huntington's Disease: From Pathology and Genetics to Potential Therapies. *Biochem. J.* 412:191–209.

Jamwal, Sumit, Kumar, Puneet. 2016. L-theanine, a Component of Green Tea Prevents 3-Nitropropionic Acid (3-NP)-Induced Striatal Toxicity by Modulating Nitric Oxide Pathway. *Mol Neurobiol.*

Jamwal S., Kumar P. 2016. Neuroprotective Potential of L-Theanine Against Excitotoxic Neuronal Death Induced by Quinolinic Acid: Possible Neurotransmitters and Nitric Oxide Modulation Mechanism [abstract]. *Mov Disord.* 2016, 31 (suppl 2). 20th *International Congress.* 1108.

Jang, Sujeong, Jeong, Han-Seong, Park, Jong-Seong, Kim, Yeong-Seong, Jin, Chun-Yan, Seol, Myung B, Kim Beyong- Chae, Lee, Min-Cheols. 2010. Neuroprotective Effects of (−)-Epigallocatechin-3-Gallate against Quinolinic Acid-Induced Excitotoxicity via PI3K Pathway and NO Inhibition. *Brain Research* 1313: 25–33.

Johri, Ashu and Beal, Flint. 2012. Antioxidants in Huntington's disease. *Biochimica et Biophysica Acta* 1822:664–674.

Juneja, LekhR, Chu, Djong-Chi, Okubo, Tsumoto, Nagato, Yukiko, Yokogoshi, Hidehiko. 1999. L-Theanine—A Unique Amino Acid of

Green Tea and Its Relaxation Effect in Humans. *Trends in Food Science & Technology.* 10(6–7):199–204.

Kulasekaran, Gopinath, Dharmalingam, Prakash, Ganapasam, Sudhandhiran. 2011. Neuroprotective Effect of Naringin, a Dietary Flavonoid against 3-Nitropropionic Acid-Induced Neuronal Apoptosis. *Neurochemistry International* 59:1066–1073.

Kumar P., Padi S. S. V., Naidu P. S., Kumar A. 2007. Possible Neuroprotective Mechanism of Curcumin in Attenuating 3-Nitropropinic Acid Neurotoxicity. *Methods Find Exp Clin Pharmacol* 29(1): 19.

Kumar, Puneet and Kumar, Anil. 2009. Effect of Lycopene and Epigallocatechin-3-Gallate against 3-Nitropropionic Acid Induced Cognitive Dysfunction and Glutathione Depletion in Rat: A Novel Nitric Oxide Mechanism. *Food and Chemical Toxicology* 47: 2522–2530.

Kumar P., Kalonia H. and Kumar A. 2010. Huntington's Diseases: Pathogenesis to Animal Models. *Pharmacological reports.* 62:1-14.

Kumar, Puneet, Kalonia, Harish, Kumar, Anil. 2009. Lycopene Modulates Nitric Oxide Pathways against 3-Nitropropionic Acid-Induced Neurotoxicity. *Life Sciences*: 711–718.

Kumar, Puneet, Kumar, Anil., 2010. Protective Effect of Hesperidin and Naringin against 3-Nitropropionic Acid Induced Huntington's Like Symptoms in Rats: Possible Role of Nitric Oxide. *Behav. Brain Res* 206: 38–46.

Kumar, Anil, Chaudhary, Tanya, Mishra, Jitendriya. 2013. Minocycline Modulates Neuroprotective Effect of Hesperidin against Quinolinic Acid Induced Huntington's Disease-like Symptoms in Rats: Behavioral, Biochemical, Cellular and Histological Evidences. *Eur J Pharmacol* 15, 720(1-3):16-28.

Mishra, Jitendriya, Kumar, Anil. 2014. Improvement of Mitochondrial NAD$^+$/FAD$^+$-Linked State-3 Respiration by Caffeine Attenuates Quinolinic Acid Induced Motor Impairment in Rats: Implications in Huntington's Disease. *Pharmacological Reports* 1148-1155.

Menze, Esther T, Tadros, Mariana, Tawab- Abdel, Ahmed M, Khalifa, Amani E. 2012. Potential Neuroprotective Effects of Hesperidin on 3-Nitropropionic Acid-Induced Neurotoxicity in Rats. *Neuro Toxicology* 33: 1265–1275.

Miodownik, Chanoch, Maayan, Rachel, Ratner, Yael, Lerner, Vladimir, Pintov, Leonid, Mar, Maria, Weizman, Abraham, Ritsner, Michael S. 2011. Serum Levels of Brain-Derived Neurotrophic Factor and Cortisol to Sulfate of Dehydroepiandrosterone Molar Ratio Associated with Clinical Response to L-Theanine as Augmentation of Antipsychotic Therapy in Schizophrenia and Schizoaffective Disorder Patients. *Clin Neuropharmacol* 34: 155-160.

Mishra, Jitendriya, Kumar, Anil. 2014. Improvement of Mitochondrial NAD+/FAD+- Linked State-3 Respiration by Caffeine Attenuates Quinolinc Acid Induced Motor Impairment in Rats: Implications in Huntington's Disease. *Pharmacological Reports* 66: 1148–1155.

Pietta, Pier-Giorgio. 2000. Flavonoids as Antioxidants. *J. Nat. Prod* 63 (7):1035–1042.

Ramírez, Ivan C, Santamaría, Abel, Tobon- Velasco, Julio C, Orozco-Ibarra, Marisol, Gonzalez- Herrera, Irma G, Pedraza- Chaverrí, Jose, Maldonado, Perla D. 2013. Curcumin Restores Nrf2 Levels and Prevents Quinolinic Acid-Induced Neurotoxicity. *Journal of Nutritional Biochemistry* 24: 14–24.

Sharangi A. B. 2009. Medicinal and Therapeutic Potentialities of Tea (*Camellia Sinensis* L.) – A Review. *Food Research International* 42:529–535.

Sharma, Manisha, Kumar, Sunil, Sharma, Nidhi. 2012. Animal Models for Huntington's Disease: A Review. *International Research Journal of Pharmacy* 3 (10): 20-26.

Singh, Shamsher, Jamwal, Sumit, Kumar, Puneet. 2015. Piperine Enhances the Protective Effect of Curcumin against 3-NP Induced Neurotoxicity: Possible Neurotransmitters Modulation Mechanism. *Neurochem Res* 40:1758–1766.

Smith, R., Brundin, P. and Li, J. Y. 2005. Synaptic Dysfunction in Huntington's Disease: A New Perspective. *Cell. Mol. Life Sci* 62:1901–1912.

Sumathi, Thangarajan, Asha, Deivasigamani, Suganya, Natrajan S, Prasanna, Krishnan, Sandhya, Mohanan K. 2014. "Neuroprotective Activity of L-Theanine on 3-Nitropropionic Acid-Induced Neurotoxicity in Rat Striatum, *International Journal of Neuroscience*, 124:9, 673-684.

Sumathi, Thangarajan, Surekha, Ramchandran, Priya Krishnamurthy. 2016. Chrysin Exerts Neuroprotective Effects Against 3-Nitropropionic Acid Induced Behavioral Despair—Mitochondrial Dysfunction and Striatal Apoptosis vvia Upregulating Bcl-2 Gene and Downregulating Bax—Bad Genes in Male Wistar Rats. *Biomedicine & Pharmacotherapy* 84: 514–525.

Tian, Xia, Sun, Lingyan, Gou, Longshan, Ling, Xin, Feng, Yan, Wang, Ling, Yin, Xioaxing, Liu Yi. 2013 Protective Effect of L-Theanine on Chronic Restraint Stress-Induced Cognitive Impairments in Mice. *Brain Res* 1503: 24- 32.

Uzunalic- Perva, Amra, Skerget, Mojca, Knez, Zeljko, Weinreich, Bernd, Otto, Frank, Gruner, Sabine. 2006. Extraction of Active Ingredients from Green Tea (*Camellia Sinensis*): Extraction Efficiency of Major Catechins and Caffeine. *Food Chemistry* 96: 597–605.

Yamada, Takashi, Terashima, Takehiko, Wada, Keiko, Ueda, Sakiko, Ito Mitsuyo, Okubo, Tsutomu, Juneja, Lekh R, Yokogoshi Hidehiko. 2007. Theanine, R-Glutamylethylamide, Increases Neurotransmission Concentrations snd Neurotrophin mRNA Levels in the Brain during Lactation. *Life Sci 81: 1247-1255.*

Yin, Cui, Gou, Lingshan, Liu, Yi, Yin, Xiaoxing, Zhang, Ling, Jia, Genguang, Zhuang, Xuemei. 2011. Antidepressant-Like Effects of L-Theanine in the Forced Swim and Tail Suspension Tests in Mice. *Phytother Res*, 25: 1636- 1639.

Zuccato, Chiara, Valenza, Marta, Cattaneo, Elena. 2010. Molecular Mechanisms and Potential Therapeutic Targets in Huntington's Disease. *Physiol Rev* 90: 905–981.

Zukhurova, Mavdzhuda, Prosvirnina, Maria, Daineko, Anastasia, Simanenkova, Anna, Petrishchev Nikolay, Sonin, Dmitry, Galagudza, Michael, Shamtsyan, Mark, Juneja, LekhR, Vlasov, Timur. 2013. L-Theanine Administration Results in Neuroprotection and Prevents Glutamate Receptor Agonist-Mediated Injury in the Rat Model of Cerebral Ischemia-Reperfusion. *Phytother Res.* 27: 1282-7.

In: Food for Huntington's Disease
Editors: M. Mohamed Essa et al.
ISBN: 978-1-53613-854-2
© 2018 Nova Science Publishers, Inc.

Chapter 4

SPICES AND HUNTINGTON'S DISEASE

*R. Balakrishnan[1], T. Manivasagam[2], A. Justin Thenmozhi[2], M. Mohamed Essa[3,4,5] and N. Elangovan[1,]**

[1]Departmentof Biotechnology, Periyar University, Tamil Nadu,India
[2]Department of Biochemistry and Biotechnology, Annamalai University, Tamil Nadu, India
[3] Department of Food Science and Nutrition, College of Agriculture and Marine Sciences, Sultan Qaboos University, Oman
[4]Ageing and Dementia Research Group, Sultan Qaboos University, Oman
[5]Food and Brain Research Foundation, Tamil Nadu, India

ABSTRACT

Spices are used as flavouring and scrumptious agents that exhibit a wide range of pharmacological activities. The Indian spices add aroma and fragrance to foods. A few spices and contain many important

---

[*] Corresponding Author Email: elangovannn@gmail.com.

chemical constituents in the form of essential oils, oleoresin, oleogu and resins, which are used for health and medicinal purposes. Central nervous system disorders are of greater importance and it has been evident in traditional books that spices can protect and cure neuronal ailments. Many spices found in India such as turmeric, pepper, ginger, cloves, cinnamon, onion, garlic and nutmeg are used for culinary purpose and have been found to have reported specific activities against brain disorders. This review focuses on the importance of spices in therapeutics of Huntington's disease by targeting mitochondrial and proteasome dysfunction, oxidative stress, inflammation and apoptosis.

Keywords: Indian spices, mitochondrial dysfunction, oxidative stress, neurodegenerative disorders, Huntington's disease

INTRODUCTION

Huntington disease (HD) is a progressive and inherited neurodegenerative disorder that causes the progressive loss of nerve cells in the brain and usually results in movement and cognitive impairments (Nance, 1997). HD patients typically display a gradual onset of an involuntary movement disorder in which occasional adventitious movements develop into rhythmic uncontrolled motions. This appearance of rhythmic uncontrolled movements led clinicians to describe the disorder as Huntington chorea to emphasize the "dance-like" appearance of these movements. With progression of the involuntary movement disorder, the clinical course is then characterized by cognitive decline, exhibited by an inability to perform sequenced tasks, suggesting a decline in executive function. Extensive neuropathology studies of HD have been performed, which have led to a rating scale of 0 (pre symptomatic) to 4 (severe) based upon the degree and extent of neurodegenerative findings at autopsy (Vonsattel et al., 1985). Most striking is an overall loss of brain volume in HD patients, with different brain regions showing different rates of neuron loss. Significant cerebral cortex and striatal degeneration occurs, while, alamic, cerebellar and spinal cord regions are unaffected. Of particular note is that only certain populations of neurons degenerate and certain non-neural cell types, specifically skeletal muscle and adipose tissue, are affected, providing an explanation for the clinical constellation of symptoms in HD (Dayalu and Albin, 2015). HD neuropathology is notable for the selective vulnerability of the striatal medium-sized spiny neurons (MSNs) in the basal ganglia region of the midbrain. The basal ganglions are mainly involved in the regulation of involuntary movement. Striatal neurons in the putamen projecting to the *Substantia nigra* are often the first to degenerate, and their demise can even be documented in pre symptomatic HD patients. Cortical pyramidal neurons projected to the putamen in the striatum were also degenerated; hence, the death of MSNs and the cortical neurons that project to them represents the neuro-pathological hallmark of HD.

In 1993, a mutation in the CAG trinucleotide repeat expansion of the huntingtin (HTT) gene was found as the cause for etiology of HD (Huntington's, 1993). HTT glutamine repeats exceed a threshold (around 37 repeats for HD) a new pathological confirmation is adopted, yielding conformers that are resistant to the protein turnover processes, culminating in neurodegeneration. The CAG repeat size ranges established in HD are as follows: less than 35 CAGs is normal; more than 40 CAGs yields disease within the typical human lifespan; and 36–39 CAGs are indeterminate, as penetrance is reduced and may not manifest as clinical disease. The length of the mutant HTT poly Q expansions is inversely proportional to the age of disease onset and pace of disease progression. Furthermore, expanded CAG repeats in HTT are genetically unstable, leading to further expansion causing the change in next generations, such that a parent with "intermediate" allele (27–35 CAGs), or "reduced penetrance" allele (36–39 CAGs) may pass on a CAG repeat that leads to penetrant HD. This enhancement in the CAG repeats number in succeeding generations may lead to the clinical symptoms, which are found in earlier age of disease onset and more rapid progression of HD in their children and even quicker in grandchildren of affected HD patients (Walker, 2007).

THERAPY FOR HD

Till now, no disease altering therapies that fully treat HD have been discovered. Rather, treatment is purely symptomatic, typically combining a variety of medications with speech, occupational, and/or physical therapy. While some medications have been specifically tested for efficacy in HD, many have been validated in other diseases to treat symptoms that also occur in HD. Most HD patients are prescribed multiple drugs to treat their array of symptoms, but as symptoms can and do evolve with disease progression the use of a particular drug must be re-evaluated overtime. For example, rigidity and bradykinesia can be problematic upon initial disease onset, while chorea and adventitial movements predominate, as HD progresses.

COMPOUNDS THAT PRIMARILY TARGET MOTOR SYMPTOMS

Uncontrolled movements in HD are believed to stem from the over activation of the dopaminergic D2 indirect pathway circuits in the basal ganglia. Thus, neuroleptic agents are typically used to block receptors or deplete presynaptic dopamine to treat these motor aspects of HD (Schwab et al., 2015). This has become the standard of care based upon years of clinical experience (though there is little in the way of clinical trial data to support use of the most prescribed medications). A variety of other drugs can also be employed, acting to modulate glutamatergic neurotransmission, BDNF-Trk B signaling, or inflammation. In the United Kingdom, medications that bind the dopamine D2 receptor to block dopamine activation are preferred (Priller et al., 2008). Recently, tetrabenazine has emerged as an efficacious anti-chorea medication based upon clinical trial experience, and it was the first FDA-approved medication for HD. Deutetrabenazine was recently approved as the second. All other treatments are prescribed "off-label."

MODULATION OF GLUTAMATERGIC SIGNALING

Beyond the dopaminergic system, other commonly used drugs in HD target glutamate neurotransmission. There is some evidence that amantadine, a glutamate antagonist, is effective at reducing chorea with a 400 mg/day dosage, but not at lower doses (O'Suilleabhain and Dewey, 2003). Unfortunately, this drug has also been shown to worsen irritability and aggression in HD patients, which can exacerbate the behavioral problems frequently found in this population of patients and there by negatively impact quality of life. In 2002, a double-blind, placebo controlled study examined the amantadine's efficacy and safety in HD patients found that amantadine therapy was linked with a reduction of 36% in chorea score at rest versus 0% with placebo, with mean improvement of 56% for the 10 patients whose plasma drugs levels were high (Jankovic and Orman, 1988). Furthermore, amantadine was safe and well tolerated without any side effects on cognitive function. Additional clinical studies of amantadine have been performed, and one trial documented reduced dyskinesia scores in treated patients, while the other trial failed to detect any improvement in mean chorea score in patients receiving drug therapy (O'Suilleabhain and Dewey, 2003). In this latter study, ameta-analysis of amantadine therapy as a treatment for HD was conducted, and concluded that amantadine does not significantly reduce chorea in HD patients.

A number of other inhibitors of glutamatergic neurotransmission have been considered and evaluated in HD, including riluzole, which blocks a subset of sodium channels, and directly inhibits kainate and N-methyl-Daspartate (NMDA) glutamate receptors, ketamine and remacemide, which are NMDA receptor blockers, and lamotrigine, which inhibits glutamate release (Song et al., 1997). Riluzole (200 mg/day) showed an improvement in the efficacy for the selected primary outcome measure (total chorea score-UHDRS). However, safety issues arose due to a constant and significant increase in the liver enzymes ALT and AST in the riluzole group, which curtailed further investigation. 379 HD patients then completed a randomized, placebo study of riluzole at 50 mg twice daily, but no intergroup difference in primary outcome was demonstrated. Thus, efficacy for riluzole, as well as for these other NMDA inhibitors, as a treatment for HD has not been attained.

TREATMENT ALGORITHM FOR CHOREA

In summary, the choice for treating significant chorea in HD is typically between TBZ and olanzapine. Clinical evidence favors TBZ, but its side effects of depression and drowsiness are relative contra-indications in some HD patients. Furthermore, as TBZ is now approved for the treatment of HD in the USA, it now costs more than $2000 a month at the starting dose of 25 mg/day, compared with about $45 per month before it was licensed (Murphy et al., 2012). TBZ is typically prescribed in divided doses and thus must be taken several times a day, which can reduce compliance. For these reasons, many clinicians favor olanzapine as the initial choice in HD as it can be given once a day, typically at night, when its sedative side effects can counter insomnia. Other beneficial effects (mood stabilization and weight gain) of olanzapine make it an even more attractive first line therapy for HD, even though definitive clinical trial data confirming its utility in HD is still lacking. Hence, a reasonable algorithm is to initiate therapy with olanzapine, with TBZ as the second line therapy if olanzapine fails to yield a satisfactory response. Selection of another drug from the various other options discussed above should only be pursued after both olanzapine and TBZ have failed to elicit symptomatic benefit.

As current therapies mainly concentrate on symptomatic treatment, there is no cure for HD. So this chapter deals with the therapeutic benefits of a few popular Indian spices that hold various pharmacological properties.

SPICES

Spices and aromatic vegetable products that are obtained from seeds, roots, bark, and leaves for example are mainly used as flavoring agents. They enhance the taste of food. The earliest record (around 6,000 BC) on the use of spices is the four Vedas Rig, Sama, Yajur and Atharva. The Rig Veda, an ancient Hindu scripture, lists greater than a 1000 healing plants including various spices. The history of the usage of spices dates back 7000 years in the past. Even though more progress in the herbal science field has been made, spices are used as home remedies for curing disease. Some spices, such as turmeric, are considered as part of our daily diets and have been used for many years. The pharmacological properties of the spices are well suited for the treatment of human ailments and the medical field is reported to have an increased interest in them.

INDIAN SPICES AND THEIR MEDICINAL USES

Indian spices were considered as health improving agents from ancient times, since they could modify the four important humors like black bile, phlegm, blood, and yellow bile and modify moods such as choleric, sanguine, melancholic, and phlegmatic. By inducing heat in the stomach, ginger improved the digestion processes. Other spices had different benefits. For example, clove comforted the sinus; mace prevented colic and bloody fluxes or diarrhea; nutmeg benefited the spleen and relieved cold; Cinnamon, was considered to be good for digestion and sore throats. Hot pungent spices were used in winter diets or to treat cold diseases. It was believed that the rheumatism was caused by abnormal accumulation of rheum, or phlegm and an appropriate therapy would be pepper or capsaicin, a chili pepper extract. Indigestion, gas, and flatulence problems were cleared by cardamom. Cumin seeds, containing large amounts of carotene and iron, were used as a tonic for the heart and nervous system. *Crocus sativus* L., (saffron) is used as an antispasmodic, expectorant, and aphrodisiac agent in folk medicine (Zargari, 1990). Garlic (*Allium sativum*

Linn.), with varied pharmacological activities, is famous for its medicinal properties (Ross, 1999). For example, garlic may lower blood pressure, cholesterol, and the risk of cancer. Capsaicin, the major component in red peppers, has anti-cancer properties against on prostate cancer cells by inducing the apoptosis in the cancer's cell lines. Curcumin, an active component of turmeric, offers a strong antioxidant, ant- atherosclerosic, anti-inflammatory, and hepatoprotective effects. Fenugreek (*Trigonella foenum graecum*) tea was used as tonic for relief of sore throats, bronchitis, and tuberculosis. Fenugreek poultices were used as a treatment for skin irritations, swollen glands, and gout. Its seed significantly lowered the blood sugar and cholesterol levels (Misra et al., 1996).

Natural remedies can be the best candidates for curing some diseases effectively with lower side effects. It is done so traditionally in India and China. Ancient traditional practices have inspired scientists to find the new therapeutic methods. Some studies have shown the health benefits and the neuroprotective effects of Indian spices even in disease like HD. Even though some scientific experiments have been carried out, the specific phytoconstituents and pharmacological actions of the spices regarding the treatment of these deleterious nervous disorders are not fully known.

Allium Sativum L.

Garlic, *Allium sativum*, belongs to the family Amaryllidaceae and is believed to have originated from Central Asia. It is used in traditional medicine to enhance physical and mental health, and also as a flavoring agent. Garlic has earned special position in the traditions of many people and acts as an important prophylactic and therapeutic agent. The role of garlic in the treatment of tumors, heart disorders, worm bites, and other ailments has been recorded in the 35 century-old book, *Egyptian Codex Ebers*. Both Hippocrates and Pliny the Elder promoted the medicinal properties of garlic. Garlic has played a therapeutic role in AD, cardiovascular disease, cancer, infections, dermatological infections, and stress. Volatiles such as diallyl trisulfide, diallyl sulfide (DAS), methyl allyl disulfide, diallyl disulfide (DADS), 2-vinyl-1,3-dithiin, 3-vinyl-1,2-dithiin, methyl allyltrisulfide, and *E*, *Z*-ajoene are present in crushed garlic and garlic essential oil. Several garlic preparations contain nonvolatile sulfur compounds such as S-ally cysteine (SAC) and S-allyl methyl cysteine (SAMC). Intact garlic also contains essential oil, prostaglandins, steroidal glycosides, pectin, lectins, fructan, vitamins B-1, B-2, B-6, C and E, adenosine, fatty acids, biotin, phospholipids, nicotinic acid, glycollipids, flavonoids, anthocyanins, essential amino acids, and phenolics. The therapeutic effect of garlic and its constituents on HD remains to be resolved (Rahman, 2001).

Carum Carvi L.

Carum carvi belongs to family Apiaceae and has many common names, such as meridian fennel, caraway, or Persian cumin. The major phytoconstituents in *C. carvi* are carvone, α-pinene, dihydrocarveol, limonene, carveol, thymol, epoxy carvones, and myrcene. Minor compounds are the limonene, α-Pinene, and carvacroldihydrocarvone. These constituents are reported to have anti-alzherimeric effects, but their role in HD is yet to be investigated.

Crocus Sativus L.

The dried red stigma of *Crocus sativus* L. (Family: Iridaceae) is widely cultivated in Iran, India, and Greece. It is commonly called as saffron and reported to contain approximately 150 aroma and volatile compounds, but mainly terpene alcohol, terpenes, and their esters. Its bitter taste and hay or iodoform like fragrances is caused by the presence of safranal and picrocrocin. This flower possesses numerous medicinal activities such as antioxidant, antidepressant, antigenototoxic, anti-inflammatory, anti-convulsant, antitussive and cytotoxic effects, anti-nociceptive, anxiolytic aphrodisiac, relaxant activity, and antihypertensive. It improves learning and memory skills as well as improves blood flow to the retina and choroid.

Curcuma Longa L.

Curcuma longa, commonly known as turmeric (Family: Zingiberaceae), and its active component, curcumin, is the most studied medicinal plant and phytochemical worldwide. It was used traditionally in India to treat various illnesses such as microbial diseases, hepatic disorders, skin diseases, inflammations, intermittent fevers, iron chelating, constipation, and as a neuroprotectant in the treatment of various neurological diseases. Previous studies have indicated that the curcumin has potent anti-Parkinsonic and anti-Alzheimeric molecules, and has exerted its neuroprotective effects by modulating various pharmacological targets.

Capsicum Annum L. Var. Angulosum

Capsicum annuum (chili) is the most frequently consumed spice worldwide. It's use in various systems of medicine against numerous diseases and/or disorders are due to the presence of therapeutically important active components. It is used as both external and internal therapeutic agents in various systems of medicine. It is used to treat lumbago, rheumatism, neuralgia, varicose veins, as a local stimulant, counter irritant, and to treat blisters externally. Creams containing capsaicin are applied topically in neuropathy, pain disorders, psoriasis, migraine, cluster headache, herpes zoster, and trigeminal neuralgia. Chili is taken internally to treat flatulence, dyspepsia, arthrosclerosis, a loss of appetite, stroke, muscle tension, and heart diseases. In addition, the chili is sometimes administered with other herbs to catalyze the activity of the other herbs (Ogunruku et al., 2014). In Unani medicine, chili is used to prevent cold, sinus infection, sore throat, and to improve digestion and blood circulation (Ogunruku et al., 2014). In folk medicine, it is recommended for the treatment of cancer, asthma, and cough. However, its regular consumption also believed to be beneficial for hemorrhoids, anorexia, varicose veins, and liver congestion. It predominantly contains variety of branched and straight-chained alkyl called vanillyl amides. They are collectively known as capsaicinoids, examples are capsaicin, nohydrocapsaicin, homodihydrocapsaicin, dihydrocapsaicin, ω-hydro-xycapsaicin, 6", 7"-dihydro-5', 5"-dicapsaicin, and homocapsaicin. It also contains threec apsinoids including capsiate, dihydrocapsiate, and nordihydrocapsiate, which are non-pungent and structurally similar to the capsaicinoids (Szabo et al., 2004). The neuroprotective effects of chili fruits and its components are not yet investigated.

Coriandrum Sativum L.

Coriandrum sativum L. has been used for more than 30 centuries (Ebers papyrus of 1550 BC) for both flavoring and medicinal purposes. It is commonly known as Coriander and is from the Apiaceae family. It is native to the Mediterranean region, but is widely cultivated in Central Europe, North Africa, Asia, and Russia. The dried fruit of coriander, also called the seeds, have as light bittersweet and spicy taste; they are globular in shape and with an aromatic smell. As a spice, it is an integral part of curry powder that can be used in minced meat stews and dishes. The young leaves of this plant are crushed to make chutneys and sauces. Due to its attractive aroma and green color, the green leaves are consumed as fresh herbs and as garnishes in salads. Its oil can be used in body care products, cosmetics and perfumes. Various parts of this plant have been reported to have numerous health improving and biological activities (Mani et al., 2011). This plant is an excellent source of petroselinic acid and an essential oil isolated from the aerial parts and seeds contain a large amount of linalool. Due to the presence of multiple bioactive constituents, it offers a wide array of pharmacological activities that include anti-oxidant, anti-inflammatory, anti-microbial, anxiolytic, anti-diabetic, anti-depressant, anti-hypertensive, anti-mutagenic, anti-epileptic, anti-dyslipidemic, diuretic, and neuroprotective. Interestingly, coriander also possesses lead-detoxifying potential. Coriander has long been used in Iranian traditional medicine as anticonvulsant, anti-depressant and for its nerve soothing, sedative and anxiolytic properties (Mani et al., 2011).

Elettaria Cardamomum L.

Elettaria cardamomum, cardamom, belongs to the ginger family (Zingiberaceae). It is called as the 'queen of spices', whereas black pepper as the 'king of spices'. Since from the 4th century BC, its dried ripe fruits were used as a spice and in medicines. In Ayurveda, cardamom is consumed to treat asthma, bronchitis, as well as urinary, stomach, and heart disorders. Traditionally, when mixed with camphor and neem, it is used as a nasal preparation to treat colds. By gargling, it can relieve sore throats, and is present in cough sweets. Its extracts show a potent anti-inflammatory response, but the active compounds responsible for this have not been identified. Its oil is rich in fatty acids such as oleic, linoleic and palmitic acids; it also contains abundant amounts of alpha terpinyl acetate and 1, 8 cineole.

Ferula Assa-Foetida L.

Ferula assa-foetida Linn belongs to the Family Apiaceae. Its gum resin is used as a condiment in India and Iran. In the Latin, ferula means "carrier" or "vehicle", Asameans "resin", and foetidus means "smelling, fetid". In Ayurvedic texts, it is categorized as sanjna-sthapakadeepniya (a hunger appetizer and consciousness restorer). It is considered a popular home medicine and its components are utilized for many prescriptions in traditional healing. Asafoetida is also used as a flavoring agent by itself as well as in spice mixtures. It is used to flavor meatballs, curries, pickles and dals. The whole plant is used as a fresh herb for cooking and even as an antidote for the effects of opium. It will counteract the effect of the opium when given in the same concentration of the opium ingested by the patient. An ethanol extract of the dried gum (20 mL) activated the CNS (Coleman, 1922).

Murraya Koenigii L.

Murraya koenigii Spreng, known commonly as the curry-leaf tree, is a bush like small aromatic tree belonging to the family Rutaceae. While native to India, only two out of the 14 species throughout the world belonging to the genus *Murraya* are available in India. These are *M. koenigii* and *M. paniculata* with *M. koenigii* being the most popular due to its large spectrum of pharmacological properties. Various parts of the plant (root, leaves, bark, and fruit) are reported to possess numerous biological activities. This plant is used in Indian systems of traditional medicine for a variety of ailments including stomachic, tonic, and carminative (Muthumani et al., 2009a). The alkaloidal extract of *M. koenigii* leaves is reported to have anti-oxidant, anti-inflammatory, anti-ulcerogenic, and analgesic effects on the CNS (Muthumani et al., 2009b).

Piper Nigrum L.

Black pepper fruits are the most widely and frequently used spices worldwide. Black, green and white pepper corns obtained from *Piper nigrum* are popularly used as a pungent and hot spice for flavoring food. Black pepper is mainly used for digestive ailments in traditional medicine. It is used as a therapeutic agent in Ayurveda, Siddha and Unani forms of medicine in South Asia. It is frequently used to increase the appetite to treat digestive system problems, and to kill parasitic worms. In Ayurveda, black pepper is used to treat colds, coughs, heart problems, diabetes, colic, piles and anaemia, as well as to improve appetite, digestion, and breathing. When mixed with castor oil, ghee or cow's urine, pepper aided the treatment of stomach ailments such as flatulence, dyspepsia, constipation and diarrhea. Black pepper when combined with other substances has also been used as a remedy for cholera and syphilis. It is used in tooth powder for toothache, and as an infusion for sore throat and hoarseness. It is chewed to reduce throat inflammation. It contains a large amount of alkaloids. Piperine, a potent alkaloid is reported to act as a CNS depressant and also have pain-relieving, anti-fever, anti-inflammatory and insecticidal effects.

Rosmarinus Officinalis L.

Rosmarinus officinalis, a perennial herb commonly known as rosemary, is a member of the family Lamiaceae. The major constituent of rosemary is *p*-cymene, rosmarinic acid, thymol and linalool. The neuroprotective effects of these pharmacological agents have not been investigated yet.

Syzygium Aromaticum L.

Clove *Syzygium aromaticum* is a valuable spice that has been used for years as food flavouring and preservative with numerous medicinal benefits. It is native to Indonesia but presently it is cultivated worldwide. It Metabolism of bilirubin is a rich source of phenolic compounds such as eugenol acetate, eugenol, and gallic acid and poses great potential for agricultural, food, cosmetic and pharmaceutical applications.

Trigonella foenum graecum L.

The common name of *Trigonella foenum graecum* (Leguminacae) is fenugreek. It is an annual herb extensively used as a spice in Mediterranean and Indian diet. It is well known for its numerous medicinal properties. Dried seeds of this plant are used as a spice, while its leaves are used as a vegetable in the Indian diet. Fenugreek seeds area rich source of omega 3 fatty acids, protein and fiber while the leaves are sources of calcium, vitamin C, β-carotene, iron, potassium and magnesium. The two major active constituents in fenugreek are diosgen in and 4-hydroxy-isoleucine. Steroidal sapogenins and mucilaginous fibers present in the seed and leaves of this legume contribute to hypocholesterolemic and anti-diabetic activities in animal studies and several human trials.

CONCLUSION

Spices are the heterogeneous collections of numerous plants that contain volatile and non-volatile compounds. A wide variety of spices are cultivated in India, due to the variety of climatic conditions and topographical features the country has. The previously discussed spices namely coriander, pepper, garlic, ginger, turmeric, and cinnamon are commonly used in Indian delicacies. These spices improve the flavor turning an ordinary meal into an extraordinary one. They contain diverse arrays of phytochemicals that have numerous pharmacological actions. As age-related degenerative disorders such as HD, are closely associated with toxic reactions involving anti-oxidant, anti-inflammatory, anti-microbial, anxiolytic, anti-diabetic, anti-depressant, anti-hypertensive, anti-mutagenic, anti-epileptic, anti-dyslipidemic and diuretic processes in the body, the use of herbs and spices as a source of phytochemicals with potent pharmacological properties warrants further attention. Therefore more focused research on specific experimental model is needed to underset and specific mechanisms of action.

REFERENCES

Coleman, D. E. (1992). The Effect of Certain Homeopathic Remedies upon the Hearing. *J Am Inst Homeopathy*, 15: 279-81.

Dayalu, P. and Albin, R. L. (2015). Huntington Disease: Pathogenesis and Treatment. *Neurologic Clinics*, 33 (1): 101-114.

Jankovic, J. and Orman, J. (1988). Tetrabenazine Therapy of Dystonia, Chorea, Tics, and Other Dyskinesias. *Neurology*, 38 (3): 391-394.

MacDonald, M. E., Ambrose, C. M., Duyao, M. P., Myers, R. H., Lin, C., Srinidhi, L., Barnes, G., Taylor, S. A., James, M., Groot, N. and Mac Farlane, H. (1993). A Novel Gene Containing a Trinucleotide Repeat That is Expanded and Unstable on Huntington's Disease Chromosomes. *Cell*, 72 (6): 971-983.

Mani, V., Parle, M., Ramasamy, K., Majeed, A. and Bakar, A. (2011). Reversal of Memory Deficits by *Coriandrum Sativum* Leaves in Mice. *Journal of the Science of Food and Agriculture*, 91(1): 186-192.

Misra, M., Alp, M. S. and Ausman, J. I. (1996). Magnetic Resonance Angiography for Anterior Midline Aneurysms. *British Journal of Neurosurgery*, 10: 621-621.

Murphy, S. M., Puwanant, A. and Griggs, R. C. (2012). Unintended Effects of Orphan Product Designation for Rare Neurological Diseases. *Annals of neurology*, 72: 481-490.

Muthumani, P., Venkatraman, S., Ramseshu, K., Meera, R., Devi, P., Kameswari, B. and Eswarapriya, B. (2009). Pharmacological Studies of Anticancer, Anti-Inflammatory Activities of *Murraya Koenigii* (Linn) Spreng in Experimental Animals. *Journal of Pharmaceutical Sciences and Research*, 17: 18.

Nance, M. A. US Huntington Disease Genetic Testing Group. (1997). Genetic Testing of Children at Risk for Huntington's disease. *Neurology*, 49 (4): 1048-1053.

Ogunruku, O. O., Oboh, G. Ademosun, A. O. (2014). Water Extractable Phytochemicals from Peppers (*Capsicum* spp.) Inhibit Acetyl-Cholinesterase and Butyrylcholinesterase Activities and Prooxidants Induced Lipid Peroxidation in Rat Brain *In Vitro*. *International Journal of Food Science*, 2014.

O'Suilleabhain, P. and Dewey, Jr. R. B. (2003). A Randomized Trial of Amantadine in Huntington Disease. *Archives of Neurology*, 60 (7): 996-998.

Priller, J., Ecker, D., Landwehrmeyer, B. Craufurd, D. (2008). A Europe-Wide Assessment of Current Medication Choices in Huntington's Disease. *Movement Disorders*, 23 (12): 1788-1788.

Rahman, K. (2001). Historical Perspective on Garlic and Cardiovascular Disease. *J Nutr*, 131: 977-979.

Ross, I. A. (2010). *Medicinal Plants of the World*, 3.

Schwab, L. C., Garas, S. N., Drouin-Ouellet, J., Mason, S. L., Stott, S. R. Barker, R. A. (2015). Dopamine and Huntington's Disease. *Expert Review of Neurotherapeutics*, 15 (4): 445-458.

Song, J. H., Huang, C. S., Nagata, K., Yeh, J.Z. Narahashi, T. (1997). Differential Action of Riluzole on Tetrodotoxin-Sensitive and Tetrodotoxin-Resistant Sodium Channels. *Journal of Pharmacology and Experimental Therapeutics*, 282 (2): 707-714.

Szabó, B., Hori, K., Nakajima, A., Sasagawa, N., Watanabe, Y. and Ishiura, S. (2004). Expression of Amyloid-β1–40 and 1–42 Peptides in *Capsicum Annum Var. Angulosum* for Oral Immunization. *Assay and Drug Development Technologies*, 2 (4): 383-388.

Vonsattel, J. P., Myers, R. H., Stevens, T. J., Ferrante, R. J., Bird, E. D. and Richardson, E. P. (1985). Neuropathological Classification of Huntington's Disease. *Journal of Neuropathology & Experimental Neurology*, 44 (6): 559-577.

Walker, F. O. (2007). Huntington's Disease. *The Lancet*, 369, (9557): 218-228.

Zargari, A. (1990). *In Medicinal Plants*. Tehran University Publications, Tehran 4, 574-8.

In: Food for Huntington's Disease ISBN: 978-1-53613-854-2
Editors: M. Mohamed Essa et al. © 2018 Nova Science Publishers, Inc.

Chapter 5

PROBIOTICS, PREBIOTICS, AND SYNBIOTICS ON NEUROLOGICAL DISORDERS: RELEVANCE TO HUNTINGTON'S DISEASE

C. Saravana Babu[1,], N. Chethan[1],
B. Srinivasa Rao[2], A. Bhat[1], R. Bipul[1], A. H. Tousif[1],
M. Mahadevan[3], S. Sathiya[4], T. Manivasagam[5],
A. Justin Thenmozhi[5], M. Mohamed Essa[6,7]
and K.S. Meena[8]*

[1]Department of Pharmacology, JSS College of Pharmacy,
JSS Academy of Higher Education and Research,
SS Nagar, Mysore, KA, India
[2]Department of Anatomy, College of Medicine, Imam Abdulrahman
Bin Faisal University, Damam, Kingdom of Saudi Arabia
[3]Department of Sirappu Maruthuvam, National Institute of Siddha,
Govt. of India, Tambaram Sanatorium, Chennai, TN, India
[4]Department of Pharmacology, College of Medicine,
University of Saskatchewan, Saskatoon, SK, Canada

---

[*] Corresponding Author. Saravana Babu Chidambaram, MPharm, PhD, Associate Professor, Department of Pharmacology, JSS College of Pharmacy, JSS Academy of Higher Education and Research, SS Nagar, Mysore - 570015, KA, India. Tel: +91-9940434129; +91-9042222277; Email: csaravanababu@gmail.com.

[5]Department of Biochemistry and Biotechnology,
Annamalai University, Annamalainagar, TN, India
[6]Department of Food Science and Nutrition, CAMS,
Sultan Qaboos University, Muscat, Oman
[7]Ageing and Dementia Research Group,
Sultan Qaboos University, Muscat, Oman
[8]College of Pharmacy and Nutrition, University of Saskatchewan,
Saskatoon, SK, Canada

ABSTRACT

Food has an undeniable impact on the overall functioning of the human body, affecting various physiological and developmental processes based on its nutritive values. It plays an important part in development, maturation and functioning of the brain. The major impact of our diet on the brain is coordinated through the Gut-Brain axis (GBA). The Gut-Brain axis is an arrangement of networks communicating between gut and the brain. The commensal gut microbiota present in the gastro-intestinal tract (GIT) are involved in aiding the process of food metabolism; they have their own impact on the functioning of the GBA and also use the GBA as a route to communicate with brain. Interestingly, the gut microbiome have a pivotal role in the normal function and development of the brain, and in some instances it is even responsible for the development of neurodegerative diseases due to dysbiosis or unfavorable alterations. Probiotics and prebiotics are live microorganisms that are fermentable and are non-digestible oligosaccharides respectively; together they are referred to as synbiotics. This review is meant to highlight the promising health benefits of probiotics, prebiotics, and synbiotics and their ability to improve the life style and alleviate the existing symptoms of patients suffering from various neurodegenerative diseases such as Huntington's disease, which has a both genetic and non-genetic origin.

INTRODUCTION

Gut Microbiota

Amidst the several microbial communities inhabiting the human body, the gut microbiome is seen as a key factor that influences the health of human beings [1]. Within the human intestine are found around 100 trillion essential bacteria for healthy living. During the process of metabolism, the breakdown of complex polysaccharides ingested is assisted by these organisms, which are also vital in the function and development of normal immune systems [2]. The approach to the process of identifying and tracking these organisms' role in health and disease has completely changed in over the last few years [3]. Friedrich Escherich investigated stool samples from healthy individuals by culturing and characterizing the *Bacterium coli commune*, today it is known as *Escherichia coli*, a highly sought out species of microorganism in molecular biology [4]. Over the past few decades many new commensal microorganisms were isolated and characterized. But the current implementation of advanced high-output genetic profiling has given us a comprehensive insight into the universe of intestinal microorganisms. Gut bacteria create a broad-ranging, lively microbial community that is involved in many processes of the host organism and responds to changes in the physiology of host.

Joshua Lederberg an American molecular biologist who coined the term "microbiota" to illustrate this complex microbial population and defined it as the ecological neighborhood of commensal, symbiotic, and pathogenic microorganisms that take shelter in us [5]. The collective genome of these symbiotic microorganisms is referred to as the "microbiome"; interestingly, their collective number of genes is higher than that found in the human genome [6]. It has been shown that the microbiota structure is affected by basic temporal and spatial factors. The human fetal gut starts out as sterile, with colonization beginning instantaneously after birth. The major influence to colonization are the route of delivery, maternal transfer, diet, environmental stimuli, and antibiotic usage [7]. Recently it was shown that even before breastfeeding, the amniotic fluid, placenta, and meconium of newborns all contain small counts of bacteria [8].

The microbiota of the infants and elderly individuals is highly dynamic and unstable until the age of 2 years and above the age of 55 years respectively [8]. The adult gut microbiota population is composed of four major phyla: *Bacteroidetes*, *Firmicutes*, *Actinobacteria*, and *Verrucomicrobia* [9]. With age, the composition of microbial population is altered, shifting to a greater proportion of *Bacteroides* spp. and distinct abundance patterns of *Clostridium* groups are also identified in elderly individuals compared to younger adults [10].

The gut microbiota is made up of a diverse community of bacteria existing in symbiotic relationship with the host's intestine. Most of the microbiota belong to the phylum Firmicutes (~51%). Firmicutes coexists with the *Clostridium coccoides* and *Clostridium leptum* groups as well as the very familiar *Lactobacillus genera* and the phylum Bacteroidetes (~48%), which includes the genera *Bacteroides* and *Prevotella* [11]. The phyla Proteobacteria, Actinobacteria, Fusobacteria, Spirochaetes, Verrucomicrobia, and Lentisphaerae constitute to the remaining 1% [12]. Among the total 10^{13}–10^{14} microorganisms that reside in the gut microbiota, only around 1000 species have been identified and nearly 7000 strains of bacteria have been characterized [13]. The composition of microbiota has been found to vary for each individual; while the function of the microbiota remains the same, entitling it as a major player in the maintenance of basic set of physiological functions [14]. The gut microbiota is practically an organ itself, playing a major part in various physiological activities such as host metabolism, immune regulation, neurological development, vitamin synthesis, energy homeostasis, and digestion [15].

The gut bacteria modulate the immune system, aid in the development of the nervous system, and also act as a main source of vitamin K and vitamin B [16, 17]. It has been acknowledged by many researchers that the composition of gut microbiota has its own part in the development of human diseases such as inflammatory bowel disease [18], diabetes [19], cancer [20], and disorders pertaining to nervous system, for example pain syndromes [21], Parkinson's disease [22], spinal cord injury [23], autism [24], and stroke [25]. Recently even ageing was reported to have large impact on gut microbiome composition and its involvement in various physiological processes. The data generated from various clinical and even non-clinical studies has shown that there is a drastic increase in the number of neurological disorders that originate from the commensal microbiota in gut. Henceforth, the microbiome is a very important subject of interest in the field of Neuroscience [3].

GUT BRAIN AXIS

The connection between the gut and brain, i.e., the GIT and the nervous system, is a bidirectional neuro-endocrine system otherwise defined as the Gut Brain Axis [26]. The Gut Brain Axis (GBA) is a complex reflexive network of efferent and afferent fibers between the GI tract and the CNS. It acts as a bidirectional communication along hormonal, neural, and immune pathways that allow the CNS to affect motor, sensory, and secretory functions of the GI tract, and vice versa [8].

The autonomic system consists of both the sympathetic and parasympathetic limbs together, conducting the afferent signals generated from the lumen of the gut and then sending these signals to the CNS through enteric spinal and vagal nerve pathways and the efferent signals from CNS to the intestinal wall. The main efferent axis that synchronizes all the types of stressors with adaptive responses is the Hypothalamic Pituitary Adrenal (HPA) axis [27]. HPA axis, being a segment of the limbic system in the brain, is mainly concerned with memory and emotional reactions. The HPA axis is triggered by environmental stress through elevated concentrations of systemic pro-inflammatory cytokines, stimulating the hypothalamus to release corticotropin-releasing factor (CRF), and further initiating the release of the adrenocorticotropic hormone (ACTH) from pituitary gland, sequentially leading to the release of the major stress hormone cortisol from the adrenal glands. Cortisol has its effects on many human organs; the most vital among the organs is brain. In this fashion, with the neural and hormonal communication lines in co-existence, the brain controls the functions of the intestinal effector cells, such as immune cells, epithelial cells, enteric neurons, smooth muscle cells, interstitial cells of Cajal, and enterochromaffin cells. These are the cells, whose role in the brain-gut bidirectional communication under the influence of the gut microbiota has been demonstrated [28].

The gut physiology can be altered by the autonomic nervous system and the HPA axis that control the CNS and viscera, having an impact on motility, epithelial permeability, and secretion, in addition to systemic hormones that affect the host-microbiome interface at the mucosae and niche environments for microbiota [29]. Santos et al. (2001) discovered that stress caused flaws in epithelial barrier with subsequent activation of the mucosal mast cell [30]. An early life stress, such as maternal separation, resulted in an increase in the systemic corticosterone level and immune responses comorbid within distinct fecal microbiota of the test animals [31]. Murine gut microbiota were seen to be altered through immune system activation when they were co-housed with aggressive littermates, a condition referred to as social disruption [32]. In addition, the release of cytokines and anti-microbial peptides (AMPs), which are the signaling molecules into the gut lumen by neurons, immune cells, enteroendocrine cells, and Paneth cells through the direct or indirect CNS signaling is speculated to alter the gut microbiota immediately [33].

The afferent signaling pathways in the vagal and spinal afferent nerves communicate the information from the intestinal mucosa to nucleus, arcuate nucleus, tractus solitarius, and thalamic center of satiety [34]. The satiation-signaling peptides are mainly produced in the GI tract but are also synthesized within brain [35]. Beyond that, the CNS can influence the gut microbiome through neural and endocrine pathways in both direct and indirect manners.

Food intake, gastric emptying, and the stimulation of pancreatic secretion are affected by the stimulation of the afferent vagal nerves. The origin of these afferent nerves is very close to the basolateral membrane of enteroendocrine cells, yet they are unable to reach the gut lumen [36]. The afferent nerves are indirectly activated by the contents of the lumen under the regulation of paracrine factors released by enterocytes. It is understood that the GIT functions are affected greatly by CCK and serotonin (5-hydroxytryptamine, 5-HT) acting through vagal afferents [37].

ROLE OF MICROBIOTA IN GBA

Many studies have been performed to characterize the mechanisms and to explain the process of the generation of signals from luminal microorganisms and their influence on the gut epithelium, such as by bipeptides or tripeptides, like N-formylmethionyl–eucyl–phenylalanine and Toll like receptor signaling [33]. The enteric microbiota has a major effect on the GBA, not just locally with ENS and intestinal cells but also through neuroendocrine and metabolomics with the CNS, which was evident in both clinical and experimental studies [38].

The most common mechanism through which the pathogenic bacteria inhibit the intestinal secretions is by signaling the via α2 adrenergic receptors, and thereby inhibiting the expulsion of the pathogen by the host [39]. Many studies depict the ability of microbiota to influence behaviors like anxiety and depression, as well as impact dysbiosisin autism. Patients suffering from autism were found to exhibit specific microbial population changes depending on the severity of the disease [28]. Various preclinical models have been used to study the influence of gut microbiota on behavior and brain functions by using GF (germ free) mice treated with pre-biotics, pro-biotics, antibiotics, fecal microbiota transplant, and deliberate material infection [8].

The central regulation of satiety has a crucial role in the CNS-gut-microbiome signaling. There is a serious impact on the availability of nutrition and the composition of gut microbiota when there are changes in the dietary pattern through the influence of the CNS. This downhill signaling process is controlled by the Satiation-signaling peptides acting as the key molecular intermediates. The peptide YY, is transported to brain through blood postprandial in order to exert its impact on satiety [36].

In the normal physiological state it was observed that the gut microbiome plays a crucial role in the maturation of the CNS. The prenatal and postnatal brain development was seen to be altered due to various external cues derived from the indigenous commensal microbiota [40, 41]. The CNS upward regulation by the microbiome was evident through various mechanisms involving neural, metabolic, immunological, and endocrine pathways [7].

Evidence has suggested that microbiome dysbiosis can influence the initial onset and progression of various neurological diseases [42]. The manipulation of the gut microbiome with short chain fatty acid (SCFA) producing bacteria modulated the neuroimmune system activation. The activation of microglia, the chief player in the neuroimmune system, is controlled by gut microbiota [43]. This correlation elucidated the neurodegenerative diseases were co-morbid with gastrointestinal disease like microbial dysbiosis, diarrhea, constipation, vitamin deficiencies, diabetes, and obesity [44]. These co-morbidities gave a clear picture of the functional relationship between the GBA and Neurodegeneration [45]. The relative balance as well as the metabolic and genomic expression of the microbiota is altered by changes in its physiology through endocrine signaling, metabolism, and innervations in the host as a reply to oxidative stress, a common environmental stressor [46].

ROLE OF MICROBIOTA IN BRAIN

A variety of microbiota dependent effects on the brain have been reported such as anxiety-like behavior, depression-like behavior, nociceptive responses, stress responsiveness, feeding behavior, taste preferences, and metabolic consequences in numerous clinical and pre-clinical studies [21].

It has been shown that the development and maturation of the CNS and the ENS were heavily dependent on the colonization of gut bacteria in studies on GF animals. The altered genomic expression and neurotransmitter production were found in both the CNS and the ENS in an absence of microbial colonization [47]. When the gut sensory-motor function is altered, the reveals the role of the microbiome in delayed gastric emptying and a reduced intestinal transit migrating motor complex cyclic recurrence as well as distal propagation and enlarged cecal size [48]. There was an evident decrease in genetic expression of enzymes that are vital in the synthesis and transport of neurotransmitters resulting in neuromuscular abnormalities and diminishing the level of muscular contractile proteins. The bacterial species specific colonization was shown to alleviate of all these abnormalities [28].

Decreased levels of Adrenocorticotropic Hormone (ACTH) and cortisol and an improved response to stress like anti-anxiety was recorded in studies conducted on GF mice [49, 50]. The modulation of the seretonergic system was also observed in GF mice, resulting in an increased serotonin turnover [28]. These GF animal studies have also showed decrease in memory due to alterations in the brain derived neurotropic factor BDNF expression.

Selective modification of the gut microbiota is possible with the use of antibiotics. Mice were less prone to autoimmune diseases using the Experimental autoimmune encephalomyelitis (EAE) when they were pre-treated with antibiotics. The amelioration of the EAE produced an increase in the IL-13 and IL-10, and a decrease in the IFNγ and IL-17 [51, 52]. Even iNKT cells were found to have protection against EAE [53]. The usage of various antibiotic agents has shown variation in the populations of the gut microbiome in the EAE studies, elucidating the variability of immune mechanisms. These studies provide evidence regarding the beneficial role of antibiotics in the treatment of neuro-behavioral disorders. Treatment with antibiotics increased the exploratory behavior in mice and reduced the stress responses; they also provided an immediate benefit to regressive-onset autism in children [7]. Changes in the CNS signals, i.e., hippocampal expression of BDNF and fall in luminal LPS concentration (reduced chronic inflammation), serve as the primary mechanisms involved in behavioral alterations in mice by antibiotics [7, 54, 55]. The antibiotics were able to retune the altered immune and neuro-hormonal condition caused by the commensal microbiome, which in the long run would have led to the development of various CNS disorders.

The presence of neurotransmitter receptors on bacteria acts as a communication link between the CNS effectors and bacteria. Recent studies have revealed that the bacteria in the gut have receptors which provide binding sites for enteric neurotransmitters that are produced by the host, which in turn influence the function of the gut microbiota, leading to an increased predisposition of infection stimuli and inflammatory factors [39]. *Pseudomonas fluorescens* have a binding site for GABA similar to the binding sites in brain [56]. *Escherichia coli* O157:H7 was found to possess a receptor for adrenaline/nor-adrenaline; various adrenaline antagonists were able to bind to this bacterial receptor and block it [57].

MICROBE-TO-HOST SIGNALING BY MICROBIAL SIGNALING MOLECULES

Numerous signaling molecules have been identified by which the gut microbiome communicates with its host neuronal networks, the ENS and the CNS. The immune cells, enteroendocrine cells, and nerve endings in the gut lumen are influenced by Quorum-sensing molecules that help microbes communicate such as metabolites and neurotransmitter homologs that are recognized by the host cells. The microbes in the gut can signal the host through receptors on the local cells in the gut through the metabolites synthesized by them along with SCFAs, bile acid metabolites, and neuroactive substances like precursors and metabolites of tryptophan, GABA, catecholamines, and serotonin, as well as free metabolites [58]; cytokines are released as an immune response to microbes [32]. Alternative signaling pathways involve signaling by neurocrine, the afferent vagal signals with spinal pathways and endocrine mechanisms targeting well past the GI tract, along with the vagal afferents in the portal vein and up to receptors present in brain. Acetate, propionate, butyrate are a few examples of fermentable carbohydrates which upon passing through the colon they are converted into SCFAs, which is a well-elucidated example of a metabolite derived from the microbiome. A reduction in the consumption of food, an improved glucose tolerance, the modulation of neutrophil and lymphocyte functions leads to the activation of signaling through epithelial cells [59].

There are numerous, well explained, and hypothetical mechanisms through which the microbiota co-ordinates communication between the gut and nervous system. Thus, modification to the microbial community is expected to have a direct impact on the gut and brain bidirectional communication network.

GUT MICROBIOTA IN PATHOGENESIS OF VARIOUS NEUROLOGICAL DISORDERS

Autism Spectrum Disorder

Autism is frequently referred to as a neurodevelopmental syndrome, characterized by low social responsiveness, communication, and by odd constrained repetitive behaviors. Autism normally develops in the first three years after birth, especially during infancy. There is no clear theory to explain the development of Autism and other autism spectrum disorders (ASDs). Many etiological theories have been put forward to explain autism. One among of such theories stated that autism resulted due to faulty child rearing. However, this theory was rejected as various researchers proved that there are multiple factors responsible for development of Autism, and one among them is genetic defect [60].

Clinical studies have shown that problems related to gut in early childhood may contribute to development of autism in children [61]. The disorder is characterized by an abnormal HPA response as well as altered microbiome and metabolic profiles [61, 62]. The gut microbiota of ASD children was found to have higher rates of Proteobacteria and Bacteroidetes while Firmicutes and bifidobacteria were found in lower proportions when compared with healthy controls [1]. The Clostridia class of bacteria belonging to the phyla Firmicutes was found at elevated numbers in children suffering from autism and with a history of GI problems [63].

The spores of clostridium are pH, antibiotic, and temperature-resistant, with an ability to sporulate the endotoxin-producing bacteria [55]. Leaky gut syndrome is a condition where large numbers of pathogenic bacteria that produce neuro and endo-toxins expose the mucosa and sub-mucosa of the intestine to bacterial infection [55]. This intrusion of an aseptic environment by the bacteria results in the up-regulation of pro-inflammatory cytokines like IL-1β and TNFα, and an activation of the immune system. This cascade of inflammatory responses gives rise to an inflammatory cycle as a result of the increased barrier permeability. One of the theories put forward to explain the etiology of autism stated that in a subgroup of children, a disturbance of the normal gut microbiota was thought to encourage colonization by one or more neurotoxin-producing bacteria, which could be a possible mechanism, at least in a part, in the future onset of autism [55]. Later it was also discovered that with an exposure to a broad spectrum antibiotic followed by chronic continuous diarrhea, features resembling autism appeared along with the deterioration of skills acquired in the past [55].

Parkinson's Disease (PD)

The mechanism through which the gut microbiome exerts its impact in the development of chronic neurodegenerative disease like Parkinson's is still unclear. GI deregulation is observed even some years before the diagnosis of PD. One hypothesis states that PD initially begins in the Gut and then travels to brain through the vagal and the spinal pathway of the gut-brain axis [64]. The dorsal motor nucleus (DMVX) was recognized to be the origin of parasympathetic vagal nerve fibers that innervate the intestine [64]. The alpha-synuclein and ubiquitin which form the protein aggregates know as lewy bodies, are recognized as the major traits in Parkinson's; They were identified in the enteric nervous system of patients, who were found to be at the beginning stages of PD [64]. In the postmortem of PD patients, these protein aggregates were further observed in the spinal cord, prefrontal cortex, mid brain region, and DMVX as the disease progressed; their locations were found linked with the increasing stages of PD [1].

In order to study the above mentioned mechanism, alpha-synuclein was injected in the intestinal wall of rats, they were then sacrificed and the brain histopathology showed the migration of alpha-synuclein from gut to brain through vagus nerve at the rate of 5-10 mm/day in a prion like fashion or by initiating inflammation and oxidative stress [65]. When the colonic biopsies of PD patients were compared with the biopsy samples of control patients, elevated levels of pro-inflammatory mRNA expression was observed [66], followed by a reduction in the anti-inflammatory butyrate producing bacteria (*Roseburia* and *Faecalibacterium* spp.) and a rise in pro-inflammatory Proteobacteria species [67]. This explains the blood brain barrier leakiness, the activation of immune cells and their infiltration, which consequently lead to neuro-inflammation in the CNS, all of which were triggered by chronic low-grade inflammation in the GIT.

The variance in the composition of the gut microbiota was studied in order to understand its role in the older patients suffering from neurodegenerative disorders. In one such study, a bacterial metabolite named indican, recognized as one of the intestinal dysbiosis markers, was found to be elevated in Parkinson's patients; a clear picture of bacterial dysbiosis [68]. A study was conducted on PD and healthy subjects, 72 each, which showed a 77.6% reduction in Prevotellaceae class bacteria [22]. Prevotellaceae is recognized to have a major role in the production of mucin, a glycosylated protein that forms a barrier on the intestinal epithelial wall in order to protect the epithelium from invading pathogens [22]. An increase in enterobacteriaceae class was found, a class of organisms directly related with the postural instability, a characteristic feature of PD [22].

As discussed earlier SCFAs are able to alter the ENS. In PD patients, it was observed that there was a reduction in level of fecal SCFAs, which was assumed to be responsible for reduction of GI motility [69]. A notable reduction of sodium butyrate, a histone deacetylase (HDAC) inhibitor that up-regulates neurotrophic factors including brain-derived growth factor and glial cell line-derived neurotrophic factor and shields dopaminergic neurons from degeneration, was observed in PD patients [70, 71]. Metagenomic studies have shown lower counts of metabolic genes stemming from a setback in metabolism in PD patients [67].

A study was conducted where the fecal samples from healthy individuals were transplanted into the gut of PD patients, resulting in alleviation of the motor and non-motor PD symptoms, which gives rise to a new therapeutic approach by altering the gut microbiota [26]. As a confirmatory study, an experiment was done on the α-Syn overexpressing GF mice. The study revealed that germ-free α-Syn over-expressing mice were able to maintain higher physical coordination when compared to the wild-strain, leading us to infer that the microbiota plays a part in the expression of physical symptoms in PD [72]. Considering the complex microbiota, α-Syn mice were observed to develop the similar physiological effects and physical impairments as those found in germ-free PD mice. On the other hand, the effects were significantly postponed by almost 12 weeks. The study also depicted that the microbes present in the experimental model promoted the microglia activation in PD brains with the influence on α-Syn, in turn worsening the disease by promoting inflammation [72].

Cyanobacteria, existing in the GI tract in very low numbers, produces β-N-methylamino-L-alanine (BMAA), an excitotoxin that activates the metabotropicglutamate receptor 5 that is found in the brains of AD, PD, and amyotrophic lateral sclerosis (ALS) patients in increased levels. BMAA depletes the antioxidant glutathione leading to oxidative damage in brain by ROS and RNS [73]. The misfolding of proteins and their aggregation that is observed in PD, AD and ALS are also among the various destructive roles of BMAA [73].

Alzheimer's Disease

Alois Alzheimer identified Alzheimer's disease in 1906. Alzheimer's disease is a progressive brain disorder characterized by cognitive impairment. It is the most common cause of dementia, affecting over 24 million people worldwide, with around 4.6 million new cases every year [74]. The presence of amyloid β plaques and neurofibrillary tangles of the tau protein are the primary characteristics of an Alzheimer's disease [74].

Many bacteria are identified with the ability of producing or elevating the amyloid β (Aβ) plaques, such as *B. subtilis*, *E. coli*, *Klebsiella, Pneumonia, Salmonella* spp., s*taphylococcus aureus, Mycobacterium* spp., and *streptococcus* spp. [75]. Increased proportions of Gram-negative bacteria were identified in the gut of AD patients followed by a mucosal disruption as a response to dysbiosis [26].

Many theories exist to explain the role of the gut microbiome in AD. One among them is the histamine theory. Histamine is a potential target in neurodegenerative diseases like MS and AD [76]. Histamine is a biogenic mono-amine synthesized from enterochromaffin cells of the GIT. The release of histamine was also observed from certain *Lactobacillus* spp. Histamine was recently found to be a metabolite resulting from the gut microbial metabolism [77]. *Lactobacillus, Lactococcus, Streptococcus, Pediococcus,* and *Enterococcus* spp. contain a gene called histidine decarboxylase aiding them in the production of histamine [77]. Histamine can act as either a pro- or an anti-inflammatory mediator depending the receptor it acts on [76, 78]. In the brain, histamine was notably found with the induction of allergic responses leading to inflammation by producing pro-inflammatory cytokines IL-1α, IL-1β, IL-6, and chemokines [79]. Elevated levels of histamine were found to be associated with AD by producing neuroinflammation through the elevation of nitric oxide levels [79].

MODULATION OF THE GUT MICROBIOTA BRAIN AXIS (GBA) FOR A HEALTHY BRAIN

The link between microbiota and brain health and disorders raises the question of how to amend and re-calibrate the gut microbiota compositions that were altered by brain disorders. Now let's look into the ability of probiotics, prebiotics, and synbiotics to normalize the dysbiotic microbiota involved with neurological disorders.

Probiotics

Probiotic, comes from a Greek word, meaning "for life". Probiotics can be defined as "The live organisms that are able to provide health benefits upon ingestion in adequate amounts" [80]. Elie Metchnikoff correlated the longevity of Bulgarians to their consumption of fermented milk. This initiated the idea of probiotics in early 20th century. Bacteria belonging to genera *Lactobacillus* and *Bifidobacterium* produce lactic acid and are the most familiar and widely used probiotics. Other genera, such as *Enterococcus* and *Streptococcus*, are also used [80]. The consumption of probiotics is considered to provide many health benefits including serving as medicine in many disorders [80, 81].

Molecular and genetic studies have unveiled the mechanisms through which the probiotics are able to exert the following health benefits:

- They antagonize pathogens by producing antimicrobial substances [82].
- Probiotics compete with pathogenic microbes for nutrients and adhesion to the gut epithelium [83].
- They modulate the immune system of the host [84].
- They inhibit the production of toxins from pathogenic bacteria [85].

The first two benefits involve a direct effect of the probiotics on the other microorganisms. Probiotics play a pivotal role both in a prophylactic approach as well as a treatment for infections. They help to maintain the gut microbiome balance of the host. Probiotic bacteria act by binding to the gut epithelium thus blocking the binding sites for pathogenic bacteria and initiate an immune response cascade [83].

In some cases the release of soluble components by probiotic bacteria has been seen to elucidate the activation of immunological cells by the epithelium itself [83]. This provides an opportunity for a radical approach in the prevention and treatment of various contagious and chronic inflammatory diseases of the alimentary tract. One theory even states that probiotics have the ability to cure cancer [83].

Table 1. Probiotics clinical trials (ongoing) on various neurological diseases (www.clinicaltrials.gov)

S.No	Title	Conditions	Interventions	Location
1	Probiotics and the Microbiome: Clinical Intervention Trial for Anxiety and Depression	• Anxiety • Depression	• Other: Probiotics • Drug: Placebo	Acadia University, Wolfville, Nova Scotia, Canada
2	A Study of Protein Metabolism, Microbiome and Investigational Probiotic Use in Patients With ALS	• Amyotrophic Lateral Sclerosis • ALS	• Dietary Supplement: probiotic	Avera Medical Group Neurology Sioux Falls, Sioux Falls, South Dakota, United States
3	Probiotic on Psychological and Cognitive Effects	• Aging	• Dietary Supplement: Probiotic - Lactobacillus Rhamnosus GG • Other: Placebo	Kent State University, Kent, Ohio, United States
4	Effects of Probiotics on Gastrointestinal Symptoms and on the Immune System in Patients With Systemic Sclerosis	• Systemic Sclerosis • Scleroderma	• Other: Probiotic • Other: Placebo	Systemic Sclerosis Outpatient Clinic, Hospital São Paulo, São Paulo, SP, Brazil
5	Probiotics to Prevent Relapse After Hospitalization for Bipolar Depression	• Bipolar Depression	• Biological: Probiotic Supplement • Biological: Inert Compound	Sheppart Pratt Health System, Towson, Maryland, United States
6	Clinical Trial of Probiotics in Systemic Sclerosis Associated Gastrointestinal Disease	• Systemic Sclerosis	• Dietary Supplement: Vivomixx probiotics	Singapore General Hospital, Singapore, Singapore

Enhanced activity levels of immunoglobulins, interferons, macrophages, and lymphocytes can be seen as the manifestations of Probiotic-induced immunological stimulation. The cell wall constituents of the lactic acid producing bacteria stimulate the macrophages; in turn killing the pathogenic microbes by giving rise to free oxygen radicals and lysosome enzymes. The last mentioned mechanism involves the inactivation and removal of bacterial toxins [86]. The process of detoxification can involve the adsorption of toxins on their cell walls to avoid the toxins' contact with the intestinal wall, or by metabolism of mycotoxins by microorganisms [86]. Many of the probiotics used in the treatment of diarrhea are known to possess the ability to protect the host from toxins. Some of them are even able to counter the toxin release with the production of antimicrobial substances, vitamins, and native enzymes that inhibit the metabolic reactions in pathogens leading to a reduction in the toxin production [87].

Probiotics are considered to possess the ability to treat conditions like inflammatory bowel syndrome (IBS). Probiotics have been used in treatments to reducing anxiety, stress, and also as a mood elevator in patients suffering from IBS comorbid with chronic fatigue [88, 89]. A probiotic combination of *B. longum* and *Lactobacillus helveticus* displayed the ability to reduce anxiety in animals and lower serum cortisol levels. The same combination was also able to alleviate depression like behavior in rats in a post-myocardial infarction state [90]. The mechanisms behind all these effects are not clear, but a hypothesis exists explaining them to be a result of a reduction in pro-inflammatory cytokines and oxidative stress, accompanied with nutritional modifications [29].

Since a complex relationship between the gut microbiota and anxiety/depression exists, it is possible to improve anxiety and depression through probiotic modulation. For example, Bercik et al. 2010 indicated that *Bifidobacterium longum* normalized anxiety-like behavior induced by the infection of the noninvasive parasite *Trichuris muris* [91]. Bravo et al. 2011 showed that chronic treatment with *Lactobacillus rhamnosus* (JB-1) reduced anxiety and depression-related behavior in the *Trichuris muris*-infected mice [92]. Ingestion of selected probiotics also exhibits effects on brain activity in humans. After 2 months of administration of *Lactobacillus casei* strain Shirota in chronic fatigue syndrome patients, there were significantly increased levels of Lactobacillus and Bifidobacterium microbes present in the Gut microbiota as well as a significant reduction in symptoms of anxiety among those taking the probiotic versus controls [93].

Table 2. Commonly available Probiotics

Microorganisms	Use	References
L. acidophilus, L. rhamnosus GG, L. delbruckii, L. fermentum and *S. boulardi*	Reduce the incidence of antibiotic-induced diarrhea	[111]
Lactobacilli, Bifidobacteria, Enterococci and *Streptococci*	Prophylactically to prevent traveler's diarrhea	[112]
Fermented milk with *B. breve, B. bifidum* and *L. acidophilu*	Induce mild degree remission in Ulcerative colitis patients	[113]
Bifidobacterium bifidum MIMBb75	Alleviated Irritable bowel syndrome (IBS)	[114]
Escherichia coli Nissle 1917	Effective in IBS treatment, especially in patients with altered enteric microflora	[115]

Ferulic acid (FA), is a phenolic compound found in seeds of plants like rice, wheat, and oats, as well as vegetables like tomatoes and carrots, and fruits such as pineapple and orange [94]. FA possesses a highly potent ROS scavenging activity; presenting itself as a promising therapeutic regimen to treat a variety of chronic diseases affected by oxidative stress [94]. One among those conditions is neurodegeneration, where FA directly acts on neurons and stimulates both in-vitro and in-vivo proliferation of neural stem cells [95]. FA, administered orally for six months in as a treatment for AD, was not only able to improve the behavioral traits of the AD mice but also simultaneously reduced Aβ accumulation, faulty cleavage at β-carboxy-terminal of amyloid precursor protein (APP), ROS damage, and inflammation in neurons [96]. FA has been found to be a metabolite synthesized by *L. fermentum* [97] and *B. animalis* [98]; gut microbes that contain the ferulic acid esterase gene. With this we can infer that the probiotic delivery of bacteria that produce ferulic acid can be used as a potential therapeutic approach in various neurodegenerative diseases.

Prebiotics

Prebiotics are fermentable and non digestible foods that have beneficial effects on host by selective stimulation and aid in the development of one particular species of bacteria or maybe even restrict the number of bacteria in the colon [80]. Prebiotics normally are non-starch polysaccharides (NSP) or non-starch oligosaccharides (NSO); they are further characterized into fructooligosaccharides (FOS), arabinoxylan oligosaccharides, galactooligosaccharides, raffinose family oligosaccharides (RFO), among others [83]. The modulatory effect of a prebiotic is restricted to a particular strain and the prediction of that strain which can act as a prebiotic serves to be a challenge prior to administration [83]. It has been shown that many varieties of polysaccharides improve brain function in humans, animals, and in vitro studies after oral, systemic, and localized exposure. Inulin and pectin in the prebiotic form possess the ability to reduce the frequency and prevalence of diarrhea. They also reduced inflammation in IBS and are shown to elicit a protective effect against colon cancer [99]

Providing the gut microbiome with an energy source that can be utilized by a particular species has a great impact on the composition and metabolism of microbiota. The physiological effects and the type of bacteria that can utilize the prebiotic as a source of carbon and energy is directly dependent on structure of the prebiotic administered [83]. The mechanism through which prebiotics bring out the beneficial effects and immunomodulation is explained by the theories mentioned below [100]:

- With the increased production of SCFAs like propionic acid, prebiotics regulate the action of hepatic lipogenic enzymes.

- SCFAs, like butyric acid, produced as a result of fermentation modulate histone acetylation, thus increasing the availability of genes for transcription factors.
- Prebiotic based mucin production modulation.
- Prebiotics like FOS were able to increase leukocytes and lymphocytes counts in gut-associated lymphoid tissues and in the blood peripherally.
- Stimulation in the phagocytic function of intra-inflammatory macrophages was assumed to be a result from an increased IgA secretion GALTs.

Table 3. Commonly available Prebiotics

Prebiotic	Source	Reference
A low-molecular-weight polysaccharide	Agar and alginate of seaweed Gelidium CC2253	[116]
ß-glucans	*Pleurotus sp.* (pleuran) mushrooms	
Ulvan	Green algae-Ulvarigida	
Inulin-type fructans	Roots of traditional Chinese medicine *Morinda officinalis* or Indian mulberry	
Oligosaccharide	White and red-flesh pitayas (dragon fruit)	

In a murine experimental model, galactooligosaccharides were shown to possess protective effects against *Salmonella typhimurium* infections [101]. Fructooligosaccharide (FOS) showed a protective effect against both *Salmonella typhimurium* and *Listeria monocytogenes* infections [102]. Prebiotics are considered to be a novel choice to combat pathogens like *Escherichia coli* and *Salmonella enteritidis*, leading to a reduction in odiferous compounds [103]. Many reports suggest prebiotics possess anti carcinogenic properties. Results obtained from a study on rats illustrated that a prebiotic enriched diet significantly lowered the incidence of cancer [104]. The ability of butyric acid against carcinogenesis was reported by many researchers [104]. Prebiotics in the form of a chemoprotective agent provides protection against colorectal carcinoma by promoting cell differentiation [83]. In these ways prebiotics play a beneficial role in treating various GIT disorders; in the same fashion the alterations of the gut commensal bacteria by prebiotics will help to treat neurodegenerative diseases.

Synbiotics

The concept of prebiotics was introduced by GR Gibson a scientist at Dunn Clinical Nutrition Centre, Cambridge [105]. He had stated that the combination of a prebiotic with a probiotic could give rise to synbiotics, with the combined benefits of both [99]. Synbiotics are mixtures of both prebiotics and probiotics aimed at increasing the ability of probiotics to survive in the gastric pH along with the ability to stimulate *bifidobacteria* and *lactobacilli* indigenous bacteria [80]. Being a combination of both prebiotics and probiotcs, synbiotics not only improve the probiotic survival but also aid in triggering the proliferation of particular indigenous bacterial strains present in the GIT [106]. The usage of synbiotics for gut microbiome modulation in a human host has emerged to be a promising approach after taking into consideration the vast number of potential combinations.

Table 4. Commonly available Synbiotics [117–119]

Lactobacillus genus bacteria + inulin
Lactobacillus, Streptococcus and *Bifidobacterium* genus bacteria + FOS
Lactobacillus and *Bifidobacterium* genus bacteria + inulin
Lactobacillus and *Bifidobacterium* genus bacteria + oligofructose
Lactobacillus, Bifidobacterium, Enterococcus genus bacteria + FOS

Bifidobacteria spp, *S. boulardii*, *Lacbobacilli*, and *B. coagulans*, among others, are used in combination with oligosaccharides like fructo-oligosaccharide, galactooligosaccharides, xyloseoligosaccharide, and inulin, as prebiotics from natural sources in the formulation of synbiotics [99].

The combination of probiotics and prebiotics is considered to have synergistic effects. A probiotic is predominantly active in the small and large intestines, while prebiotics focus their mainstream activity chiefly in the large intestine [107]. Synbiotics portray their effects mainly through two modes [108]:

- Acting via the enhanced viability of probiotic microorganisms.
- Acting through the provision of particular health effects.

Synbiotics exert their effects by reducing the concentration of toxic metabolites along with the deactivation of nitrosamines and carcinogenic substances. The usage of synbiotics has resulted in the elevation SCFAs, carbon disulphides, ketones, and methyl acetate levels, which have a positive role in maintenance of host's health [108].

In some studies involving rats, the IgA levels were found to be elevated following the administration of a symbiotic formulation consisting of *Bifidobacterium lactis* and *Lactobacillus rhamnosus* as probiotics, and inulin and oligofructose as prebiotics. The synbiotics were able to bring down the high blood pressure and cholesterol levels [83]. Synbiotics are also able to treat hepatic conditions and aid in the absorption of essential minerals such as calcium, phosphorus, and magnesium [109]. Possibly, in the same pattern, the synbiotics can be useful in the treatment or prophylaxis of various neuronal disorders.

HUNTINGTON'S DISEASE AND PROBIOTICS

Huntington's is a genetic progressive neurodegenerative disorder predominantly characterized by movement disorders like chorea, dementia, and depression, among others. The major mechanisms involved in the development of the disease include the elevated NMDAR signaling leading to excitotoxicity, a reduction in the synaptic connectivity, and a reduction in the BDNF levels [110]. The excitotoxicity causes mitochondrial damage releasing ROS that result in neuronal damage. Many species of bacteria have the ability to produce potent antioxidants, for example *L. fermentum* and *B. animalis* produce Ferulic acid, a potent antioxidant [26]. These types of bacteria, delivered in the form of a probiotic, can serve as efficient ROS scavengers and may help in the maintenance of Huntington's disorder.

The movement disorders, such as in the case of the Huntington's disease, are mainly due to damage of dopaminergic neurons in the brain [26]. BDNF, whose levels are found to decrease in Huntington's disease, serves as a predominant protector of dopaminergic neurons. Sodium butyrate is a histone deacetylase (HDAC) inhibitor that up-regulates neurotrophic factors including BDNF [26]. *Roseburia* and *Faecalibacterium* species of bacteria are known to produce butyrate in the gut [26]. The probiotic administration of such species can also serve to reduce the movement complications of the Huntington's patients.

REFERENCES

[1] Ghaisas S, Maher J, Kanthasamy A. Gut Microbiome in Health and Disease: Linking the Microbiome-Gut-Brain Axis and Environmental Factors in the Pathogenesis of Systemic and Neurodegenerative Diseases. *Pharmacol Ther.* 2016 Feb;158:52–62.

[2] Foster JA, McVey Neufeld K-A. Gut-Brain Axis: How the Microbiome Influences Anxiety and Depression. *Trends Neurosci.* 2013 May;36(5):305–12.

[3] Winek K, Dirnagl U, Meisel A. The Gut Microbiome as Therapeutic Target in Central Nervous System Diseases: Implications for Stroke. *Neurother J Am Soc Exp Neurother.* 2016 Oct;13(4):762–74.

[4] Shulman ST, Friedmann HC, Sims RH. Theodor Escherich: The First Pediatric Infectious Diseases Physician? *Clin Infect Dis Off Publ Infect Dis Soc Am.* 2007 Oct 15;45(8):1025–9.

[5] Grice EA, Segre JA. The Human Microbiome: Our Second Genome. *Annu Rev Genomics Hum Genet.* 2012;13:151–70.

[6] Xu J, Gordon JI. Honor Thy Symbionts. *Proc Natl Acad Sci U S A.* 2003 Sep 2;100(18):10452–9.

[7] Wang Y, Kasper LH. The Role of Microbiome in Central Nervous System Disorders. *Brain Behav Immun.* 2014 May;38:1–12.

[8] Kennedy PJ, Cryan JF, Dinan TG, Clarke G. Kynurenine Pathway Metabolism and the Microbiota-Gut-Brain Axis. *Neuropharmacology.* 2017 Jan;112(Pt B):399–412.

[9] Turnbaugh PJ, Ley RE, Hamady M, Fraser-Liggett CM, Knight R, Gordon JI. The Human Microbiome Project. *Nature.* 2007 Oct 18;449(7164):804–10.

[10] Claesson MJ, Cusack S, O'Sullivan O, Greene-Diniz R, de Weerd H, Flannery E, et al. Composition, Variability, and Temporal Stability of the Intestinal Microbiota of the Elderly. *Proc Natl Acad Sci U S A.* 2011 Mar 15;108 Suppl 1:4586–91.

[11] Qin J, Li R, Raes J, Arumugam M, Burgdorf KS, Manichanh C, et al. A Human Gut Microbial Gene Catalogue Established by Metagenomic Sequencing. *Nature.* 2010 Mar 4;464(7285):59–65.

[12] Rajilić-Stojanović M, Smidt H, de Vos WM. Diversity of the Human Gastrointestinal Tract Microbiota Revisited. *Environ Microbiol.* 2007 Sep;9(9):2125–36.

[13] Human Microbiome Project Consortium. Structure, Function and Diversity of the Healthy Human Microbiome. *Nature.* 2012 Jun 13;486(7402):207–14.

[14] Mandal RS, Saha S, Das S. Metagenomic Surveys of Gut Microbiota. *Genomics Proteomics Bioinformatics.* 2015 Jun;13(3):148–58.

[15] Everard A, Cani PD. Gut Microbiota and GLP-1. *Rev Endocr Metab Disord.* 2014 Sep;15(3):189–96.

[16] Littman DR, Pamer EG. Role of the Commensal Microbiota in Normal and Pathogenic Host Immune Responses. *Cell Host Microbe.* 2011 Oct 20;10(4):311–23.

[17] Kelly D, King T, Aminov R. Importance of Microbial Colonization of the Gut in Early Life to the Development of Immunity. *Mutat Res.* 2007 Sep 1;622(1–2):58–69.

[18] Buttó LF, Haller D. Dysbiosis in Intestinal Inflammation: Cause or Consequence. *Int J Med Microbiol IJMM.* 2016 Aug;306(5):302–9.

[19] Karlsson FH, Tremaroli V, Nookaew I, Bergström G, Behre CJ, Fagerberg B, et al. Gut Metagenome in European Women with Normal, Impaired and Diabetic Glucose Control. *Nature.* 2013 Jun 6;498(7452):99–103.

[20] Bultman SJ. Emerging Roles of the Microbiome in Cancer. *Carcinogenesis.* 2014 Feb;35(2):249–55.

[21] Mayer EA, Knight R, Mazmanian SK, Cryan JF, Tillisch K. Gut Microbes and the Brain: Paradigm Shift in Neuroscience. *J Neurosci Off J Soc Neurosci.* 2014 Nov 12;34(46):15490–6.

[22] Scheperjans F, Aho V, Pereira PAB, Koskinen K, Paulin L, Pekkonen E, et al. Gut Microbiota are Related to Parkinson's Disease and Clinical Phenotype. *Mov Disord Off J Mov Disord Soc.* 2015 Mar;30(3):350–8.

[23] Gungor B, Adiguzel E, Gursel I, Yilmaz B, Gursel M. Intestinal Microbiota in Patients with Spinal Cord Injury. *PloS One.* 2016;11(1):e0145878.

[24] De Angelis M, Francavilla R, Piccolo M, De Giacomo A, Gobbetti M. Autism Spectrum Disorders and Intestinal Microbiota. *Gut Microbes. 2015*;6(3):207–13.

[25] Singh V, Roth S, Llovera G, Sadler R, Garzetti D, Stecher B, et al. Microbiota Dysbiosis Controls the Neuroinflammatory Response after Stroke. *J Neurosci off J Soc Neurosci.* 2016 Jul 13;36 (28):7428–40.

[26] Westfall S, Lomis N, Kahouli I, Dia SY, Singh SP, Prakash S. Microbiome, Probiotics and Neurodegenerative Diseases: Deciphering the Gut Brain Axis. *Cell Mol Life Sci CMLS.* 2017 Oct;74(20):3769–87.

[27] Tsigos C, Chrousos GP. Hypothalamic-Pituitary-Adrenal Axis, Neuroendocrine Factors and Stress. *J Psychosom Res.* 2002 Oct;53 (4):865–71.

[28] Carabotti M, Scirocco A, Maselli MA, Severi C. The Gut-Brain Axis: Interactions Between Enteric Microbiota, Central and Enteric

Nervous Systems. *Ann Gastroenterol Q Publ Hell Soc Gastroenterol.* 2015;28(2):203–9.

[29] Cryan JF, Dinan TG. Mind-Altering Microorganisms: The Impact of the Gut Microbiota on Brain and Behaviour. *Nat Rev Neurosci.* 2012 Oct;13(10):701–12.

[30] Santos J, Yang PC, Söderholm JD, Benjamin M, Perdue MH. Role of Mast Cells in Chronic Stress Induced Colonic Epithelial Barrier Dysfunction in the Rat. *Gut.* 2001 May;48(5):630–6.

[31] O'Mahony SM, Marchesi JR, Scully P, Codling C, Ceolho A-M, Quigley EMM, et al. Early life Stress Alters Behavior, Immunity, and Microbiota in Rats: Implications For Irritable Bowel Syndrome and Psychiatric Illnesses. *Biol Psychiatry.* 2009 Feb 1;65(3):263–7.

[32] Bailey MT, Dowd SE, Galley JD, Hufnagle AR, Allen RG, Lyte M. Exposure to a Social Stressor Alters the Structure of the Intestinal Microbiota: Implications For Stressor-Induced Immunomodulation. *Brain Behav Immun.* 2011 Mar;25(3):397–407.

[33] Rhee SH, Pothoulakis C, Mayer EA. Principles and Clinical Implications of the Brain-Gut-Enteric Microbiota Axis. *Nat Rev Gastroenterol Hepatol.* 2009 May;6(5):306–14.

[34] Li Y. Sensory Signal Transduction in the Vagal Primary Afferent Neurons. *Curr Med Chem.* 2007;14(24):2554–63.

[35] Cummings DE, Overduin J. Gastrointestinal Regulation of Food Intake. *J Clin Invest.* 2007 Jan;117(1):13–23.

[36] Romijn JA, Corssmit EP, Havekes LM, Pijl H. Gut-Brain Axis. *Curr Opin Clin Nutr Metab Care.* 2008 Jul;11(4):518–21.

[37] Li Y, Wu XY, Owyang C. Serotonin and Cholecystokinin Synergistically Stimulate Rat Vagal Primary Afferent Neurones. *J Physiol.* 2004 Sep 1;559(Pt 2):651–62.

[38] Valet P, Senard JM, Devedjian JC, Planat V, Salomon R, Voisin T, et al. Characterization and Distribution of Alpha 2-Adrenergic Receptors in the Human Intestinal Mucosa. *J Clin Invest.* 1993 May;91(5):2049–57.

[39] Hughes DT, Sperandio V. Inter-Kingdom Signalling: Communication between Bacteria and Their Hosts. *Nat Rev Microbiol.* 2008 Feb;6(2):111–20.

[40] Al-Asmakh M, Anuar F, Zadjali F, Rafter J, Pettersson S. Gut Microbial Communities Modulating Brain Development and Function. *Gut Microbes.* 2012 Aug;3(4):366–73.

[41] Douglas-Escobar M, Elliott E, Neu J. Effect of Intestinal Microbial Ecology on the Developing Brain. *JAMA Pediatr.* 2013 Apr;167(4):374–9.

[42] Catanzaro R, Anzalone M, Calabrese F, Milazzo M, Capuana M, Italia A, et al. The Gut Microbiota and Its Correlations with the Central Nervous System Disorders. *Panminerva Med.* 2015 Sep;57(3):127–43.

[43] Dinan TG, Cryan JF. Gut Instincts: Microbiota as a Key Regulator of Brain Development, Ageing and Neurodegeneration. *J Physiol.* 2017 Jan 15;595(2):489–503.

[44] Bekkering P, Jafri I, van Overveld FJ, Rijkers GT. The Intricate Association Between Gut Microbiota and Development of Type 1, Type 2 And Type 3 Diabetes. *Expert Rev Clin Immunol.* 2013 Nov;9(11):1031–41.

[45] Rao M, Gershon MD. The Bowel and Beyond: The Enteric Nervous System in Neurological Disorders. *Nat Rev Gastroenterol Hepatol.* 2016 Sep;13(9):517–28.

[46] Ley RE, Hamady M, Lozupone C, Turnbaugh PJ, Ramey RR, Bircher JS, et al. Evolution of Mammals and Their Gut Microbes. *Science.* 2008 Jun 20;320(5883):1647–51.

[47] Clarke G, Grenham S, Scully P, Fitzgerald P, Moloney RD, Shanahan F, et al. The Microbiome-Gut-Brain Axis During Early Life Regulates the Hippocampal Serotonergic System in a Sex-Dependent Manner. *Mol Psychiatry.* 2013 Jun;18(6):666–73.

[48] Husebye E, Hellström PM, Sundler F, Chen J, Midtvedt T. Influence of Microbial Species on Small Intestinal Myoelectric Activity and Transit in Germ-Free Rats. *Am J Physiol Gastrointest Liver Physiol.* 2001 Mar;280(3):G368-380.

[49] Neufeld KM, Kang N, Bienenstock J, Foster JA. Reduced Anxiety-Like Behavior and Central Neurochemical Change in Germ-Free Mice. *Neurogastroenterol Motil Off J Eur Gastrointest Motil Soc.* 2011 Mar;23(3):255-64, e119.

[50] Sudo N, Chida Y, Aiba Y, Sonoda J, Oyama N, Yu X-N, et al. Postnatal Microbial Colonization Programs the Hypothalamic-Pituitary-Adrenal System For Stress Response in Mice. *J Physiol.* 2004 Jul 1;558(Pt 1):263-75.

[51] Ochoa-Repáraz J, Mielcarz DW, Haque-Begum S, Kasper LH. Induction of a Regulatory B Cell Population in Experimental Allergic Encephalomyelitis by Alteration of the Gut Commensal Microflora. *Gut Microbes.* 2010 Mar;1(2):103-8.

[52] Ochoa-Repáraz J, Mielcarz DW, Ditrio LE, Burroughs AR, Foureau DM, Haque-Begum S, et al. Role of Gut Commensal Microflora in the Development of Experimental Autoimmune Encephalomyelitis. *J Immunol Baltim Md* 1950. 2009 Nov 15;183(10):6041-50.

[53] Yokote H, Miyake S, Croxford JL, Oki S, Mizusawa H, Yamamura T. NKT Cell-Dependent Amelioration of a Mouse Model of Multiple Sclerosis by Altering Gut Flora. *Am J Pathol.* 2008 Dec;173(6):1714-23.

[54] Ait-Belgnaoui A, Durand H, Cartier C, Chaumaz G, Eutamene H, Ferrier L, et al. Prevention of Gut Leakiness by a Probiotic Treatment Leads to Attenuated HPA Response to an Acute Psychological Stress in Rats. *Psychoneuroendocrinology.* 2012 Nov;37(11):1885-95.

[55] Sandler RH, Finegold SM, Bolte ER, Buchanan CP, Maxwell AP, Väisänen ML, et al. Short-Term Benefit From Oral Vancomycin Treatment of Regressive-Onset Autism. *J Child Neurol.* 2000 Jul;15(7):429-35.

[56] Guthrie GD, Nicholson-Guthrie CS. Gamma-Aminobutyric Acid Uptake by a Bacterial System with Neurotransmitter Binding Characteristics. *Proc Natl Acad Sci U S A.* 1989 Oct;86(19):7378-81.

[57] Clarke MB, Hughes DT, Zhu C, Boedeker EC, Sperandio V. The QseC Sensor Kinase: A Bacterial Adrenergic Receptor. *Proc Natl Acad Sci U S A.* 2006 Jul 5;103(27):10420–5.

[58] Chey WY, Jin HO, Lee MH, Sun SW, Lee KY. Colonic Motility Abnormality in Patients with Irritable Bowel Syndrome Exhibiting Abdominal Pain and Diarrhea. *Am J Gastroenterol.* 2001 May;96(5):1499–506.

[59] Mayer EA, Tillisch K, Gupta A. Gut/Brain Axis and the Microbiota. *J Clin Invest.* 2015 Mar 2;125(3):926–38.

[60] Lord C, Cook EH, Leventhal BL, Amaral DG. Autism Spectrum Disorders. *Neuron.* 2000 Nov;28(2):355–63.

[61] Kaneko M, Hoshino Y, Hashimoto S, Okano T, Kumashiro H. Hypothalamic-Pituitary-Adrenal Axis Function in Children with Attention-Deficit Hyperactivity Disorder. *J Autism Dev Disord.* 1993 Mar;23(1):59–65.

[62] Ming X, Stein TP, Barnes V, Rhodes N, Guo L. Metabolic Perturbance in Autism Spectrum Disorders: A Metabolomics Study. *J Proteome Res.* 2012 Dec 7;11(12):5856–62.

[63] Song Y, Liu C, Finegold SM. Real-Time PCR Quantitation of Clostridia in Feces of Autistic Children. *Appl Environ Microbiol.* 2004 Nov;70(11):6459–65.

[64] Braak H, de Vos RAI, Bohl J, Del Tredici K. Gastric Alpha-Synuclein Immunoreactive Inclusions in Meissner's and Auerbach's Plexuses in Cases Staged for Parkinson's Disease-Related Brain Pathology. *Neurosci Lett.* 2006 Mar 20;396(1):67–72.

[65] Holmqvist S, Chutna O, Bousset L, Aldrin-Kirk P, Li W, Björklund T, et al. Direct Evidence of Parkinson Pathology Spread From the Gastrointestinal Tract to the Brain in Rats. *Acta Neuropathol (Berl).* 2014 Dec;128(6):805–20.

[66] Devos D, Lebouvier T, Lardeux B, Biraud M, Rouaud T, Pouclet H, et al. Colonic Inflammation in Parkinson's Disease. *Neurobiol Dis.* 2013 Feb;50:42–8.

[67] Keshavarzian A, Green SJ, Engen PA, Voigt RM, Naqib A, Forsyth CB, et al. Colonic Bacterial Composition in Parkinson's Disease. *Mov Disord Off J Mov Disord Soc.* 2015 Sep;30(10):1351–60.

[68] Cassani E, Barichella M, Cancello R, Cavanna F, Iorio L, Cereda E, et al. Increased Urinary Indoxyl Sulfate (Indican): New Insights into Gut Dysbiosis in Parkinson's Disease. *Parkinsonism Relat Disord.* 2015 Apr;21(4):389–93.

[69] Unger MM, Spiegel J, Dillmann K-U, Grundmann D, Philippeit H, Bürmann J, et al. Short Chain Fatty Acids and Gut Microbiota Differ Between Patients with Parkinson's Disease and Age-Matched Controls. *Parkinsonism Relat Disord.* 2016 Nov;32:66–72.

[70] Kidd SK, Schneider JS. Protection of Dopaminergic Cells from MPP+-Mediated Toxicity by Histone Deacetylase Inhibition. *Brain Res.* 2010 Oct 1;1354:172–8.

[71] Wu X, Chen PS, Dallas S, Wilson B, Block ML, Wang C-C, et al. Histone Deacetylase Inhibitors Up-Regulate Astrocyte GDNF and BDNF Gene Transcription and Protect Dopaminergic Neurons. *Int J Neuropsychopharmacol.* 2008 Dec;11(8):1123–34.

[72] Sampson TR, Debelius JW, Thron T, Janssen S, Shastri GG, Ilhan ZE, et al. Gut Microbiota Regulate Motor Deficits and Neuroinflammation in a Model of Parkinson's Disease. *Cell.* 2016 Dec 1;167(6):1469–1480.e12.

[73] Brenner SR. Blue-Green Algae or Cyanobacteria in the Intestinal Micro-Flora May Produce Neurotoxins Such as Beta-N-Methylamino-L-Alanine (BMAA) Which May Be Related to Development of Amyotrophic Lateral Sclerosis, Alzheimer's Disease And Parkinson-Dementia-Complex in Humans and Equine Motor Neuron Disease in Horses. *Med Hypotheses.* 2013 Jan;80 (1):103.

[74] Irvine GB, El-Agnaf OM, Shankar GM, Walsh DM. Protein Aggregation in the Brain: The Molecular Basis for Alzheimer's and Parkinson's Diseases. *Mol Med.* 2008;14(7–8):451–64.

[75] Friedland RP. Mechanisms of Molecular Mimicry Involving the Microbiota in Neurodegeneration. *J Alzheimers Dis JAD.* 2015;45 (2):349–62.

[76] del Rio R, Noubade R, Saligrama N, Wall EH, Krementsov DN, Poynter ME, et al. Histamine H4 Receptor Optimizes T Regulatory Cell Frequency and Facilitates Anti-Inflammatory Responses within the Central Nervous System. *J Immunol Baltim Md* 1950. 2012 Jan 15; 188(2):541–7.

[77] Landete JM, De las Rivas B, Marcobal A, Muñoz R. Updated Molecular Knowledge About Histamine Biosynthesis by Bacteria. *Crit Rev Food Sci Nutr.* 2008 Sep;48(8):697–714.

[78] Dong H, Zhang W, Zeng X, Hu G, Zhang H, He S, et al. Histamine Induces Upregulated Expression of Histamine Receptors and Increases Release of Inflammatory Mediators From Microglia. *Mol Neurobiol.* 2014 Jun;49(3):1487–500.

[79] Alvarez XA, Franco A, Fernández-Novoa L, Cacabelos R. Blood Levels of Histamine, IL-1 Beta, and TNF-Alpha in Patients with Mild to Moderate Alzheimer Disease. *Mol Chem Neuropathol.* 1996 Dec;29(2–3):237–52.

[80] Quigley EMM. Prebiotics and Probiotics; Modifying and Mining the Microbiota. *Pharmacol Res.* 2010 Mar;61(3):213–8.

[81] Ducatelle R, Eeckhaut V, Haesebrouck F, Van Immerseel F. A Review on Prebiotics and Probiotics for the Control of Dysbiosis: Present Status and Future Perspectives. *Anim Int J Anim Biosci.* 2015 Jan;9(1):43–8.

[82] Vandenbergh PA. Lactic Acid Bacteria, Their Metabolic Products and Interference with Microbial Growth. *FEMS Microbiol Rev.* 1993 Sep 1;12(1–3):221–37.

[83] Markowiak P, Śliżewska K. Effects of Probiotics, Prebiotics, and Synbiotics on Human Health. *Nutrients.* 2017 Sep 15;9(9).

[84] Isolauri E, Sütas Y, Kankaanpää P, Arvilommi H, Salminen S. Probiotics: Effects on Immunity. *Am J Clin Nutr.* 2001 Feb;73(2 Suppl):444S–450S.

[85] Brandão RL, Castro IM, Bambirra EA, Amaral SC, Fietto LG, Tropia MJ, et al. Intracellular Signal Triggered by Cholera Toxin in *Saccharomyces Boulardii* and *Saccharomyces Cerevisiae*. *Appl Environ Microbiol.* 1998 Feb;64(2):564–8.

[86] Schatzmayr G, Zehner F, Täubel M, Schatzmayr D, Klimitsch A, Loibner AP, et al. Microbiologicals for Deactivating Mycotoxins. *Mol Nutr Food Res.* 2006 May;50(6):543–51.

[87] Oelschlaeger TA. Mechanisms of Probiotic Actions - A Review. *Int J Med Microbiol IJMM.* 2010 Jan;300(1):57–62.

[88] Aziz Q, Thompson DG. Brain-Gut Axis in Health and Disease. *Gastroenterology.* 1998 Mar;114(3):559–78.

[89] Logan AC, Katzman M. Major Depressive Disorder: Probiotics May Be an Adjuvant Therapy. *Med Hypotheses.* 2005;64(3):533–8.

[90] Arseneault-Bréard J, Rondeau I, Gilbert K, Girard S-A, Tompkins TA, Godbout R, et al. Combination of *Lactobacillus helveticus* R0052 and *Bifidobacterium longum* R0175 Reduces Post-Myocardial Infarction Depression Symptoms and Restores Intestinal Permeability in a Rat Model. *Br J Nutr.* 2012 Jun;107(12):1793–9.

[91] Bercik P, Verdu EF, Foster JA, Macri J, Potter M, Huang X, et al. Chronic Gastrointestinal Inflammation Induces Anxiety-Like Behavior and Alters Central Nervous System Biochemistry in Mice. *Gastroenterology.* 2010 Dec;139(6):2102–2112.e1.

[92] Bravo JA, Forsythe P, Chew MV, Escaravage E, Savignac HM, Dinan TG, et al. Ingestion of *Lactobacillus* Strain Regulates Emotional Behavior and Central GABA Receptor Expression in a Mouse via the Vagus Nerve. *Proc Natl Acad Sci U S A.* 2011 Sep 20; 108(38): 16050–5.

[93] Liu X, Cao S, Zhang X. Modulation of Gut Microbiota-Brain Axis by Probiotics, Prebiotics, and Diet. *J Agric Food Chem.* 2015 Sep 16;63(36):7885–95.

[94] Hu C-T, Wu J-R, Cheng C-C, Wang S, Wang H-T, Lee M-C, et al. Reactive Oxygen Species-Mediated PKC and Integrin Signaling Promotes Tumor Progression of Human Hepatoma HepG2. *Clin Exp Metastasis.* 2011 Dec;28(8):851–63.

[95] Yabe T, Hirahara H, Harada N, Ito N, Nagai T, Sanagi T, et al. Ferulic Acid Induces Neural Progenitor Cell Proliferation *In Vitro* and *In Vivo*. *Neuroscience*. 2010 Jan 20;165(2):515–24.

[96] Mori T, Koyama N, Guillot-Sestier M-V, Tan J, Town T. Ferulic Acid Is A Nutraceutical B-Secretase Modulator That Improves Behavioral Impairment and Alzheimer-Like Pathology in Transgenic Mice. *PloS One*. 2013;8(2):e55774.

[97] Tomaro-Duchesneau C, Saha S, Malhotra M, Coussa-Charley M, Kahouli I, Jones ML, et al. Probiotic Ferulic Acid Esterase Active *Lactobacillus Fermentum* NCIMB 5221 APA Microcapsules for Oral Delivery: Preparation and *in vitro* Characterization. *Pharm Basel Switz*. 2012 Feb 16;5(2):236–48.

[98] Szwajgier D, Dmowska A. Novel Ferulic Acid Esterases From *Bifidobacterium* Sp. Produced on Selected Synthetic and Natural Carbon Sources. *Acta Sci Pol Technol Aliment* [Internet]. 2010 [cited 2018 Jan 1]; Available from: http://agris.fao.org/agris-search/search.do?recordID=DJ2012054676

[99] Pandey KR, Naik SR, Vakil BV. Probiotics, Prebiotics and Synbiotics- A Review. *J Food Sci Technol*. 2015 Dec;52(12):7577–87.

[100] Schley PD, Field CJ. The Immune-Enhancing Effects of Dietary Fibres and Prebiotics. *Br J Nutr*. 2002 May;87 Suppl 2:S221-230.

[101] Asahara T, Nomoto K, Shimizu K, Watanuki M, Tanaka R. Increased Resistance of Mice to *Salmonella Enterica* Serovar Typhimurium Infection By Synbiotic Administration of *Bifidobacteria* and Transgalactosylated Oligosaccharides. *J Appl Microbiol*. 2001 Dec;91(6):985–96.

[102] Buddington KK, Donahoo JB, Buddington RK. Dietary Oligofructose and Inulin Protect Mice From Enteric and Systemic Pathogens and Tumor Inducers. *J Nutr*. 2002 Mar;132(3):472–7.

[103] Cummings JH, Macfarlane GT. Gastrointestinal Effects of Prebiotics. *Br J Nutr*. 2002 May;87 Suppl 2:S145-151.

[104] Scheppach W, Weiler F. The Butyrate Story: Old Wine in New Bottles? *Curr Opin Clin Nutr Metab Care*. 2004 Sep;7(5):563–7.

[105] Gibson GR, Roberfroid MB. Dietary Modulation of the Human Colonic Microbiota: Introducing the Concept of Prebiotics. *J Nutr.* 1995 Jun;125(6):1401–12.

[106] Gourbeyre P, Denery S, Bodinier M. Probiotics, Prebiotics, and Synbiotics: Impact on the Gut Immune System and Allergic Reactions. *J Leukoc Biol.* 2011 May;89(5):685–95.

[107] Hamasalim HJ. Synbiotic as Feed Additives Relating to Animal Health and Performance. *Adv Microbiol.* 2016 Apr 7;06(04):288.

[108] Manigandan T, Mangaiyarkarasi SP, Hemalatha R, Hemalatha VT, Murali NP. Probiotics, Prebiotics and Synbiotics – A Review. *Biomed Pharmacol J.* 2015 Apr 26;5(2):295–304.

[109] Pérez-Conesa D, López G, Abellán P, Ros G. Bioavailability of Calcium, Magnesium and Phosphorus in Rats Fed Probiotic, Prebiotic and Synbiotic Powder Follow-Up Infant Formulas and Their Effect on Physiological and Nutritional Parameters. *J Sci Food Agric.* 2006 Nov 1;86(14):2327–36.

[110] Milnerwood AJ, Raymond LA. Early Synaptic Pathophysiology in Neurodegeneration: Insights From Huntington's Disease. *Trends Neurosci.* 2010 Nov;33(11):513–23.

[111] McFarland LV. Meta-Analysis of Probiotics for the Prevention of Antibiotic Associated Diarrhea and the Treatment of Clostridium Difficile Disease. *Am J Gastroenterol.* 2006 Apr;101(4):812–22.

[112] McFarland LV. Meta-Analysis of Probiotics for the Prevention of Traveler's Diarrhea. *Travel Med Infect Dis.* 2007 Mar;5(2):97–105.

[113] Sheil B, Shanahan F, O'Mahony L. Probiotic Effects on Inflammatory Bowel Disease. *J Nutr.* 2007 Mar;137(3 Suppl 2): 819S–24S.

[114] Guglielmetti S, Mora D, Gschwender M, Popp K. Randomised Clinical Trial: *Bifidobacterium Bifidum* Mimbb75 Significantly Alleviates Irritable Bowel Syndrome and Improves Quality of Life-- A Double-Blind, Placebo-Controlled Study. *Aliment Pharmacol Ther.* 2011 May;33(10):1123–32.

[115] Kruis W, Chrubasik S, Boehm S, Stange C, Schulze J. A Double-Blind Placebo-Controlled Trial to Study Therapeutic Effects of Probiotic *Escherichia Coli* Nissle 1917 in Subgroups of Patients

With Irritable Bowel Syndrome. *Int J Colorectal Dis.* 2012 Apr;27(4):467–74.

[116] Saulnier DMA, Spinler JK, Gibson GR, Versalovic J. Mechanisms of Probiosis and Prebiosis: Considerations for Enhanced Functional Foods. *Curr Opin Biotechnol.* 2009 Apr;20(2):135–41.

[117] Crittenden R, Playne MJ. Prebiotics. In: Lee YK, Salminen S, editors. *Handbook of Probiotics and Prebiotics* [Internet]. John Wiley & Sons, Inc.; 2008 [cited 2018 Jan 2]. p. 533–81. Available from: http://onlinelibrary.wiley.com/doi/10.1002/9780470432624.ch7/summary.

[118] Olveira G, González-Molero I. An Update on Probiotics, Prebiotics and Symbiotics in Clinical Nutrition. *Endocrinol Nutr Organo Soc Espanola Endocrinol Nutr.* 2016 Nov;63(9):482–94.

[119] Sáez-Lara MJ, Robles-Sanchez C, Ruiz-Ojeda FJ, Plaza-Diaz J, Gil A. Effects of Probiotics and Synbiotics on Obesity, Insulin Resistance Syndrome, Type 2 Diabetes and Non-Alcoholic Fatty Liver Disease: A Review of Human Clinical Trials. *Int J Mol Sci.* 2016 Jun 13;17(6).

In: Food for Huntington's Disease
Editors: M. Mohamed Essa et al.
ISBN: 978-1-53613-854-2
© 2018 Nova Science Publishers, Inc.

Chapter 6

NUTRACEUTICALS: A NOVEL NEUROPROTECTIVE APPROACH AGAINST HUNTINGTON'S DISORDER

*N. J. Dar[1] and R. S.Yadav[2],**

[1]Neuropharmacology Laboratory,
CSIR-Indian Institute of Integrative Medicine,
Jammu (J&K) 180 001, India
[2]Department of Criminology and Forensic Science,
School of Applied Sciences, Dr. Harisingh Gour Vishwavidyalaya
(A Central University), Sagar – 470 003 (MP), India

ABSTRACT

Neurodegenerative diseases are one of the most devastating conditions that are typically associated with mutated genes, accumulation of abnormal proteins, enhanced oxidative stress and like. The mechanisms underlying neurodegenerative disorders are multifactorial and complex. Huntington disease is one such inherited condition that

---

* Corresponding Author: Dr. Rajesh Singh Yadav, Assistant Professor, Department of Criminology and Forensic Science, School of Applied Sciences, Dr. Harisingh Gour Vishwavidyalaya, (A Central University), Sagar – 470 003 (MP), India, Email: razitrc@gmail.com, Phone: +91-07582-264122, Mobile: +91-9179444557.

causes progressive degeneration of neurons in the brain. Escalating interests are focused on determining the protection against the progression of such devastating conditions through natural compounds. Nutraceuticals have recently gained importance owing to their safe use and multifaceted effects. In the present chapter, an attempt has been made to demonstrate the potential of coenzyme Q10, curcumin, resveratrol, α-lipoic acid and epigallocatechin 3-gallate in restoring the mitochondrial machinery by acting as highly strong anti-oxidant agents and modulating the pro-survival or pro-apoptotic signalling pathways. These food based compounds are believed to target multiple pathways in a slow but more physiological manner without causing any relentless adverse effects such as generation of ATP through participation in mitochondrial respiratory chain, SIRT1 activation, COX-1 inhibition, anti-protein aggregation, anti-inflammatory cascade, restoration of mitochondrial membrane, trans-location of NF-kB and restoration of Keap1/Nrf pathway leading to mitochondrial biogenesis, etc. All these effects of the nutraceuticals have attracted many research groups to focus on them so that potential therapeutic candidates against neurodegenerative disorders such as Huntington's disease can be developed to combat such alarming ailments.

Keywords: Huntington disease, coenzyme Q10, curcumin, resveratrol, α-lipoic acid, epigallocatechin 3-gallate, neutraceuticals

INTRODUCTION

The brain is a very complex organ of any individual's body. It is the control centre of our body which regulates various physiological and pharmacological functions. The brain along with the spinal cord and neurons constitutes the nervous system. Memory, sensations, and behaviour can be affected if the brain is damaged or injured, or in case of disease or disorder. Neurological disorders are the disorders of the nervous system that can occur due to structural, biochemical, or signal abnormalities in the brain, spinal cord and neurons. There are more than 600 diseases associated with brain; a few important examples are epilepsy, Parkinson's disease, Huntington's disease, Alzheimer's disease, multiple scelerosis, among others. Neurodegenerative diseases are can be quite debilitating and their fundamental mechanisms are complex and multifactorial. Huntington's disease (HD), is caused by genetic mutations encoding the huntingtin protein (*HTT*) in which some DNA base pairs are repeated multiple times. The disease produces physical, emotional, cognitive, and behavioral disturbances that are linked with mental deterioration and uncontrolled movements (Bonelli et al., 2007). Due to this, the caretakers and their physicians are willing to try almost any potential treatment to slow down its progression. Past and ongoing studies have reconstructed the evolutionary history of the affected gene to find out the exact cause of its progression and the mechanism behind the uncontrolled movements. The mutant huntingtin protein has been found to cause death of specific brain regions including caudate, putamen, and cerebral cortex (Aylward, 2007). The disturbances that are associated with different parts of the brain may vary depending upon the progression of disease as well as other factors. As the brain cells die, symptoms will appear in each of the three associated components (physical, cognitive and emotional). These include:

- **Physical Symptoms:** Impact on patient ability to work, involuntary jerking or movements (chorea), weight loss, poor coordination, trouble walking, talking, and swallowing.
- **Cognitive Symptoms:** Difficulty in organizing and task oriented behaviour, recall of information, and making decisions, impaired learning.
- **Emotional Symptoms:** Obsessive behaviour, irritability, depression, anxiety, and apathy.

The disease prevalence has been estimated to 10.6–13.7 individuals per 100,000 in Western populations (Bates et al., 2015). However, the occurrence of this disorder appears to be less in the populations of Chinese, Japanese, and African countries. In South Africa, lower rates are seen in black populations compared to white and mixed populations. The difference in disease prevalence across ethnic groups relates to genetic differences in the *HTT* gene; populations with a high prevalence have longer average CAG repeats. For example, those of European ancestry have an average of 18.4 – 18.7, whilst those of Asian ancestry have an average of 16.9 – 17.4 (Bates et al., 2015). Numerous research and clinical trials have been carried out by various health scientists but no effective therapy or drugs are available to slow the progression of this disease. However, there are some drugs that may provide temporary relief from the symptoms. In 2015, the first human trial of a huntingtin lowering drug (IONIS-HTTRx) was led by Professor Sarah Tabrizi at the UCL Institute of Neurology; the results of the trial were of revolutionary importance for the patients and their families. They reported that the drug is safe and well-tolerated and has the ability to lower toxic protein levels in the brain. They further demonstrated that IONIS-HTTRx produced a significant dose-dependent reduction of the level of *HTT*. However, detailed mechanistic studies are warranted before its FDA approval. There is also a need for a novel class of neuroprotective compounds to be explored to combat Huntington's Disease and other neurodegenerative disorders.

Nutraceuticals have received great attention in recent years due to their potential nutritional and therapeutic effects with little risk of side effects. Nutraceuticals are dietary supplements or pharmacological agents with a great medicinal value that are used for enhancing health, boosting immunity, and slowing down the development of various diseases (Hardy et al., 2003). As Hippocrates correctly emphasized "Let food be your medicine and medicine be your food". It has been observed that mitochondrial and metabolic dysfunction, defective autophagy lysosomal function, transcriptional dysregulation, impaired ubiquitin proteasome activity, abnormal protein-protein interaction, and oxidative stress play important roles in the pathogenesis of HD (Li et al., 2004). Moreover, the brain contains fatty acids that are more susceptible to oxidative damage than other types of cells. Nutraceuticals have strong antioxidant potential, great tolerance levels at higher doses, and an ability to act on multiple cellular pathways, which could make them well suited for long term use in treatments of chronic diseases like HD. Recently, nutraceuticals have received substantial global interest for their use against disease conditions. This chapter will be focussed on the anti-oxidant potential and the role certain nutraceuticals, such as coenzyme Q10 (ubiquinone), curcumin, resveratrol, α-lipoic acid, and Epigallocatechin 3-Gallate have in slowing down the progression of HD.

COENZYME Q10 (UBIQUINONE) AND HUNTINGTON'S

Coenzyme Q10 (CoQ10) is a substance that helps to convert food into energy. It is a powerful antioxidant that consists of quinone ring and a 10-isoprene unit tail. It is distributed in all cellular membranes and therefore serves as a valuable co-factor of the electron transport chain (ETS) (accepts electrons from complexes I and II).

Initially, it is reduced to the semi-ubiquinone radical and transfers one electron to complex III of the ETS at a time (Flint et al., 2003). It mediates some of its antioxidant effects through interactions with alpha-tocopherol neutralizing free radicals and thereby reduces or even helps in preventing some of the damage they cause. It also contributes to the generation of ATP through participation in the mitochondrial respiratory chain. With energy failure and oxidative stress being a part of the pathogenesis in HD, and CoQ10 being safe and readily available, The Huntington study group (HSG), a non-profit group of clinical investigators from the United States, Canada, Europe, and Australia, set out to evaluate CoQ10 for safety, tolerability, availability and possible benefits. In an open-label dose-escalating trial, the HSG investigators found a trend of protection after 20 weeks of high doses of CoQ10 administration. CoQ10 has also been found to be very effective against mitochondrial dysfunctions. The oral administration of CoQ10 has been found to produce neuroprotective effects against striatal lesions produced by malonate (mitochondrial toxin) and amino-oxyacetic acid in dose-dependent manner. Further, it has demonstrated to increase the lactate concentrations and attenuate the toxic levels of malonate thereby rescuing the ATP levels (Beal et al., 1988). They further suggested that, pre-treatment with α-tocopherol caused no neuroprotective effect in an animal model of HD (Beal et al., 1988), while high doses of α-tocopherol was effective only in patients in early stages of the disease (Peyser et al., 1995). Studies have revealed significant attenuation by CoQ10 in the depletion of dopamine levels induced by MPTP in mice. Kasparov et al., (2006) studied the 3-nitropropionic acid induced animal model of HD to assess the mitochondrial respiratory chain and creatine kinase activity in the brain of aged rats. They suggested that the antioxidants CoQ10 and Vitamin E maintain the level of CoQ10 in brain tissue, but affect the function of the respiratory chain. Moreover, the oral administration of CoQ10 for one week prior to co-administration of 3-nitropropionic acid demonstrated significant protection against the 3-nitropropionic acid induced neurotoxicity (Matthews et al., 1998). Studies have indicated patients with HD have a significant increase in lactate concentrations in the basal ganglia and other areas of the cerebral cortex. Showing its therapeutic potential, the administration of CoQ10 results in a significant reduction of the lactate levels in the occipital cortex in HD patients (Koroshetz et al., 1997). It has also been shown to reduce the damage to the nigrostriatal dopaminergic system in one-year old mice treated with MPTP (Spindler et al., 2009). The administration of CoQ10 for treatment of neurodegenerative disease showed promising results helping to slow down the progression of these disorders in a preliminary study (Flint et al., 2003). Further, since it has been suggested that CoQ10 acts as an antioxidant and is also a component of electron transport chain, it could be used as to prevent neurodegeneration against, oxidative stress, mitochondrial dysfunctions, and as a treatment for other neurodegenerative diseases (Shannon and Fraint, 2015; Yang et al., 2016).

CURCUMIN AND HUNTINGTON'S DISEASE

Curcumin, the active ingredient in turmeric, has long been used in traditional Indian and Chinese systems of medicine. It shows beneficial effects as a treatment for multiple disease conditions and also for neurodegenerative processes similar to those happening in HD.

Most of therapeutic effects of curcumin are associated to it being a robust antioxidant, anti-inflammatory, and anti-protein aggregation candidate. Curcumin has demonstrated beneficial effects on inflammation, cystic fibrosis, gastric ulcers, liver diseases, arthritis, and neurological diseases including Alzheimer's disease (Aggarwal et al., 2009).

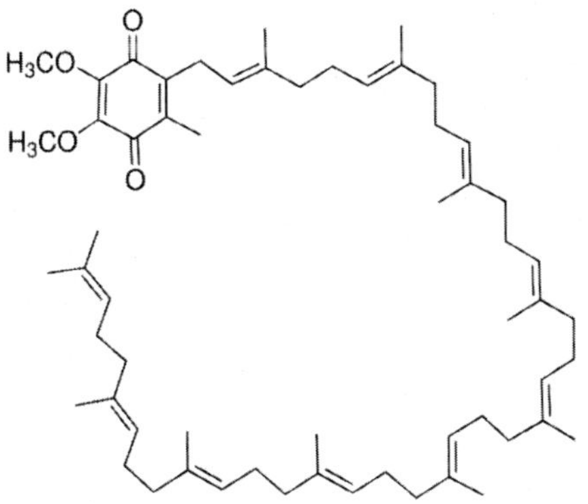

Figure 1. Chemical structure of Coenzyme Q10.

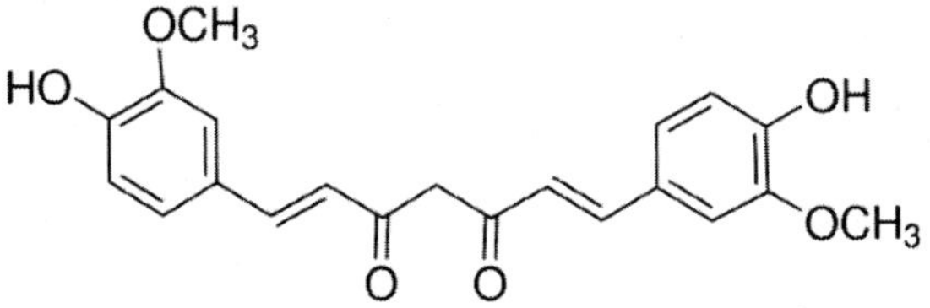

Figure 2. Chemical structure of Curcumin.

The neuroprotective potential of curcumin is due to its potential antioxidant and free radical scavenging properties (Yadav et al., 2009; 2012). Curcumin has significantly improved the neuropathology related defects in a mouse model of HD; this effect was primarily due to its anti-inflammatory and anti-oxidative activities (Choudhary et al., 2013) The MPTP induced neurodegeneration of the nigrostriatal tract, linked with glutathione depletion and enhanced lipid peroxidation in mice, has been found to be prevented by curcumin. In addition, the catalase and SOD activities were rescued in the striatum and midbrain of MPTP treated mice (Rajeswari, 2006). As stated earlier, HD is caused by an abnormal expansion of the polyglutamine (polyQ) repeat within the *HTT* protein. Recently, studies have demonstrated that curcumin was able to suppress the polyQ mediated photoreceptor neuron degeneration and internal eye dysmorphology. It also showed a protective effect in polyQ induced rough eye phenotype and pigment loss in the *Drosophila* model of HD. Furthermore, it ameliorated the polyQ-mediated locomotor dysfunction and reduced polyQ-induced cytotoxicity and cell death in *Drosophila* (Chongtham et al., 2016). Moreover, curcumin ameliorated 6-hydroxy-dopamine-induced neurotoxicity in MES23.5 cells by restoring the mitochondrial membrane potential ($\Delta\Psi m$), the translocation of NF-κB, and reduced the oxidative stress.

Singh and Kumar's (2016) study on quinolinic acid induced Huntington's Disease like symptoms in animals and humans suggested that curcumin treatment could have a beneficial effect against induced motor deficit, biochemical, and neurochemical abnormalities in rats. Since the bioavailability of curcumin is low, combining it with piperine showed significant protection. Due to the low bioavailability of curcumin, studies have also been carried out on nanocurcumin and similar analogs. In one study, Sandhir et al. (2014) demonstrated the ameliorating effect of curcumin encapsulated solid lipid nanoparticles (C-SLNs) against 3-nitropropionic acid induced HD in rats. They further reported significant improvement in neuromotor coordination in 3-nitropropionic acid induced HD by C-SLN in rats and suggested its applicability as a promising therapeutic tool to attenuate mitochondrial dysfunctions in HD. In an interesting study by Hickey et al. (2012), a diet containing curcumin since conception showed decreased huntingtin aggregates and increased striatal DARPP-32 and D1 receptor mRNAs. It also showed protection against rearing deficits in the knock-in mouse model of HD. Although, curcumin showed some motor impairment in these mice, the overall findings support a net positive effect of curcumin in HD.

RESVERATROL AND HUNTINGTON'S DISEASE

Resveratrol, 3,5,4′-trihydroxy-trans-stilbene, is a stilbenoid product which is produced by several plant species in response to a pathogen attack or stress conditions such as exposure to UV radiation. It is a natural phenol found in red grapes, mulberries, peanuts, wines, and tea. Additionally, it can be extracted from red wine during fermentation of grape skin.

Resveratrol is a naturally occurring polyphenol has been been found to be associated with the protective effect on aging, neurotoxic conditions, metabolic disorders, neurotoxic diseases, inflammation, and cancer in animal models (Pasinetti et al., 2011). It has antioxidant properties and is involved in the activation of the SIRT1, a NAD^+-dependent histone deacetylase that further enhance the peroxisome proliferator-γ-activated receptor coactivator-1α (PGC-1α) and FOXO activity. The neuroprotective and anti-adipogenic actions of resveratrol are found to be regulated through SIRT1 activation. Resveratrol has been observed to be a potent neuroprotective agent in several models of HD (In animals and alternate animal models). Resveratrol has shown pragmatic results against 3-nitropropionic acid induced neurotoxicity in HD; as 3-nitropropionic acid is an inhibitor of complex II of the electron transport chain leading to HD's like symptoms in different animal models. It inhibits cyclo-oxygenase I activity significantly and thereby improves motor and cognitive impairments in the 3-nitropropionic acid-induced model of HD (Kumar et al., 2007). Resveratrol has a potential to directly interpose in mitochondrial oxidation through its antioxidant effects and can counteract impaired mitochondrial function through the activation of the SIRT1-PGC1α pathway (Feng et al., 2013). It has rescued neurons from the cytotoxicity of the mutant polyglutamine *HTT*, intervening through SIRT1 activation. It has also been found to induce an indirect inhibition of p53 and protects the cells against the toxic effects of the m-*HTT* potentiating SIRT1 activity (Desquiret-Dumas et al., 2013). Imparting further substance for resveratrol neuroprotection, studies have shown its beneficial effect in the mouse models of Alzheimer's disease and amyotrophic lateral sclerosis (Song et al., 2014) Resveratrol is a multi-target compound with a number of neuroprotective roles; it is an intriguing candidate for its potential application in the treatment of neurological impairments. Resveratrol has an immense role improving the mitochondrial functions and biogenesis through the SIRT1/AMPK/PGC1α pathway; this highlights that its benefits are not only limited to the antioxidant and anti-inflammatory properties.

In a recent study, Vidoni et al. (2017) found that HD patients also have Parkinsonian like motor deficits that are linked with the abnormal dopamine neurotransmission associated with the impaired autophagy clearance of the polyQ-HTT aggregates. They demonstrated that resveratrol reduces oxidative stress, restores the level of ATG4, allows the lipidation of LC3, facilitates the degradation of polyQ-HTT aggregates, showed protection against dopamine toxicity in the cells and therefore slows down the progression of HD (Vidoni et al., 2017). The protective potential of a micronised proprietary resveratrol formulation (SRT501) in the N171-82Q transgenic mouse model of HD was also investigated (Ho et al., 2010). In their Study, Ho et al. (2010) reported that SRT501 had beneficial anti-diabetic effects on these mice. Studies have suggested that the activation of ERK pathway might be a novel therapeutic target for the treatment of HD and other neurological diseases (Maher et al., 2011). Further, it was also reported that fisetin, a polyphenol and resveratrol, also activates the ERK pathways and could be used as a potential drug for the treatment of HD (Maher et al., 2011).

ALPHA-LIPOIC ACID AND HUNTINGTON'S DISEASE

Alpha-lipoic acid is an antioxidant derived from caprylic acid (octenoic acid). Alpha-lipoic acid is synthesized in the body and involved in aerobic metabolism. It is a mitochondrial fatty acid that is associated in the process of energy metabolism. Its functioning is regulated by the mitochondria and it participates in the body's natural anti-oxidant defence system. Additionally, it has a potential anti-aging property as it can reverse some of the oxidant damage cause by free radicals related to the effects of aging. It has been shown to restore vitamin E and C levels and can improve the function and synaptic transmission between neurons in the case of diabetes (Andreassen et al., 2001; Johri and Beal 2012).

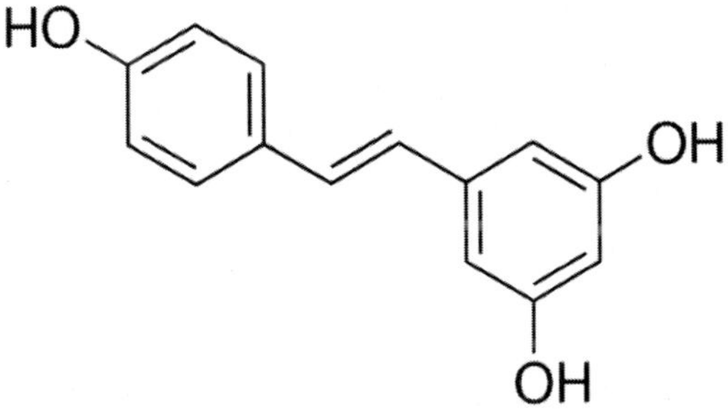

Figure 3. Chemical structure of Resveratrol.

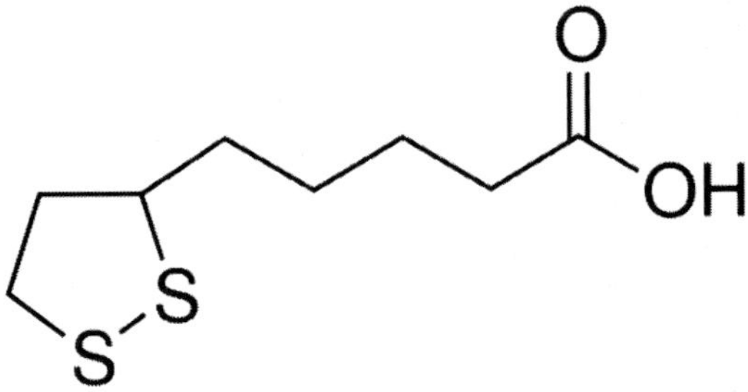

Figure 4. Chemical structure of alpha-lipoic acid.

Alpha-lipoic acid has shown to significant increase the survival rate in the R6/2 and N171-82Q transgenic mouse models of HD by restoring the mitochondrial machinery. Mitochondrial dysfunctions, oxidative stress, histologic alterations, behavioural deficits, and neuropathological changes similar to those observed in HD induced by 3-nitropropionic acid have been found to be restored by the combined treatment of alpha-lipoic acid with acetyl-l-carnitine (Mehrotra et al., 2015). The protective effect is due to the reduced oxidative stress, the mitochondrial dysfunctions, and decreased anti-apoptotic protein expression. These effects of α-lipoic acid are indicators of protection to the brain under cell damage or injury conditions and suggests the protective efficacy of these two compounds in combination in the management of HD. Numerous clinical trials have been initiated for α-lipoic acid in patients with diabetic neuropathy, some have very interesting findings. Alpha-lipoic acid has shown to chelate toxic metals both directly and indirectly by its capability to enhance intracellular glutathione (GSH) levels (Tibullo et al., 2017). It has demonstrated abilities to up-regulate the activities of oxidative phosphorylation complexes, diminish acrylamide induced distinction in AMPK/GSK3β, Ca^{2+} disturbance, and ATP depletion, as well as recover the Keap1/Nrf2 pathway leading to the mitochondrial biogenesis (Song et al., 2017).

EPIGALLOCATECHIN 3-GALLATE (EGCG) AND HUNTINGTON'S DISEASE

Epigallocatechin 3-Gallate (EGCG) is the major antioxidant compound found in large amounts in the dried leaves of green tea and black tea which also contain polyphenol flavonoids. It is used in many dietary supplements as a potential antioxidant to benefit human health. Green tea as a popular drink consumed by millions of people around the world. Studies have reported that green tea has water soluble polyphenol compounds which possess antioxidant, anticancer, neuroprotective activities that are beneficial to almost every organ of the body.

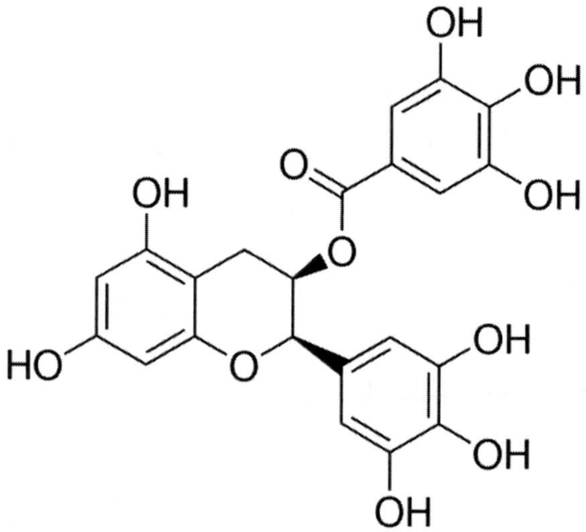

Figure 5. Chemical structure of Epigallocatechin 3-Gallate.

Since 2014, seventeen clinical trials are being conducted to study the beneficial effect of EGCG against several clinical conditions; they are still ongoing. EGCG shows neuroprotective efficacy in pre-clinical and *in vitro* studies in which therapeutic effects have been observed in cell and animal models of HD. It was taken further in phase II clinical trials and evaluated for efficacy and tolerability. EGCG has been shown to attenuate the mitochondrial oxidative stress and intrinsic apoptosis by increasing the expression levels of anti-apoptotic proteins in cultured rat cerebellar granule neurons (Schroeder et al., 2009). It has mitigated the enhanced oxidative stress and neuronal apoptosis induced by hydrogen peroxide, MPTP, MPP+, and other neurotoxins in motor neurons (Schroeder et al., 2009). Moreover, EGCG also improves motor function and reduces photoreceptor degeneration in a *Drosophila* model of Huntington's disease (Ehrnhoefer et al., 2006).

CONCLUSION

The fundamental mechanisms that are involved in neurodegenerative disorders are complex and multifactorial, currently there is lack of effective treatment options. The disappointing upshots of several phase III clinical trials against these disorders always warrants a novel and potent candidate to treat such ailments. Since, Huntington's Disease stands as a serious problem by disturbing the physical, emotional and cognitive state of an individual there, is an immediate need to find out novel, potent, safe, and tolerable therapeutic agents. Presently nutraceuticals are attaining distinction for their use against neurodegenerative disorders like Alzheimer's disease, Parkinson's disease, and HD due to their potential ability to restore the mitochondrial machinery by acting as strong anti-oxidant agents and modulating the pro-survival or pro-apoptotic signalling pathways. Numerous nutraceuticals have found their way into clinical trials. Currently compounds like CoQ10, curcumin, resveratrol, and epigallocatechin 3-gallate are being evaluated against different neurodegenerative disorders. The use of nutraceuticals in clinical trials has significantly increased in recent years, but important pharmaceutical and clinical issues need to be addressed through further research into the bioavailability of some nutraceuticals and their penetrability through blood brain barrier. By utilizing different nano-technological approaches these impediments can be overcome. The future use of nutraceutical antioxidants is very promising to provide therapeutic benefits for patients, provided the mechanistic basis of their action are fully understood. Currently there is an immediate need to explore the potential of these novel entities utilizing diverse disease model systems in order to take the full advantage of what they have to offer.

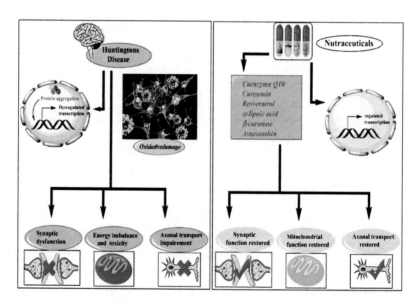

Figure 6. Schematic diagram illustrating different cell degrading events like protein aggregation, synaptic dysfunction, energy imbalance and mitochondrial dysfunction in Huntington's disease and their restoration by different nutraceutical.

REFERENCES

Aggarwal, BB; Sung, B. Pharmacological Basis for the Role of Curcumin in Chronic Diseases: An Age-Old Spice with Modern Targets. *Trends in Pharmacological Sciences*, 2009, 30, 2, 85-94.

Andreassen, OA; Ferrante, RJ; et al. Lipoic Acid Improves Survival in Transgenic Mouse Models of Huntington's Disease. *Neuroreport*, 2001, 12(15), 3371-3373.

Aylward, EH. Change in MRI Striatal Volumes as a Biomarker in Preclinical Huntington's Disease. *Brain Res Bull.*, 2007, 72, 152–158.

Bates, GP; Dorsey, R; Gusella, JF; et al. Huntington Disease. *Nat Rev Dis Primers*, 2015, 1, 1–21.

Bonelli, RM; Hofmann, P. A Systematic Review of the Treatment Studies in Huntington's Disease Since 1990. *Expert Opin Pharmacother.*, 2007, 8, 141–153.

Chongtham, A; Agrawal, N. Curcumin Modulates Cell Death and Is Protective in Huntington's Disease Model. *Scientific reports*, 2016, (6), 18736.

Choudhary, S; Kumar, P; Malik, J. Plants and Phytochemicals for Huntington's Disease. *Pharmacognosy reviews.*, 2013, 7(14), 81.

Desquiret-Dumas, V; Gueguen, N; Leman, G; Baron, S; Nivet-Antoine, V; et al. Resveratrol Induces a Mitochondrial Complex I-Dependent Increase in NADH Oxidation Responsible For Sirtuin Activation in Liver Cells. *Journal of Biological Chemistry*, 2013, 288, 51, 36662-36675.

Ehrnhoefer, DE; Duennwald, M; Markovic, P; Wacker, JL; Engemann, S; et al. Green Tea (−)-Epigallocatechin-Gallate Modulates Early Events in Huntingtin Misfolding and Reduces Toxicity in Huntington's Disease Models. *Human Molecular Genetics*, 2006, 15, 18, 2743-2751.

Feng, X; Liang, N; Zhu, D; Gao, Q; Peng, L; et al. Resveratrol Inhibits β-Amyloid-Induced Neuronal Apoptosis Through Regulation of SIRT1-ROCK1 Signaling Pathway. *PloS one*, 2013, 8, 3, e59888.

Flint Beal, M; Clifford, W. Shults. Effects of Coenzyme Q10 in Huntington's Disease and Early Parkinson's Disease. *Biofactors*, 2003, 18, (1-4), 153-161.

Hardy, G; Hardy, I; Ball, PA. Nutraceuticals--A Pharmaceutical Viewpoint: Part II. *Curr. Opin. Clin. Nutr. Metab. Care*, 2003, 6(6), 661-671.

Hickey, MA; Zhu, C; Medvedeva, V; Lerner, RP; Patassini, S; et al. Improvement of Neuropathology and Transcriptional Deficits in CAG 140 Knock-In Mice Supports a Beneficial Effect of Dietary Curcumin in Huntington's Disease. *Mol Neurodegener.*, 2012, 4, 7, 12.

Ho, DJ; Calingasan, NY; Wille, E; Dumont, M; Beal, MF. Resveratrol Protects Against Peripheral Deficits in a Mouse Model of Huntington's Disease. *Exp Neurol.*, 2010, 225(1), 74-84.

Johri, A; Beal, MF. Antioxidants in Huntington's disease. *Biochimica et Biophysica Acta (BBA)-Molecular Basis of Disease.*, 2012, 1822(5), 664-674.

Kasparová, S; Sumbalová, Z; Bystrický, P; Kucharská, J; et al. Effect of Coenzyme Q_{10} and Vitamin E on Brain Energy Metabolism in the Animal Model of Huntington's Disease. *Neurochem. Int.*, 2006, 48, p. 93-99.

Koroshetz, WJ; Jenkins, BG; Rosen, BR; Beal, MF. Energy Metabolism Defects in Hiuntington's Disease and Effects of Coenzyme Q10. *Ann. Neurol.*, 1997, 41, 160-165.

Kumar, P; Padi, SS; Naidu, PS; Kumar, A. Cyclooxygenase Inhibition Attenuates 3'nitropropionic Acid Induced Neurotoxicity in Rats: Possible Antioxidant Mechanisms. *Fundamental & Clinical Pharmacology*, 2007, 21, 3, 297-306.

Li, SH; Li, XJ. Huntingtin–Protein Interactions and the Pathogenesis of Huntington's Disease. *TRENDS in Genetics*, 2004, 20, 3, 146-154.

Maher, P; Dargusch, R; Bodai, L; Gerard, PE; et al. ERK Activation by the Polyphenols Fisetin and Resveratrol Provides Neuroprotection in Multiple Models of Huntington's Disease. *Hum Mol Genet.*, 2011, Jan 15, 20(2), 261-70.

Matthews, RT; Yang, L; Browne, S; Baik, M; et al. Coenzyme Q10 Administration Increases Brain Mitochondrial Concentrations and Exerts Neuroprotective Effects. *Proceedings of the National Academy of Sciences*, 1998, 95, 15, 8892-8897.

Mehrotra, A; Kanwal, A; Banerjee, SK; Sandhir, R. Mitochondrial Modulators in Experimental Huntington's Disease: Reversal of

Mitochondrial Dysfunctions and Cognitive Deficits. *Neurobiol Aging.*, 2015, 36(6), 2186-200.

Pasinetti, GM; Wang, J; Marambaud, P; Ferruzzi, M; Gregor, P; Knable, LA; Ho, L. Neuroprotective and Metabolic Effects of Resveratrol: Therapeutic Implications For Huntington's Disease and Other Neurodegenerative Disorders. *Exp Neurol.*, 2011, 232(1), 1-6.

Peyser, CE; Folstein, M; Chase, GA; Starkstein, S; Brandt, J; et al. Trial of D-a-Tocopherol in Huntington's Disease. *Am. J. Psychiat.*, 1995, 152, p. 1771-1775.

Rajeswari, A. Curcumin Protects Mouse Brain From Oxidative Stress Caused by 1-methyl-4-phenyl-1, 2, 3, 6-Tetrahydro Pyridine. *European Review For Medical and Pharmacological Sciences*, 2006, 10, 4, 157.

Sandhir, R; Yadav, A; Mehrotra, A; Sunkaria, A; Singh, A; Sharma, S. Curcumin Nanoparticles Attenuate Neurochemical and Neurobehavioral Deficits in Experimental Model of Huntington's Disease. *Neuromolecular Med.*, 2014, 16(1), 106-18.

Schroeder, EK; Kelsey, NA; et al. Green tea Epigallocatechin 3-Gallate Accumulates in Mitochondria and Displays a Selective Antiapoptotic Effect Against Inducers of Mitochondrial Oxidative Stress in Neurons. *Antioxidants & redox signalling*, 2009, 11(3), 469-480.

Schroeder, EK; Kelsey, NA; Doyle, J; Breed, E; Bouchard, RJ; et al. Green Tea Epigallocatechin 3-Gallate Accumulates in Mitochondria and Displays a Selective Antiapoptotic Effect Against Inducers of Mitochondrial Oxidative Stress in Neurons. *Antioxidants & redox signaling*, 2009, 11, 3, 469-480.

Shannon, KM; Fraint, A. Therapeutic Advances in Huntington's Disease. *Mov Disord.*, 2015, 15, 30(11), 1539-46.

Singh, S; Kumar, P. Neuroprotective Activity of Curcumin in Combination with Piperine against Quinolinic Acid Induced Neurodegeneration in Rats. *Pharmacology.*, 2016, 97(3-4), 151-60.

Song, G; Liu, Z; Wang, L; Shi, R; Chu, C; Xiang, M; et al. Protective Effects of Lipoic Acid Against Acrylamide-Induced Neurotoxicity:

Involvement of Mitochondrial Energy Metabolism and Autophagy. *Food & function*, 2017, 8, 12, 4657-4667.

Song, L; Chen, L; Zhang, X; et al. Resveratrol Ameliorates Motor Neuron Degeneration and Improves Survival in SOD1G93A Mouse Model of Amyotrophic Lateral Sclerosis. *Bio Med research international*, 2014.

Spindler, M; Beal, MF; Henchcliffe, C. Coenzyme Q10 Effects in Neurodegenerative Disease. *Neuropsychiatric Disease and Treatment.*, 2009, 5, 597.

Tibullo, D; Volti, G; Giallongo, C; Grasso, S; Tomassoni, D; et al. Biochemical and Clinical Relevance of Alpha Lipoic Acid: Antioxidant and Anti-Inflammatory Activity, Molecular Pathways and Therapeutic Potential. *Inflammation Research*, 2017, 66, 11, 947-959.

Vidoni, C; Secomandi, E; Castiglioni, A; Melone, MAB; Isidoro, C. Resveratrol Protects Neuronal-Like Cells Expressing Mutant Huntingtin From Dopamine Toxicity by Rescuing ATG4-Mediated Autophagosome Formation. *Neurochem Int.*, 2017, pii: S0197-0186(17)30243-7. doi: 10.1016/j.neuint.2017.05.013.

Yadav, RS; Chandravanshi, LP; Shukla, RK; Sankhwar, ML; Ansari, RW; Shukla, PK; Pant, AB; Khanna, VK. Neuroprotective Efficacy of Curcumin in Arsenic Induced Cholinergic Dysfunctions in Rats. *Neurotoxicology.*, 2011, 32(6), 760-8.

Yadav, RS; Sankhwar, ML; Shukla, RK; Chandra, R; Pant, AB; Islam, F; Khanna, VK. Attenuation of Arsenic Neurotoxicity by Curcumin in Rats. *Toxicol Appl Pharmacol.*, 2009, 1, 240(3), 367-76.

Yang, X; Zhang, Y; Xu, H; Luo, X; Yu, J; Liu, J; Chang, RC. Neuroprotection of Coenzyme Q10 in Neurodegenerative Diseases. *Curr Top Med Chem.*, 2016, 16(8), 858-66.

In: Food for Huntington's Disease
Editors: M. Mohamed Essa et al.
ISBN: 978-1-53613-854-2
© 2018 Nova Science Publishers, Inc.

Chapter 7

MANAGEMENT OF HUNTINGTON'S DISEASE: PERSPECTIVES FROM THE SIDDHA SYSTEM OF MEDICINE

C. Saravana Babu[1,], M. Mahadevan[2], B. Srinivasa Rao[3], V. Ranju[4], R. Bipul[1], A. Bhat[1], N. Chethan[1], A. H. Tousif[1], T. Manivasagam[5], A. Justin Thenmozhi[5] and M. Mohamed Essa[6,7]*

[1]Department of Pharmacology, JSS College of Pharmacy, JSS Academy of Higher Education and Research, SS Nagar, Mysore, KA, India
[2]Department of Sirappu Maruthuvam, National Institute of Siddha, (An Autonomous Body under the Ministry of AYUSH), Govt. of India, Tambaram Sanatorium, Chennai, TN, India
[3]Department of Anatomy, College of Medicine, Imam Abdulrahman Bin Faisal University, Damam, Kingdom of Saudi Arabia

---

[*] Corresponding Author: Saravana Babu Chidambaram, Associate Professor, Department of Pharmacology, JSS College of Pharmacy, JSS Academy of Higher Education and Research, SS Nagar, Mysore - 570015, KA, India, Tel: +91-9940434129; Email: csaravanababu@gmail.com.

[4]Department of Biotechnology, Dr. M.G.R. Educational and Research Institute University, Chennai, TN, India
[5]Department of Biochemistry and Biotechnology, Annamalai University, Annamalai nagar, TN, India
[6]Department of Food Science and Nutrition, CAMS, Sultan Qaboos University, Muscat, Oman
[7]Ageing and Dementia Research Group, Sultan Qaboos University, Muscat, Oman

ABSTRACT

Readers are requested to read the chapter patiently without bouncing fast as it carries traditional and cultural rich medical proofs on treating many neurological diseases using simple life-style modifications and dietary supplements. Huntington's disease (HD), an inherited neurodegenerative disorder, being incurable and progressive, its management also remains highly complicated. Currently, only symptomatic drugs available for HD management and HD patients mainly depend on these drugs and support therapies in order to lead a better quality of life. Recently high interest shown by researchers towards herbs as an alternative option for the management of HD. *Siddha medicine system* also called as *Tamil Medicine* is in vogue since time immemorial and it is widely practiced in the Southern part of India particularly in Tamil Nadu and Kerala. This system has very old history with richest evidences on the efficacy and safety of the medicines used in different neurological diseases. Interestingly, Siddha system recommends different herbs, food and life style changes as the major therapeutic strategy to patients depending upon their body's humor type (vaatham, pitham or kabam) and five elements (water, earth, air, fire and sky) composition. As the most common saying, Siddha system denotes *Food is Medicine,* stringent dietary manipulations will be recommended for patients, which should be practiced during the entire duration of the treatment period. Five thousand years before, Siddha medicine system categorised HD as a central nervous system disease and is classified under *Nadukku Vaatham.* Many evidences regarding the practical use of various herbs, vegetables, fruits, seeds, cereals and functional foods to treat HD are also obtained from ancient times and routine use of these edibles are highly recommended for HD patients. This chapter briefs about the use of herbs, and dietary supplements by HD patients as per the Siddha system of Medicine.

HUNTINGTON'S DISEASE – HISTORICAL PERSPECTIVES

Huntington's disease (HD) is an autosomal dominant, a progressive neurodegenerative disease, usually characterised by an involuntary movement of the face and body along with psychological problems and dementia [1]. Hen Paracelsus was the first scientist who coined the term "Chorea" for involuntary episodes of writhing movement under movement disorders, even many years before the clinical cases of HD are reported. First case report on HD was clinically presented by Charles Oscar Waters in 1841. Furthermore, George Huntington was the first American physician to provide a detailed description on the pathophysiology of HD in his paper on "Chorea" in 1872. HD research milestones were accomplished when chromosomal linkage in HD was established in 1983 [2] and the gene responsible for HD pathology was also identified. Advancement in this research field lead to the discovery of intracellular mutant huntingtin (mHTT) aggregates [3] in neurons.

HUNTINGTON'S DISEASE – CLINICAL SYMPTOMS

HD usually manifests as movement, cognitive and psychiatric disorders with a broad variety of signs and symptoms. Although most of the HD patients exhibit similar physical symptoms, but the onset, progression, and degree of cognitive and behavioural symptoms vary distinctively between each and every individual [4]. HD is a predominating neurodegenerative condition caused by a CAG/polyglutamine repeat growth. Common symptomatic features of HD are involuntary movements of the face and body; abnormalities in gait, posture and balance; obsessive-compulsive behaviour, and dementia [1]. Main psychomotor dysfunction "chorea" may present primarily as general restlessness, poor coordination, small unintentional movements or delayed saccadic eye movements, while rigidity, writhing motions or abnormal posturing appear clearly in the advanced stages [5]. However, chorea is not considered to be a prominent marker of disease progression as the incidence and intensity of it varies from person to person. Lack of muscle control and coordination results in abnormal facial expression, physical instability, slurred speech, and difficulties in chewing and swallowing [6]. Sleep disturbances, seizures, neuropsychiatric issues and cognitive impairments including difficulties in planning, abstract thinking, cognitive flexibility, are also associated symptoms of HD [7, 5]., whereas memory deficits appear as the disease progresses resulting ultimately in dementia in the advanced stages [8]. During the advanced stages of disease, other motor dysfunctions such as dystonia and bradykinesia are widely documented [9].

HUNTINGTON'S DISEASE – GENETIC PATHOLOGY

HD is also known as poly-glutamine disease, as the striking neuropathological feature is the abnormal accumulation of intra cellular huntingtin (*HTT*) protein (HTT) due to the presence of elongated tri-nucleated cytosine-adenine- guanine (CAG) repeat, which encodes glutamine (also called as poly-Q) [10]. The role of HTT is not well elucidated, however it was reported that it has prominent roles in embryonic development, regulation of gene expression and cell survival [11]. HTT also act as an anti-apoptotic agent and controls the production of brain-derived neurotrophic factor (BDNF), a protein which protects neurons and regulates neuronal formation. It is facilitator in vesicular trafficking and synaptic transmission and it can able to control the gene transcription in neurons [12].

Abnormal HTT accumulation leads to selective neuronal death mainly in the cortex and medium spiny neurons of the striatum, and common consequences are cognitive, psychiatric and motor impairments [13]. In addition, polyglutamine repeat in HTT is also a crucial and detrimental factor for disease inheritance and severity. It means, rise in the number of

CAG repeats results in superior HTT aggregates leading to increased neurotoxicity [14].

Due to its varied clinical manifestations, HD is often misdiagnosed for various other neurodegenerative diseases like Huntington's Disease-like 2 [15, 6]. Molecular characterisation of CAG repeat length is one of the prominent diagnostic markers and molecular diagnosis will be conducted for patients expressing various clinical manifestations associated with HD or for those who are at higher risk with a family history of HD [4].

CURRENT TREATMENT STRATEGIES

Presently, no treatment options in allopathic system are available to attain complete cure or to change the course of HD. Symptomatic treatment alternatives for HD fall under three major scopes namely treatment for motor dysfunction, psychiatric disturbances and neurodegeneration [16]. Treatments targeted towards motor dysfunction are mainly anti-psychotic drugs such as tetrabenazine and haloperidol [17]. Although these drugs improved motor function, they posed constant side effects which limited their clinical use.

Other strategies related with combating the psychiatric disturbances and neurodegeneration also causes unwanted side effects and the progression of disease can't be stoppable [18].

ALTERNATIVE THERAPEUTIC STRATEGIES

An alternative treatment strategy was aimed to improve mitochondrial function in HD. Coenzyme Q10, an integral component of mitochondrial electron transport chain, was found to be effective against disease progression in transgenic mouse models [19]. In clinical trials, coenzyme Q10 was found to slow the progression of motor and cognitive decline. Creatinine was reported to improve brain ATP levels and attenuate DNA injury in HD patients [16]. On the contrary, creatinine intake for one year did not improve motor function or cognitive deficits in a double-blind placebo-controlled study.

Apart from these, stem cell therapy, trans-glutamine inhibitors, human single chain FV antibodies and ubiquilin are other upcoming therapeutic choices. However, development of these treatment strategies requires more specific attentions [20].

A single therapy has not been elucidated to combat all the symptoms associated with HD. To address the myriad of devastations in HD, combination of agents that targets the pathological aspects are commonly considered [21].

SIDDHA SYSTEM OF MEDICINE AND HD

Introduction to Siddha Medicine System

In process of evolution, the means to lead healthy longevity made man to fine tune medical knowledge and life style disciplines. These factors ultimately lead to attain mastery over nature. Those who have dedicated themselves to these tasks were great Yogis otherwise called as "Siddhars"

As per the Indian mythology, Lord Shiva taught the knowledge of medicines to his wife Lordess Parvathi. Lordess Parvathi taught this medical knowledge to Nandi, the gate-guardian deity of Lord Shiva. Nandhi shared the knowledge to eight disciples of Nandinatha Sampradaya - Sanaka, Sanatana, Sanandana, Sanatkumara, Tirumular, Vyagrapada, Patanjali and Sivayoga Muni and they were sent to eight directions to spread the wisdom of Shaivam and medical knowledge. According to the Tamil mythology, there are 18 Siddhars: Nandi, Agasthyar, Thirumular, Punnakkesar, Pulasthiyar, Poonaikannar, Idaikkadhar, Pulikaisar, Karuvurar, Konjanavavar, Kalangi, Sattinathar, Azhugganni Agappai, Pubatti, Thoraiyar and Kudhambai and Dhanvanthri.

The medical system and life style disciplines preached and complied by Siddhars is called as "Siddha system of Medicine/" Siddhars shared their knowledge with the world through their writing in scriptures. On the other means, Siddhi means the process of attainment of divine super natural powers or being divine human. The Siddha science is a traditional treatment system found to be emerged from Tamil culture. Agathiyar, commonly believed as the first one as well as considered as the father of the *Siddha medicine system,* laid the first foundation of this efficient medicinal system [25]. By practising years of periodic fasting and meditation, Siddhars focus on attainment of "Ashtamaha Siddhi," the eight-main supernatural power, to acquire the supreme wisdom and overall immortality. Achievement of Siddhi confers immortal state which possesses any of the eight classes as mentioned below.

Siddhis are:

- Anima: shaping as tiny as an atom
- Mahima: shaping as large as possible
- Laghima: becoming light which is enough to float in the air
- Garima: Capable of expansion
- Prapti: Power to obtain any desired object
- Prakamyam: Irresistible will to perform
- Ishitvam: Lording over everything
- Vashivtam: Power of subduing anyone/anything.

Basics of Siddha Medicine System

Siddha system of medicine holds a complicated scientific basis which has in-store, various theories yet to be discovered. The five basic elements namely space, air, fire, water and earth are the building blocks of all physical and subtle bodies, existing in the whole universe by an eminent process called Pancheekaranam (mutual intra inclusion). Human body is one among them. The physiological units of human body are Vaatham (Creative force; formed by air and space), Pitham (Force of preservation; formed by fire) and Kabam (Destructive force; formed by earth and water). These units are also called as life forces. In healthy state, the physiological units of these three exists in 4:2:1 ratio. Disturbances in this equilibrium by factors such as dietary habits, life style changes (both physical and mental), and environmental changes leads to the derangement of five elements which in turn affects three life forces and these changes will be obviously reflected in the seven physical constituents of the body

Diagnosis of Diseases in Siddha System of Medicine

As per Siddha system of medicine, diet and lifestyle play a major role in health. Imbalance or derangement between vaatham, pitham, and kabam, leads to sickness/diseases. Siddha system of medicine has fine art of diseases diagnosis ways. There are eight examinations tools which are based on the three humours:

1. *Nadi* (Pulse)
2. *Kan* (Eyes)
3. *Na* (Tongue)
4. *Varna* (Colour of skin)
5. *Sparism* (Touch)
6. *Svara* (Voice)
7. *Neer* (Urine)
8. *Mala* (Stool).

Vaatham

Vaatham mainly refers to "Vayu" (air). Vayu forms the vital force of the body and it travels in a rapid current thereby helps to keep various tissues in healthy state. Vaatham types: Pranan, abaanan, uthanan, vyaanan, samaanan, naagan, koorman, kirukaran, devathathan and thananjeyan (Table 1). Of these, the first five play an important role in the physical and mental functions.

According to Siddha literature, locomotor and neurological components are mainly governed by "vaatham" humor. Impairment in vaatham affects normal balance and leads to disease state. Among these ten vaatham types, the first five play an important role in the preservation of the physical body.

Table.1. Types of vaatham

Pranan (Life air)	Regulates respiratory system and helps the digestive system
Abaanan (Downward air)	It takes part in excretory functions and controls the sphincters of anal canal.
Uthaanan (Upward air)	It is responsible for the physiological reflex actions like vomiting, hiccups, and cough, etc. Regulates higher functions in brain like speech.
Vyaanan (Centrifugal air)	Maintains circulation, ventilation and body heat, and also helps in the movements of both movable and immovable parts of the body
Samaanan (Digestive air)	It helps in proper digestion by neutralising the other vayus, six tastes, water and food.
Naagan (Intellectual air)	It is responsible for intelligence of the individual such as learning and memory, skill in arts, and signing etc. Regulation of eye lid movements and formation of new hair, hair follicle, and fixation of hair follicle in hair shaft etc.
Koorman (Visual air)	It is responsible for yawning, shedding of tears, and vision etc.
Kirugaran (Secretory air)	It is responsible for salivation and nasal secretion. It helps in meditation.
Dhevathathan (Tiresaome air)	It is responsible for laziness, quarrelling, arguing, and also anger. It helps movements of the eyeball in various directions and is present in genital and anal region.
Dhananjeyan (Intracranial air)	It is present in nose and responsible for swelling of the body and tinnitus. It leaves the body via cranial cavity only on the third day after death.

Factors That Vaatham Humor

- Dietary factors - increased intake of bitter, astringent, and spicy tastes; and higher intake of kodo millet, foxtail millet, ghee, old boiled rice, and tubers.

- Behavior - Hypersexuality, egocentrism, aggression, compulsive behavior, increased food starvation, wicked mindedness, and disrespectful acts.
- Life style - Living in higher altitudes, increased exposure to chill weather, day time sleeping and staying back at nights.

Impact of Vaatham on Neurological Diseases

As per the Siddha scripts, neurological disorders are classified under Vaatham-Kabam diseases. The major causative factor for neurological diseases occurs due to vitiation of Vaatham and the co-morbid symptoms are due to vitiation of Kabam humor.

In Paanikkamba vaatham, the primary humour affected is vaatham. Vitiation of vaatham is accompanied by vitiation of kabam, often. This is clearly indicated in verse by sage Theraiyar (Verse 1/Figure 1). The poem means that vaatham is the prime indicator of health.

With respect to the present chapter, clinical signs and symptoms of Huntington's chorea can be correlated to imbalance in vaatham humor and so on the neurological disorders. These evidences are shown here with the help of few verses written in Siddha scripts.

"வாதமலாது மேனிகெடாது"

Figure 1. Theraiyar Verse [26].

Correlating Huntington's Diseases with Vaatham Vitiation

The Siddha scripts mentioned below clearly explains the primary correlation between the alterations in vaatham humor with the onset and progression of neurological diseases. Interestingly, this vaatham vitiation and neurological diseases are explained way back 10000 years back which shows the immense collection of pathological information and extrapolating to humor factors and documentation. Vitiation of Kabam affects the functions of certain types of Kabam namely Avalambakam, Kilethakam, Bothagam and Santhikam resulting in indigestion, tasteless in mouth, and difficulty in extension, flexion and movement of joints etc.

Verses describing the correlation between Vaathamand neurological functions (Verse 2; Figure 2):

"மார்க்கமாய் வாய்வுமாய் மெய்நி றைந்து
வயிறுதனிற் பசியிலா தூணு மற்று
நார்க்கமாய் ஞாலத்து நடக்கை யற்று
நடுக்கமாங் கையிரண்டுந் திமிருண்டகும்
ஊர்க்கமா யுறக்கமில்லா துணர்ச்சியற்று
உதறியே சரீரமெங்கு முலர்ந்து காணும்
பார்க்கமாய் வாய்விட்டு அலத்தலாகும்
பாணிக்கம்ப வாதத்தின் பாங்குதானே"

Figure 2. Correlation between Vaatham and Neurological functions [27].

Meaning of the Verse (2)

Vitiation of vaatham leads to bloating, loss of appetite, fatigue, tremors in hands and difficulty in walking. Along with this numbness of hands, lack of sleep, dryness of skin with blabbering are also seen in "Paanikamba vaatham", a type of vaatham. Verse 3 (Figure 3)

"கம்பவாதம் செப்பியிடின் கைகால் தலைநடுக்கம்
வெம்புமுட லும்சுழலும் மெய்நோவாம்- அம்புவியில்
தூக்கம் இரவின்றித் தூபகாய மோவிளைக்கும்
அக்கமின்றி யேபுலம்பு மாம்"

Figure 3. [27].

Meaning of the Verse (3)

The alteration in vaatham precipitates tremors in limbs, head and also general body ache and discomfort. Vaatham vitiation produces dizziness, sleep loss, and lamentation presentation without any logical reasoning.

Verse 4 (Figure 4):

"திடுக்கமுறவே உடல் நடுக்கமுறும் வாதமிது செய்யுமது தன்மைகேளு
கெணிதமுறவே பெரும் நரம்பதுகள் வெட்டியே உடல் கிடுக்கும்நடுக்கும்
வெடுக்குரிய கைகாலு திமிரமாகியே வரும் விறைகடும்பெலம்குன்றியே
விதமான நாக்கு அசையாது வாய் பேசிடாது விறைத்தும் தேகம் வெட்டும்
நடுக்க முடியாதும் குளிரதிம மாகுமே வயிறு பொருமியே வீக்கம்
நளினமொடு தலை குனிந்துடல் தலை வேர்க்கும் நயனமது ஒளிகுறையுமே
திடுக்கிடு முடல் அபரும் அங்கமது மேனியுமே திடமகலு முடலுமெலியும்
தேகமதிலே பிணமாக நடையாச்சுமே தொனிவாகுமே இது பாரு நீ!

Figure 4. [28].

Meaning of the Verse (4)

This type of Vaatham vitiation causes abnormal jerky movement on excitation such as sudden and sharp limb flexion and extension; followed by numbness of the affected limbs, whole body tremor, speech difficulty, abnormal gait, reduced vision, abdominal bloating, and mental depression. It also produces flatulence, hypothermia, fatigue and emaciation.

Verse 5 (Figure 5):

உதறியே சரீரமுற்று மொக்கவே நடுக்க முண்டாய்
கதறவே யுளைந்து குத்திக் கால்கையுந் திமிருண்டாகும்
சிதறவே யுறைந்து மிண்டித் தியங்கவே யுவாதி செய்யும்
பதறவே யுதறுவாதஞ் செய்குணம் பகருங்காலே
நடுக்கிடும் பதறு மேனி நலங்கிட வுதறித்தள்ளித்
திடுக்கிட நடுக்க மிண்டித் தியங்கிட கைகால் சோடும்
விடுத்திட கடுத்து நொந்து விசைகொடு தள்ளி வீழ்த்தும்
மடக்கிடப் பதறுவாத குணமிது மாறாதென்றார்.

Figure 5. [26].

Meaning of the Verse (5)

Vaatham vitiation produces physical symptoms like sharp, abnormal and uncontrollable writhing movements, medically termed as chorea. It also causes numbness in legs and hands with pain, slowed saccadic movements of limbs including eye lids and expression less face. It also causes agitation and cognitive decline.

Inference from the Above Verses

- From the above verses in the literature of Siddha, it is clear that neurological diseases occur mainly due to vitiation of vaatham. It can be understood that vaatham play key role in sensory impulses conduction between organs and limbs. It plays an important role in psychomotor functions.
- Abnormal functions of vaatham leads to involuntary and abnormal muscle movements, tremors, and numbness or paralysis of the limb and/or muscle wasting, etc.
- It also causes sleep disturbances, depression, and decreased excretion of stools and urine.
- Vaatham controls several higher intellectual and cognitive functions of the brain, and gives energy to perform all physical and mental activities.

Bowel and Bladder Problems in Huntington's Disease

Inflammation in oesophagus and stomach is the frequent clinical finding in HD patients. In a recent study of 68 HD patients, it was reported that 32% of cases suffered from esophagitis (inflammation of the oesophagus), and almost 30-32% had gastritis (inflammation of the stomach) using upper gastrointestinal (UGI) endoscopy. Most of the HD patients had both esophagitis and gastritis [16]. These results revealed that

UGI inflammation appears more commonly in advanced disease state. It is unclear that the swallowing problems of HD might contribute to UGI inflammation. Using transgenic mouse (R62) model of HD, [23] confirmed the occurrence of lower GI problems. Moreover, abnormalities found in the villi cells of the GI tract leads to poor absorption of nutrients and minerals resulting in malnutrition. Furthermore, the role of inflammatory modulators such as anti-gliadin antibodies is found to contribute to GI distress in HD patients [24]. In many HD cases, GI distress is majorly contributed due to the toxic effects of medications used and sedentary lifestyle.

Description of GI Dysfunctions in Neurological Diseases - Siddha Perspectives

Certain extrinsic and intrinsic cells and humoral factors are said to be the causative factors, which alters vaatham, pithtam, and kabam equilibrium and results in diseases.

Verse 6 (Figure 6):

"வளிதரு காய்கிழங்கு வரைவிலா தயிலல் கோழை
முளி போன்மிகுக்கு முறையிலா வுண்டி கோடல்
குளிர்தரு வளியிற் றேகங் குனிப்புற வுலவல் பெண்டிர்
குளிதரு முயக்கம் பெற்றோர் கடிசெயல் கருவியாமால்"
- சித்த மருத்துவம்- சபாபதி கையேடு

Figure 6. GI dysfunction and Neurological diseases [30].

Meaning of the Verse (6)

Excessive intake of tubers, chilled foods, living in cold climates and hilly regions, and increased sexual indulgence are the major causatives for vaatham vitiation. Vaatha diseases show genetic inheritance and

Management of Huntington's Disease

sometimes may play a crucial role in triggering neurological diseases.

Verse 7 (Figure 7):

> வாதமே கதித்த போது வாய்வு மெழும்பி மீளும்
> வாதமே யிருமலாகித் தொடர்ந்திடுஞ் சன்னி வாதம்
> பேதமே செய்கிராணி பெருவயி றுதாதோஷம்
> போதவே தோன்று மென்றுவ்பொருத்தவே முனிவர் சொன்னார்
> வாதமே முதலா நாடி வாதமே தூலகாயம்
> வாதமே பெலவானாகும் யழலை வேண்டும்
> வாதமே மந்தம் பற்றும் வாதமே சீதகாலம்
> வாதமே யுடற்கு ளிர்ச்சி வாதமே மூலமாமே
> வாதமே வாயுவாகும் வாதமே காலிற் சேரும்
> வாதமே நன்னியோடு மருவிடில் வலியுமுண்டாம்
> வாதமே விடியப்பத்து வாதமே சாயங்காலம்
> வாதமே புளிப்பு வாங்கும் வாதமுந் தளர்ச்சி காலம்

Figure 7. [31].

Meaning of the Verse (7)

Deranged vaatham causes continuous cough, delirium, bloating, flatulence with diarrhoea, rigors, piles, pain in the legs and also fatigue.

Verse 8 (Figure 8):

> மேவியவாதஞ் செய்யுங் குணந்தனை வியம்பக் கேளாய்
> தாவியே வயிறு மந்தஞ் சந்துகள் பொருந்து நோவாஞ்
> சீவிய தாதுநாசஞ் செறுத்துடன் சிறுநீர் வீழுங்
> காவியங் கண்ணி னாளே மலமது கருகி வீழும்
> வாதத்தின் குணமேதென்னில் வயிறது பொருமிக்கொள்ளுந்
> தாதுகளுலர்ந்த கைகால் சந்துகள் கடுப்புத் தோன்றுந்
> தீதுற்றுச் சிறுநீர்தானுஞ் சிறுத்துடன் கடுத்து வீழும்
> போதுற்ற வாதமென்று புகன்றனர் முனிவர் தாமே

Figure 8. (28).

Meaning of the Verse (8)

According to Agasthiyar vaidhiya kaviyam, the vitiated vaatham produces constipation and flatulence, abdominal discomfort, pain in joints and oliguria with painful micturition.

All the verses mentioned above clearly indicates the crucial role of vaatham in regulating GI and neurological functions. Verse 9 (Figure 9):

"தானென்ற கசப்போடு துவர்ப்பு றைப்பு
சாதகமாய் மின்சுகிலும் சமைத்த வன்னம்
ஆனென்ற வாறினது புசித்த லாலும்
ஆகாயத் தேறலது குடித்த லாலும்
பானென்ற பகலுறக்க மிரா விழிப்பு
பட்டினியே மிகவுறுதல் பார மெய்தல்
தேனென்ற மொழியார் மேற் சிந்தையாதல்
சீக்கிரமாய் வாதமது செனிக்குந் தானே"

Figure 9. [27].

Meaning of the Poem

Excessive consumption of food items like bitter, astringent and pungent taste, drinking rain water without purification, altered sleep pattern, undue starving, lifting or carrying heavy loads and sexual indulgence can cause vaatham diseases.

Siddha system recommends that the following diet could be avoided to overcome neurological illness:

- Diets which are sour and astringent taste should be avoided.
- All sea foods except small prawns should be avoided.
- Details of other diets to be avoided in given in the table.

Table 2. Recommended diets in vaatham vitiation and neurological diseases - Herbs those can be used in edible form

Herb	English name	Which part and How to use	Frequency
Glycyrrhiza glabra	Liquorice	Dried root, 2 gm powdered form with honey	Morning and evening for 48 days
Withania somnifera	Winter cherry	Dried root powder, 3 gm with palm sugar along with cow's milk	Morning and evening for 48 days
Argyreia nervosa	Wood rose	Dried root powder soaked in *asparagus racemosus* juice for 7 days, 2 to 3 gm with butter	Morning and evening for 40 days
Terminalia chebula	Myrobalans	Dried powder, 1 to 2 gm with ghee	Morning and evening for 48 days
Mucuna prurieus	Velvet bean	Seed powder, 3 to 5 gm with milk	Morning and evening for 48 days
Sida cordifolia	Country mallow	Oil for bath	Weekly twice
Cuminum cyminum	Cumin seeds	2 to 5 gm with ghee	Morning and evening for 48 days
Semecarpus anacardium	Marking nut	Ghee prepared from nut, 3 to 5 gm with warm water.	Morning and evening for 48 days
Herpestis monniera	Water hyssop	Ghee preparation of this plant, 3 to 5 gm with milk.	Morning and evening for 48 days
Hydrocotyle asiatica	Water pennywort	Leaf powder, 2 gm with milk.	Morning and evening for 48 days

Table 3. Diets recommended in Siddha system of Medicine in neurological disorders

Diets	Botanical name	English name
Tender vegetables	*Solanum melongena*	Tender Brinjal
	Ficus racemosa	Crattock
	Dolichos lablab	Tonga bean
Green leaves	*Cardiospermum halicacabum*	Baloon plant
	Alternanthera sessilis	Sessile joyweed
	Solanum trilobatum	Climbing brinjal
Pulses	*Cajanus cajan*	Red gram
Dairy products		Cow buttermilk
Meat diet		White goat meat

Table 4. Other diets recommended in Siddha system of Medicine in neurological disorders

Diet	English name
Lagenaria siceraria	Long melon
Luffaacut angula	Vegetable gourd
Cucumis sativus	Cucumber
Trichosanthes cucumerina	snake gourd
Vigna unguiculata	Cow pea
Vigna mungo	Black gram
Macrotyloma uniflorum	Horse gram
Brassica juncea	Mustard

Other advice given by Siddha medicine:

- To practice and involve in regular exercises
- Breathing exercises (Pranayamam)
- Herbal rejuvenation therapies
- Avoiding cold atmosphere, sleeping on cold floor, and living on high altitudes.

CONCLUSION

Modern medicine system states that HD is incurable and only symptomatic management is the only available option for the patients. So far, the current conventional treatment strategy provides only a transient symptomatic relief in HD patients [18]. Even though, clinical progression of the HD could be controlled to some extent with the help of drugs, improvement in overall and general health is not guaranteed [19]. Widely, these therapeutic regimens (pharmaceuticals and other supporting therapies) provide partial improvement of the clinical condition in patients, but also cause many side effects. In many HD cases, treatments with different drugs cause many adverse events like GI inflammation, difficulty in swallowing and poor nutritional absorption, ultimately resulting in malnutrition [20]. Thus, the quality of life in HD patients' declines with the current allopathic/pharmaceutical therapy, as on one side, betterment of the symptoms causes serious side effects on other side [22]. However, Siddha medicine system on the ground of rich scientific background of the body type and composition, analyses the derangement in the physiological and elemental system of the body in HD patients. This system scrutinizes the causative, triggering and/or precipitating factors of the disease, and tries to alleviate the symptoms by restoring the equilibrium of the basic five elements in their right proportion. Siddha system prescribes mainly traditional herbs, life style changes and functional foods as the major therapeutics to treat any kind of disease including HD. Depending upon the onset, duration, progression and intensity of the disease as well as on the age and body type of the patient, the quantities and durational usage of herbs along with life style habitual alterations are recommended. Though this traditional therapy takes longer period of time to heal the disease, the improvement in both clinical conditions and general health without side effects always proven to be better and wise option. This medical system targets mainly on the root cause of the ailments rather than alleviating the disease-associated clinical symptoms. Restoring the balance of deranged factors in HD patients improves the clinical condition of the patient with mere or no side effects. Overall health of the patients also improves which help them significantly to lead a better quality of life.

REFERENCES

[1] Bertram L, Tanzi RE. The Genetic Epidemiology of Neurodegenerative Disease. *J Clin Invest.* 2005 Jun 1;115(6):1449–57.

[2] Gusella JF, Wexler NS, Conneally PM, Naylor SL, Anderson MA, Tanzi RE, et al. A Polymorphic DNA Marker Genetically Linked to Huntington's Disease. *Nature.* 1983 Nov 17;306(5940):234–8.

[3] Mangiarini L, Sathasivam K, Seller M, Cozens B, Harper A, Hetherington C, et al. Exon 1 of the HD Gene with an Expanded

CAG Repeat Is Sufficient to Cause a Progressive Neurological Phenotype in Transgenic Mice. *Cell.* 1996 Nov 1;87(3):493–506.
[4] Kremer B, Goldberg P, Andrew SE, Theilmann J, Telenius H, Zeisler J, et al. A Worldwide Study of the Huntington's Disease Mutation. The Sensitivity and Specificity of Measuring CAG Repeats. *N Engl J Med.* 1994 May 19;330(20):1401–6.
[5] Walker FO. Huntington's Disease. *Lancet.* 2007 Jan;369(9557): 218–28.
[6] Greenstein PE, Vonsattel JPG, Margolis RL, Joseph JT. Huntington's Disease Like-2 Neuropathology. *Mov Disord.* 2007 Jul 30;22 (10):1416–23.
[7] Gagnon J-F, Petit D, Latreille V, Montplaisir J. Neurobiology of Sleep Disturbances in Neurodegenerative Disorders. *Curr Pharm Des.* 2008;14(32):3430–45.
[8] Montoya A, Price BH, Menear M, Lepage M. Brain Imaging and Cognitive Dysfunctions in Huntington's Disease. *J Psychiatry Neurosci.* 2006 Jan;31(1):21–9.
[9] Perez-De La Cruz V, Santamaria A. Integrative Hypothesis For Huntington's Disease: A Brief Review of Experimental Evidence. *Physiol Res.* 2007;56(5):513–26.
[10] Evans-Galea MV, Hannan AJ, Carrodus N, Delatycki MB, Saffery R. Epigenetic Modifications in Trinucleotide Repeat Diseases. *Trends in Molecular Medicine.* 2013 Nov 1;19(11):655–63.
[11] Reiner A, Dragatsis I, Dietrich P. Genetics and Neuropathology of Huntington's Disease. *Int Rev Neurobiol.* 2011;98:325–72.
[12] Cattaneo E, Zuccato C, Tartari M. Normal Huntingtin Function: An Alternative Approach to Huntington's Disease. *Nat Rev Neurosci.* 2005 Dec;6(12):919–30.
[13] Miller BR, Bezprozvanny I. Corticostriatal Circuit Dysfunction in Huntington's Disease: Intersection of Glutamate, Dopamine and Calcium. *Future Neurol.* 2010 Sep;5(5):735–56.
[14] Arrasate M, Mitra S, Schweitzer ES, Segal MR, Finkbeiner S. Inclusion Body Formation Reduces Levels of Mutant Huntingtin and the Risk of Neuronal Death. *Nature.* 2004 Oct 14;431(7010):805–10.

[15] Rudnicki DD, Pletnikova O, Vonsattel J-PG, Ross CA, Margolis RL. A Comparison of Huntington Disease and Huntington Disease-Like 2 Neuropathology. *J Neuropathol Exp Neurol.* 2008 Apr 1;67(4): 366–74.

[16] Frank S. Treatment of Huntington's Disease. *Neurotherapeutics.* 2014 Jan; 11(1):153–60.

[17] O'Suilleabhain P, Dewey RB. A Randomized Trial of Amantadine in Huntington Disease. *Arch Neurol.* 2003 Jul;60(7):996–8.

[18] Bonelli RM, Wenning GK, Kapfhammer HP. Huntington's Disease: Present Treatments and Future Therapeutic Modalities. *Int Clin Psychopharmacol.* 2004 Mar;19(2):51–62.

[19] Ondo WG, Mejia NI, Hunter CB. A Pilot Study of the Clinical Efficacy and Safety of Memantine For Huntington's Disease. *Parkinsonism Relat Disord.* 2007 Oct;13(7):453–4.

[20] Videnovic A. Treatment of Huntington's Disease. *Curr Treat Options* Neurol. 2013 Aug;15(4):424–38.

[21] Abdulrahman GO. Therapeutic Advances in the Management of Huntington's Disease. *Yale J Biol Med* [Internet]. 2011 Sep [cited 2018 Apr 14];84(3):311–9. Available from: Https://www.ncbi. nlm.nih.gov/pmc/articles/PMC3178862/.

[22] Andrich JE, Wobben M, Klotz P, Goetze O, Saft C. Upper Gastrointestinal Findings in Huntington's Disease: Patients Suffer But Do Not Complain. *J Neural Transm (Vienna).* 2009 Dec; 116(12):1607–11.

[23] van der Burg JMM, Bacos K, Wood NI, Lindqvist A, Wierup N, Woodman B, et al. Increased Metabolism in the R6/2 Mouse Model of Huntington's Disease. *Neurobiol Dis.* 2008 Jan;29(1):41–51.

[24] Bushara KO, Nance M, Gomez CM. Antigliadin Antibodies in Huntington's Disease. *Neurology.* 2004 Jan 13;62(1):132–3.

[25] Tiwari L. (2013) *Siddha Medicine. Its Basic Concepts* (http:/www. infinityfoundation.com/mandala/tes/testiwarsiddha.htm).

[26] Shanmugavelu MT. *Siddha Maruthuva Noi Naadal Noi Mudhanaadal Thirattu,* Part I, Tamilnadu Siddha Medical Council, 1987.

[27] Mohan RC. Yugi Vaidhiya Sindhamani-800, 2nd ed. *Thamarai Noolagam*, 2013.
[28] Anandhan A. *Agasthiyar Vaidhiya Sindhamani*, 1st ed., Indian Medicine-Homeopathy department, 2008.
[29] Vaatha Nithanam - 800. *Siddha Maruthuvam*, Tamilnadu Siddha Medical Council, Chennai, 1987.
[30] Mudhaliyar KNK. *Siddha Maruthuvam*, Tamilnadu Siddha Medical Council, Chennai, 1987.
[31] Sekaram P, Ezhalai, Iyyer Sudhesa, Pillai Ponnaiya. *Agasthiyar Dispensary and Pharmacy*, 1999.

In: Food for Huntington's Disease
Editors: M. Mohamed Essa et al.
ISBN: 978-1-53613-854-2
© 2018 Nova Science Publishers, Inc.

Chapter 8

ASCDIANS AS BIOACTIVE SOURCES FOR HUNTINGTON DISEASE

V. Manigandan[1,*], J. Nataraj[2,*], V. Arumugam[4,*], S. Srivarshini[3,*], K. Ramachandran[1], S. Aruna Devi[2], S. Umamaheshwari[4], T. Manivasagam[2], A. Justin Thenmozhi and R. Saravanan[1,†]

[1]Department of Medical Biotechnology,
Faculty of Allied Health Sciences, Chettinad Academy of Research and Education, Kelambakkam, Chennai, Tamil Nadu, India
[2]Department of Biochemistry and Biotechnology,
Annamalai University, Chidambaram, Tamil Nadu, India
[3]Department of Medical Gentics, Faculty of Allied Health Sciences, Chettinad Academy of Research and Education, Kelambakkam, Chennai, Tamil Nadu, India
[4]Department of Environmental Biotechnology,
Bharathidasan University, Tiruchirappalli, Tamil Nadu, India

---

[*] All authors contributed equally to this chapter.
[†] Corresponding Author Email: saranprp@gmail.com.

ABSTRACT

Huntington disease (HD) is an inherited dominant autosomal neurological disorder which directs to the breakdown of nerve cells mainly in basal ganglia. The incidence of HD is less in Asia when compared to the Europe, Australia and North America. This disease is caused by the CAG triplet repeat of variable length which is located on the chromosome 4 in the Huntingtin (HTT) gene. The normal CAG repeat is from 10-26 and the mutated abnormal CAG repeat is from 36 to more than 120 times. The symptom of HD has been occurring between the age of 30-50 which includes dementia, impairment of cardiovascular system, depression, and weight loss. Numerous shortcoming associated with the present conventional therapeutic strategies have forced researchers venture to alternate natural sources for effective compounds. The present chapter was focused towards the potentials of bioactive compounds from marine derived ascidians for the treatment of the genetic neurologic disorder - HD.

Keywords: neurological disease, Huntington's disease, marine environment, nutritive value, ascidians

INTRODUCTION

Huntington disease (HD) was discovered in 1872 by a 22 year old American doctor George Huntington, who published a study on Medical and Surgical Reporter of Philadelphia which is related to Huntington's chorea (Imarisio et al., 2008). It is a progressive inherited autosomal dominant neurological late onset disease which consequences in the breakdown of nerve cells in the brain especially damage in the basal ganglia. The basal ganglia in HD is characterized by marked depletion of Gamma-Aminobutyric Acid (GABA). HD was originally called Huntington's chorea (Chorea=dancing) in Greek (Walling et al., 1998). The Symptoms of HD usually arise between the ages of 30-50 and worsen over a 10 to 25 year period. Due to this impairment occur in the peripheral tissues like cardiovascular system, blood cells and skeletal muscles (Chen et al., 2015). HD affects all races, ethnic groups, both the sexes and they are not prevalent to a particular population. A less common form of HD is juvenile form which begins from the childhood or adolescence and is associated with other health implications (Roos, 2010). The clinical features and the symptoms of HD includes progressive motor dysfunction and psychiatric disturbance leads to neuronal dysfunction and cell death, obsessive-compulsive disorder, depression weight loss and dementia. This disease affects the cerebral cortex and the stratium in the central nervous system (CNS). The diagnosis of HD is made on the basis of characteristic extra pyramidal motor signs of chorea, dystonia and incoordination in an individual at risk. The worldwide prevalence of HD is 2.71 per 100,000. The prevalence in Europe, Australia and North America is 5.70 per 100,000 whereas, in Asia it is 0.40 per 100,000 (Pringsheim et al., 2012). It also shows that more than tenfold difference between regions across the world. The prevalence of HD is lower in Asian countries when compared to North America, Europe, and Australia.

GENETIC FACTOR INDUCED HD

HD is cause due to the mutation in the HTT gene positioned on the short (p) arm of chromosome 4 at position 16.3. The HTT gene affords information for synthesizing a cytoplasmic protein called Huntingtin. The Huntingtin protein plays a key role in the functioning of neurons in the brain. HD is one among the eight inherited neurodegenerative diseases which involves a DNA segment called CAG trinucleotide repeat in the first exon of the HTT gene which has been mutated (Alberch, 2003, Christopher A Ross et al., 2011, Chen et al., 2015). Within the gene, normally the CAG segment is repeated from 10 to 26 times, whereas in people with HD the CAG segment is repeated 36 to more than 120 times (Myers et al., 2004).

There will be no development of signs and symptoms of HD with the people who have 36 to 39 CAG repeats, but people with 40 or more repeats almost always develop the disorder. The production of an abnormally long version of mutant Huntingtin (mHTT) protein is due to an increase in the size of the CAG repeats. The elongated protein is cut into smaller, which become as toxic fragments and they bind together and accumulate in neurons and it also increases the decay rate of the certain types of neurons. The expansion of CAG repeats leads to the production of abnormal protein which causes dysfunction of brain cells and neuronal cell death in the basal ganglia and also in the cerebral cortex (Ailsa Brotherton et al., 2012). The dysfunction and eventual death of the neurons leads to the signs and symptoms of HD.

Huntingtin Protein and Its Functions

Huntingtin is a protein which has anti-apoptotic properties (Borrell-Pages et al., 2006). HD is mainly caused by the expansion of a polyglutamine tract within the N-terminal domain of the protein known as Huntingtin. The expansion of polyglutamine tract results in the gain of toxicity which causes the Huntingtin protein to interact abnormally (Shi-Hua Li et al., 2004). This protein does not affect cellular transcription or translation (Walling et al., 1998). The protein contains a repeating sequence of 11 to 35 glutamine residues, the expansion of number of glutamines in this part of protein, known as polyglutamine region, which causes HD. It is essential for human development and for the normal brain function (Zheng et al., 2011, White et al., 1997). Huntingtin protein is mostly found in the neurons and in the glial cells of the brain, in male testes and in the neurons of central nervous system (Schulte et al., 2011). The primary focus of atrophy is located in the striatum and in the cerebral cortex of the brain. The Huntingtin protein also participates a role in embryonic development and particularly in neurogenesis (Walling et al., 1998). The cellular toxic effects involve both the cell autonomous and cell-cell interaction mechanism.

Symptoms and Causes of HD

The symptoms vary from person to person and it can be divided or classified into three stages. HD is classified into five pathological status, they are from 1 to grade 4 in which most of the status shows loss of brain mass which leads to neuronal cell death which is related to the severity of the disease. Atrophy is less severe in the cerebral cortex, thalamus of the brain.

Early Stage

At the early stage of this disease, the individuals having HD will have lower body mass index when compared to the normal (Djousse et al., 2002). Some of the symptoms may include cognitive, motor and behavioural changes. Still people can maintain a normal lifestyle and can live independently.

Middle Stage

Behavioral symptoms occur even in the middle stage of HD which arises before the onset of motor symptoms. The affected individuals also experience problems in sexual behavior, shuddering motor control, and lack of motivation (Kirkwood et al., 2001). Eating becomes challenging, as the affected individual face the difficulty in swallowing due to their muscular movements. Speech and walking becomes difficult leading to choking at any time in some individuals (Roos, 2010).

Late Stage

In the later stage of the disease, the affected individuals even become mute (Roos, 2010). Most of the patients have trouble in urinating or become constipated. They eventually fall in death due to choking and heart failure. The affected individual will not be able to live independently (Table 1).

Table 1. Stages of Huntington's Disease

Stages	Symptoms
Early stage	Progressive emotional, psychiatric, weight loss, disturbance in wake-sleep cycle.
Middle stage	Alterations in sexual behavior, lack of motivation, problem in speech and walking.
Late stage	Progressive dementia, memory problems, poor dietary intake.

Diagnosis

The diagnosis for HD is based on neurological examinations which include predictive testing and neuroimaging and the affected individuals begin the signs and the symptoms before many years of diagnosing. Since the diagnosis can be made at several times, the symptoms during the early stage cannot be defined. The main symptoms includes motor symptoms, sensory symptoms, psychiatric symptoms and neuropsychological testing. The knowledgeable genetic test results, and the pre- and post-test counselling are essential components of HD diagnosis (Margolis et al., 2003). Positron Emission Tomography (PET) is useful in early diagnosis of HD. Patients with minimal neurologic symptoms and no obvious CT changes may be differentiated from normal persons with high accuracy by PET (Hayden et al., 1986). Presymptomatic diagnosis of several genetic disorders is now possible. It is used to determine whether an person is at greatly enhanced the risk of having inherited the gene for a particular disorder many years before symptoms are expected to arise and it can be performed on adults, children and even fetus in the womb (Brandt et al., 1989).

ANIMAL MODEL FOR HD

Animal model for HD have been used for the past two decades which is used to mimic the neuropathological and behavioural changes that is associated to the disease. The important models are the excitotoxic and 3-nitropropionic acids in which cognitive changes and motor have been reported. The major disadvantages are neurochemically induce lack of progressive changes which are the feature of HD. A transgenic mouse model for HD (R6/2 line) was developed in 1996. The R6/2 mouse carries the human HD gene with the expansion of 141-157 CAG repeats and these results in progressive neurologic phenotype. This includes stereotypic hind limb grooming and dyskinesias. These symptoms got poorer over following weeks with premature death reported over 10-13 weeks. The mouse shows neuropathological features such as development of intranuclear inclusions. This study indicates that the neuronal cell death cannot be indicated until late in the disorder. Therefore, the mouse is used not only for the study of neuropathology of HD, but also for testing the treatment for this disease.

CURRENT TREATMENT FOR HUNTINGTON DISEASE

Tetrabenazine (TBZ) is a dopamine depleting agent that is one of the powerful agents for reducing chorea (Frank et al., 2014). Speech or language therapy will be helpful for treating the problems relation to speech or swallowing. Occupational or physical therapy helps the individual to learn to control their movements. Fetal neural allografts could be associated with motor functional and cognitive improvements in patients with HD (Bachoud-Lévi et al., 2000). Olanzapine is a dopamine antagonist which is used for the treatment of motor and behavioural symptoms. High-dose Olanzapine is useful in grave choreatic attacks (Bonelli et al., 2002). The pathogenic pathways of HD are to be unravelled and offers target for the treatments. Amantadine is an anti-Glutamatergic drugs N-methyl-D-aspartic acid (NMDA) receptor antagonist and is commonly used in the treatment of extrapyramidal symptoms. It is recommended to start these drugs with a low dose and increase the dose with close monitoring of any side effects (Coppen et al., 2017). Recently, many of them have been focusing on anti-immunomodulatory and anti-inflammatory agents to fight against HD.

DISADVANTAGES OF CURRENT TREATMENT

Currently, available treatment is limited for suppressing chorea, the involuntary, irregular movements of the arms and legs that accompany HD, till now battling the mood altering aspects of the disorder with no disease modifying treatments available. The common side effects of TBZ include drowsiness, insomnia, and akathisia (Emma et al., 2000). It is prominent that the side effects vary slightly among different age groups: Younger patients experience more insomnia and even depression than the elderly patients and the older patients are more likely to develop Parkinsonism. The rare side effect includes diarrhea, hallucinations, headache, confusions, dizziness, hypotension, blurred vision, panic attack, etc. The extrapyramidal side effects of TBZ include Parkinson's disease, acute dystonia rarely neuroleptic malignant and syndrome akathisia (Diana et al., 2007).

Alternate Therapeutic Strategies

Conventional and existing treatment strategies for HD have either been associated with adverse effects or have failed to produce remedial results. Alternative strategies using combinatorial chemistry have also declined to yield favourable outcomes. Greater proportion of HD pharmacopoeia phase out during clinical trials due to inability of transformation from preclinical promise to clinical bedside (Jaspars et al., 2016). Prospecting of lead compounds with significant potentials against neurological disorders such from natural sources has gained wide prominence due to their promise of productive amelioration and curative effects with subsided adverse effects. The marine reservoir, with its huge abode of flora and fauna coupled with the microbiota has remained a great resource for the venture of bioactive compounds with immense industrial and therapeutic potentials. The huge biodiversity of the ocean offers the immense scope towards the exploration of novel bioactive molecules with distinctive structures and novel modes of action (Reen et al., 2015). The utilization of marine derived bioactive compounds towards the treatment of various biomedical conditions dates back to 1400 BC (Leoutsakos, 2004). Every year hundreds of new compounds are being discovered with already 28,000 potential compounds from marine sources explored till date (Blunt et al., 2015). The success rate of marine derived compounds with seven clinically approved drugs from a potential 28,175 lead molecular compounds (one drug from 4025 screened natural product) is approximately 2.5 fold better than the industrial approval of 1 in 10000 screened compounds (Gerwick and Moore, 2012). The scope of marine derived therapeutic agents against neurological disorders is quite high with 2 drugs already in various phases of clinical trials for schizophrenia and AD (Mayer et al., 2010). Emerging technological innovations such as sequencing and meta-analyses and upcoming omics concepts have revolutionized the discovery and exploration of marine based bioactive compounds and has facilitated high-throughput screening of compounds, previously considered extremely difficult (Rocha Martin et al., 2014). These alternative approaches have offered immense hope towards the development of potential lead candidate compounds against HD.

Marine Environment

Ocean covers more than 70% of the earth surface with exceptional diversity of nearly 2,210,000 species out of which only 200,000 are identified till now. Specifically, marine environment get adapted to severe physical and chemical circumstances (such as extreme pressure, low light, low temperature, higher salinity and oxygen in environment) for marine organisms that force the researchers towards the increase of diverse molecules with distinctive structural features with bioactive nature. Moreover, the marine system products are unexplored and wealthy source of natural products with a large collection of value in cosmetics, nutraceutical, and distinctive pharmaceutical activities (Subramani and Aalbersberg, 2012, Saravanan, 2014, Manigandan et al., 2015).

Marine diversity procured very different and diverse types of substances. Till now more than 30,000 new compounds are isolated (Zhang et al., 2012, Manigandan et al., 2015). Marine ecosystem is an embodiment of primary and secondary metabolites which provide numerous resources for human health and nutrition when compared to the terrestrial counterpart. Major marine nutraceutical compounds are polysaccharides, proteins, fatty acids, sterols and pigments are rich in aquatic resources (Pangestuti and Kim, 2011, Lordan et al., 2011, Kumar and Kim, 2013).

Marine Ascidians

Secondary metabolites from marine invertebrates have illustrated both cytotoxic activities, antibiotic agent and hence increased research for new drugs is needed (Sri Kumaran and Bragadeeswaran, 2012). Ascidians are conspicuous of marine fouling animal and benthic communities. Ascidians have become a hot topic for research and development both at home and aboard for its numerous active substances with potential activity (Bao ju et al., 2014). Few novel compounds are isolated from marine ascidians and the majority of which are amino acid derivatives has rich source of both biological active secondary metabolites and chemical diversity. The Sac-like filter feeding ascidians have been reported to be an important source for bioactive substance drug discovery (Figure 1). The tropical, colonial benthic species have discovered as a rich source of constituents with a pronounced pharmaceutical potential (Albert Koulman et al., 1990). Ascidians and its diversity has been the source of unique chemical compounds with the potential for development as pharmaceuticals cyclic peptides, amino acid-derived alkaloids, nutritional supplements, acetogenins cosmetics, fine chemicals molecular probes, enzymes, and agrochemicals.

Ascdians as Bioactive Sources for Huntington Disease

Many researchers interested that the development in isolation and chemical entity identification with the collaboration between chemists and pharmacologist are important determinants in the development of marine natural products research (Jimenez et al., 2003). Even today; the history of research and drug discovery dates back to more than 100 years. But, there is still a large requirement for innovative drugs. Only, a one third of all diseases can be treated efficiently.

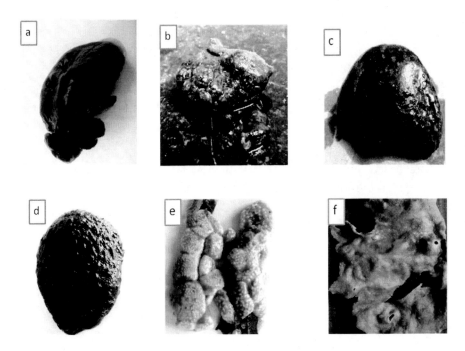

Figure 1. Some important ascidians diversity from the Gulf of Mannar, Southeast coast of India a) *Phallusia arabica* b) *Eudistoma* sp. c) *Botryllus* sp. d) *Polyglinum glabrum* e) *Didenmum* sp. f) *Lissoclinum bistratum.*

Nutritive Value of Ascidians

Tunicates have a high nutritional value and huge secondary metabolites reported from the different authors (Lee et al., 1995; Meenakshi, 2009; Choi et al., 2014). A majority number of solitary ascidians have been studied for their nutritive value, resulting that they are potentially healthy seafood high protein content and low in calories (Choi et al., 2006; Tamilselvi et al., 2010; Kang et al., 2011). Canover (1978) reported that tunicate ascidians have the high level of proteins, carbohydrates and lipids, when compared to other marine sessile benthic invertebrates. In some countries, mainly those of the far East and certain parts of the Mediterranean ascidians are consumed by man and are sufficient to merit an entry in the Food and Agricultural Organization, (FAO, 1964) year book of fisheries statistics. The commonly consumed species by the people are *Microcosmus hartmeyeri, M. sabatieri, M. vulgaris, Halocynthia aurantium, H. roretzi, Polycarpa pomaria, Pyura chilensis, Styela clava,* and *S. plicata. Halocynthia roretzi* contains a different types of vitamins like (E, B12, and C in particular), minerals (magnesium, phosphorus, iron, sodium, potassium, calcium, zinc, copper) and amino acids (folic acid, fatty acid, pantothenic acid, cholesterol). Ascidians are used as food in the form of various preparations in many parts of the world including Korea, Chile, Italy, Japan, France and other countries. The tunic of the pyurid ascidian *Microcosmus hartmeyeri* and mantle bodies of *H. auranlum* and *H. roretzi* are farmed and eaten in Japan (Nanri et al., 1992). In Europe, *Microcosmus sabatieri* and *M. vulgaris* are consumed whereas; *Pyura chilensis*is an important food item in Chile (Davis, 1995). The tunicates *Eudistoma bituminis* and *Cystodytes* violatinctus from the Indian Ocean are investigated for their phospholipid fatty acid content. The most abundant FA was the saturated ones (C10 - C18) and *Cystodytes violatinctus* contained considerable quantity of oleic acid. Both *E. bituminis* and *C. violatinctus* contained phytanic acid and Δ10-unsaturated FA, which had not previously been found in such organisms. The two tropical tunicates contained only trace amounts of PUFA which are usually predominant in this phylum (Viracaoundin et al., 2003). Kostetsky et al., 1983 discussed the Phospholipid composition of 13 Species of Tunicates. The edible ascidian *Halocynthia roretzi*, most popular in Japan and Korea, also has been studied in their FA profiles

(Kusaka et al., 1985; Vysotskii et al., 1992; Jeong et al., 1996). Several studies of phospholipids of some pelagic Tunicate of *Salpa thompsoni*, *Salpa thompsoni and Dolioletta gegenbauri* also have been undertaken (Mimura et al., 1986; Deibel et al., 1992; Pond et al., 1998). Harant (1951) reported that Microcosmus sulcatus and occasionally *Styela plicata*, *Polycarpa pomaria* are taken as food in Mediterranean, *Halocynthia roretzi* in Japan and *Styela clava* is cultured for food in Korea. Maraglino and de Stefano (1960) found that the flesh of *Microcosmus sulcatus* is almost as digestible as whole egg and has higher protein content. In Kyushu sea coast of Japan, tunic without the mantle bodies of *Microcosmus hartmeyeri* has been consumed during New Year celebrations, engagements etc. Boiling tunic is also sometimes served with vinegar. Van Name (1945) reported that *Pyura chilensis* is popular in South America as a food source.

There is rarity of information on nutritional quality of the ascidians of India. A preliminary work has been done by Meenakshi (1997) in few simple and colonial ascidians. Abdul Jaffar Ali (2004) reported the food value of simple ascidian, *Phallusia nigra.* Ananthan and co-workers in 2012 reported the high nutritive value 10 solitary and compound ascidians which showed high values of protein content of 3.8% to 20.01%, carbohydrate 2.2% to 8.29% and lipid content of 1.05% to 2.97%. Srikumaran and Bragadeeswaran, (2014) discussed the nutritional values of two the colonial ascidians *E. viride* and *D. psammathodes* are collected from southeast coast of India. In these two ascidians has a nutritional composition of carbohydrate, protein, lipid, fatty acids and amino acid of lysine, leucine, isoleucine, methionine, threonine, histidine and arginine shows high amount in *E. viride* and *D. psammathodes* tissues. Iyappan and Ananthan, (2016) reported the simple ascidian *Phallusia nigra* has contain the protein, carbohydrate, lipids discussed the different seasons and they have reported the protein content is found to be higher level. Bragadeeswaran et al., (2010) discussed *Polyclinum madrasensis* is collected from Tuticorin coast. The protein content was showed 790 µg/

mL of crude and it content clearly indicated the *P. madrasensis* have the higher amount of proteins. Meenakshi et al., (2012) reported the simple ascidians of *Microcosmus Exasperatus* were collected from southeast of India. In these study ascidians has reported vitamins D3, K water soluble vitamin riboflavin, thiamine and flavonoids are reported. It could be serving as an important source of beneficial nutrients.

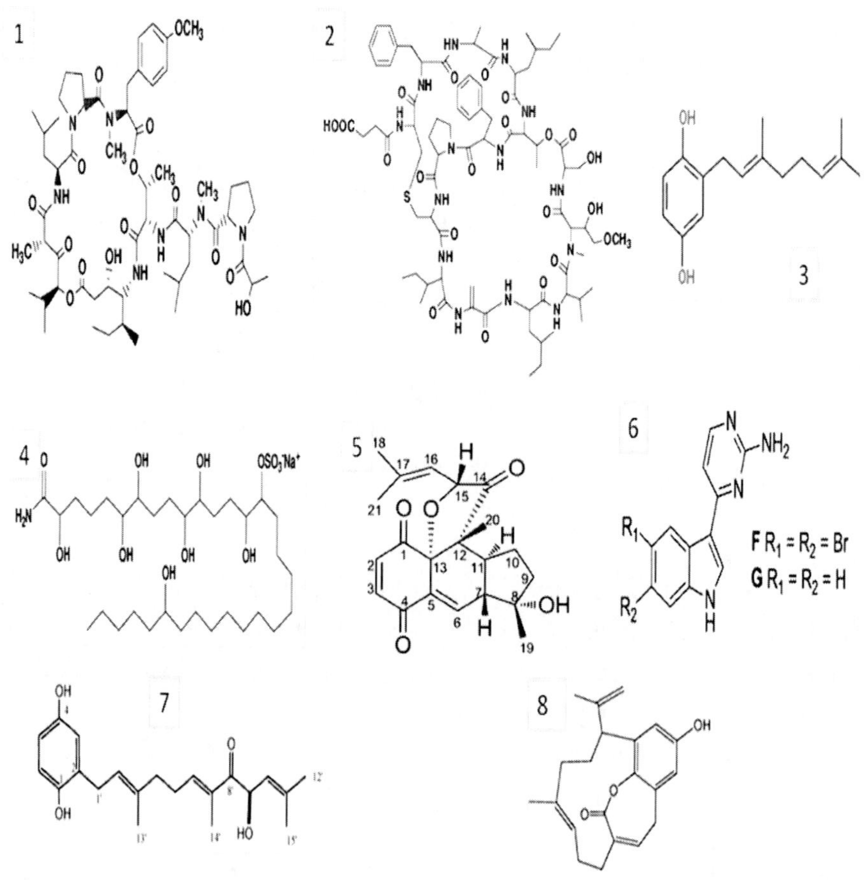

Figure 2. (Continued).

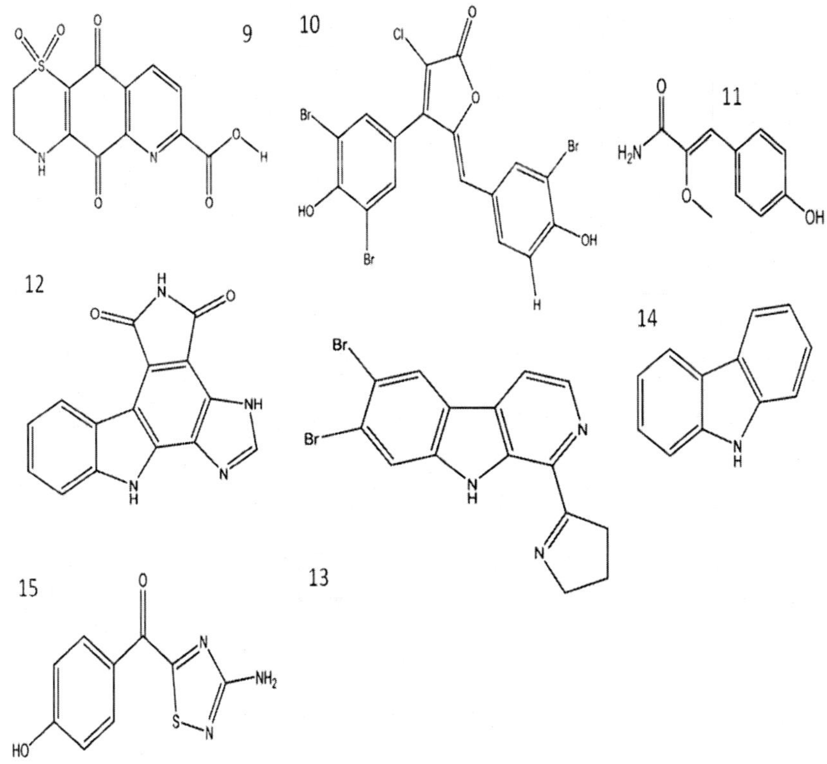

Ascdians as Bioactive Sources for Huntington Disease

Figure 2. Important chemical structure derived from ascidians 1) Didemnin B 2) Vitilevuamide 3) Geranylhydroquinone 4) Turbinamide A 5) Rossinone B 6) Meridianins F-G 7) Rossinone A 8) Floresolides B 9) Ascidiathiazone A 10) Rubrolide O 11) Botryllamide L 12) Granulatimide 13) Eudistomin V 14) β-Carboline 15) Polycarpathiamines A.

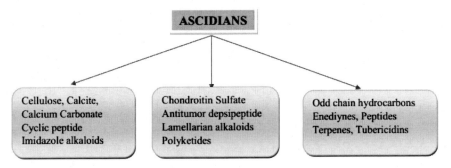

Figure 4. Important Biomaterial isolated from the ascidians.

Anti-Infective Peptides Derived from Ascidians

Halocyamine A and B are two antimicrobial tetrapeptides isolated from the ascidian *Halocynthia roretzi*. Halocyamine A has been reported to inhibit the growth of yeast, *Escherichia coli* (Azumi et al., 1990a) and the other marine bacteria *Achromobacter aquamarinus* and *Pseudomonas perfectomarinus* (Azumi et al., 1990b, Azumi et al., 1990c). A novel antimicrobial peptide, Dicunthaurin derived from hemocytes of a tunicate, *Halocynthia aurantium*. Dicynthaurin's have the broad-spectrum activity included *Escherichia coli*, *Staphylococcus aureus*, *Listeria monocytogenes*, *Pseudomonas aeruginosa* and *Micrococcus luteus*, (Lee et al., 2001). Jang et al., (2001) reported Halocidin, a new antimicrobial peptide isolated from the hemocytes of tunicate *Halocynthia aurantium*. The native peptide had a molecular weight of 3443 Da and comprised two different subunits containing 15 residues (ALLHHGLNCAKGVLA) and 18 amino acid residues (WLNALLHHGLNCAKGVLA) which were linked covalently by a single cystine disulfide bond. Halocidin, it was confirmed that congeners of the 18 residue monomer were more active than those of the 15 residue monomer against *methicillin-resistant Staphylococcus aureus* and *multidrug-resistant Pseudomonas aeruginosa*. Richard et al., (2009) reported two ascidian peptides - halocyntin and papillosin derived from *H. papillosa* active against both the gram positive and gram negative bacteria, with a higher antimicrobial activity for papillosin. New lipopeptides, peptidolipins B–F derived from the associated organisms of *Nocardia* sp. isolated from the ascidian *Trididemnum orbiculatum* (Thomas et al., 2012) and Peptidolipins B and E revealed moderate antibacterial activity against methicillin-resistant *Staphylococcus aureus* and methicillin-sensitive *Staphylococcus aureus*. Hirsch et al., 1989 reported atypical diketopiperazine peptide named Etzionin reported from an unidentified Red Sea tunicate. It is antifungal metabolite and inhibited the growth of *Aspergillus nidulans* and *C. albicans* with MIC of 3-12.5μg/ml. Clavanins A-D, α-helical AMPs of 23 residues metabolites identified in the solitary tunicate *Styela clava* and it has showed antifungal activity against *C. albicans* with MIC 5-20 μg/ml (Lee et al., 1997) and the same genus A His-rich, 23-

residue APM named clavaspirin was identified (Lee et al., 2001). A clavaspirin synthetic peptide shows the antibacterial against Gram-positive and – negative bacteria as well as antifungal against *C. albicans* with MIC ~5-10μg/ml. Cai et al., 2008 reported that Tunichromes are small peptides containing one or more dehydrodopa-derived units isolated from *Ascidia nigra* hemocytes and the similar study was done three tunichromes have also been isolated from the blood cells of *Ascidia nigra* (An-1, An-2, An-3) (Sugumaran et al., 2012). Tunichromes shows potent activity against the gram-positive human pathogen Enterococcus sp. (MICs = 0.1 μg/mL) (Cai et al., 2008). Cadiolides C–F, butenolide metabolites isolated from the tunicate *Pseudodistoma antinboja* and it has shows significant activity of Gram-positive bacteria (*B. Subtilis*, *S. epidermidis*, *S. aureus* and *Kocuria rhizophila*) MIC = 0.2–12.5 μg/mL and also methicillin-sensitive *S. aureus* (MSSA) and methicillin-resistant *S. aureus* (MRSA) ranging from 0.13 to 4 μg/mL of MICs (Wang et al., 2012).

Antioxidant and Anti-Inflammatory Properties of Ascidians

Antioxidants play a vital role in the prevention of various chronic diseases of Alzheimer disease, cancer, diabetes, heart diseases, hypertension, stroke and other diseases. The freeze-dried ascidian is well known to have antioxidant compounds such as quinone derivatives these had the superoxide scavenging activity. The freeze-dried powder of the ascidians may be useful for an addition of antioxidative assets to foods and pharmaceutical applications (Inanami et al., 2011).

Jumeri and Sang (2011) reported enzymatic hydrolysates of Alcalase (AH), pepsin (PH), Thermoase (TH), two fractions of F1 and F2 isolated from solitary tunicate, *Styela clava*. Fraction F2 with a lower molecular weight (3.6 ± 0.1 kDa) had higher ABTS and DPPH radical scavenging activities than F1 (5.0 ± 1.0 kDa), with IC_{50} values of 11.4 and 227.5 μg/mL, respectively. These solitary tunicate hydrolysates have the excellent antioxidant properties. Belmiro et al., (2009) reported the dermatan sulfate, heparin purified from the Brazilian ascidian *Styela plica* and it has showed the significantly decreased lymphocyte and macrophage recruitment as well as TNF-α, TGF-β, and VEGF production in the inflamed rat colon *in vivo* rat colitis model (8 mg/kg per day). It results indicated that the Styela plica have the anti-inflammatory properties. Two new tricyclic thiazine-containing quinolinequinone alkaloids, ascidiathiazones A and B were isolated from *Aplidium* sp., New Zealand ascidian coast. These Compounds showed a potential inhibition against human neutrophils (IC50 1.55, 0.44 µM), respectively (Pearce et al., 2007). Pearce et al., (2007a) reported a new member of the rubrolide family of Rubrolide O was isolated from the *Synoicum* sp. collected in New Zealand coast. Rubrolide O showed a significant inhibition against human neutrophil free radical release (IC_{50} 35µM).

New anti-inflammatory meroterpenoids, 2-geranyl-6-methoxy-1, 4-hydroquinone-4-sulfate, chromenol and quinol and scabellone B reported from the New Zealand ascidian *Aplidium scabellum* and it has showed a moderate potent anti-inflammatory activity (IC_{50} 21, 125, 92 and 0.2 µM), and selective ability to inhibit neutrophil respiratory burst proves that meroterpenoid sulfates may have possible for developing novel marine drugs for management of inflammation (Chan et al., 2011).

Shanmuga Priya et al., (2016) showed ethanolic extract of *Eudistoma viride* collected from the southeast coast of India and it showing the capable antioxidant potential against free radical induced oxidative damage by DPPH method. The four extracts of simple ascidian *Phallusia nigra* collected from the Tuticorin coastal waters. The extracts exhibited strong antioxidant DPPH radical scavenging activity of 0.1984 compare to the standard ascorbic acid (Shanmuga Priya et al., 2015). Sao et al., (1989) reported two novel hydroquinone and one novel chromene from the extracts of the colonial tunicate *Amaroucium multiplicatum* and it has shows the more potent than two standard antioxidants in the inhibitory effects on lipid peroxide formation in rat liver microsomes and on soybean 15-lipoxygenase antioxidants. Ticar et al., (2013) discussed ascidian tunic carotenoids results shows the mouse macrophage cell line (RAW 264.7) and the DPPH radical scavenging activity of carotenoids was 47.2% at 100 mg/mL. It also has a potential reducing power (1.025) comparable with ascorbic acid (1.584) and carotenoids have the antioxidants and anti-inflammatory properties.

Aknin et al., (1999) reported the three hydroquinone compounds were isolated the Indian ocean tunicate *Aplidium savignyi* and these compounds to be an interesting source known to be more potent antioxidants. Appleton et al., (2009) isolated two new ascidian-derived meroterpenoid metabolites Rossinones A and B from an Antarctic collection of the ascidian *Aplidium* species and anti-inflammatory activity in an *in vitro* anti-inflammatory assay with activated human peripheral blood neutrophils by inhibiting superoxide production. However, in the DPPH radical scavenging assay, 18 and 20 were found to be inactive (at doses up to 30 µM), indicating that these rossinones are considerably less effective as superoxide scavengers than as suppressors of superoxide production by neutrophils. These compounds have exhibit anti-inflammatory, antiviral and antiproliferative activities. The dihydroxystyrylguanidine alkaloid tubastrine, five new dimers, orthidines A–E and the biosynthetically unrelated 1, 14-spermine-dihomovanillamide (orthidine F,) were isolated from the New Zealand ascidian *Aplidium orthium*. Compounds tubastrine, orthidines A–C and E and orthidine F inhibited the in vitro production of superoxide by PMA-stimulated human neutrophils in a dose-dependent manner with IC_{50} of 10–36 mM and it's providing further evidence that intervention of neutrophil-mediated processes for potential anti-inflammatory agents (Pearce et al., 2008).

Meenakshi et al., (2013) discussed the GC-MS analysis of ethanolic extract of *Phallusia nigra* showed compounds with antioxidant properties like 2-Piperidinone, Benzeneacetamide, Phenol 3-pentadecyl, n-Hexadecanoic acid, (Z,Z,Z)- phenylmethyl ester of 6,9,12-Octadecatrienoic acid, Tetradecanoic acid, (z)-phenylmethyl ester of 9- Octadecenoic acid, Cholesterol, Cholestan-3-ol and 3-hydroxy-,(3a,17a)-Spiro [androst-5-ene-17,1' -cyclobutan]-2' – one and other compounds. Methanolic extract of *Phallusia nigra* collected from Tuticorin Port, Tamil Nadu and it is preliminary chemical screening showed the presence of alkaloids, terpenoids, flavonoids, glycosides, phenolic compounds, tannins etc., which may possible act as antioxidants. Further development of *Phallusia nigra* is the treatment of inflammatory diseases (Gopalakrishnan et al., 2013).

Krishnaiah et al., (2004) have reported lamellarins A,C and E and known lamellarin Alkaloids, lamellarins M, K, lamellarins U, C-diacetate,, K-diacetate, K-triacetate, I, and X-triacetates from *Didemnum obscurum* collected at southeast coast of India. Compounds, lamellarins C and K-triacetate showed a more potent activity (IC_{50} - 3.28, 2.96 mM) than isolated biomolecules. The lamellarins K, U, and I, lamellarin C-diacetate lamellarin gamma, and lamellarin gamma-monoacetate have the Antioxidant properties. Appleton et al., (2002) reported Kottamides A-D, novel 2, 2, 5-trisubstituted imidazolone-containing alkaloids, were isolated from the New Zealand endemic ascidian *Pycnoclavella kottae* and the kottamides D exhibited potent anti-inflammatory (IC_{50} 2-200µM). Rajesh and Murugan, (2013) reported the anti-inflammatory activity of methanol extracted from the ascidian *Eudistoma virde* was exhibited modest anti-inflammatory activity at a range of concentrations up to 200 mg/kg compare to the positive control Diclofenac. The ethanolic extract of simple ascidian *Phallusia nigra* and it has shows 0.60 mg/ml concentration significant reduction in weight of body. The results inhibited tumor growth by 52.69% compared to 47.12% in the standard drug and these extract reported to have the Immunomodulatory activity (Meenakshi et al., 2013). Ananthan and Iyappan (2014) discussed the ethanol extract of *Didemnum albidum* examined the human monocytic cell line (RAW 264.7.) The extract from ascidian *Didemnum albidum* showed immunomodulatory activity by activated RAW cells to produce tumor necrosis factor (TNF)-α and interleukin (IL)-1β and nitric oxide (NO). It also inhibited the growth of RAW and induce morphological changes in adherent monocytic cells into macrophages.

CONCLUSION

Neurological disorders are predominantly associated with ageing and the marine environment with its longest standing timeline could provide valuable outcomes to counter the threat of these emerging threats. The present attempt delivers an alternate strategy of marine ascidians as potential sources of bioactive compounds with biomedical applications. The ascidians and tunicates have been reported with numerous unique molecules and compounds with novel structures and proven preclinical and preliminary biomedical activities. This chapter also draws its focus towards the utilization of novel bioactive molecules from tunicates and ascidians towards the neurologic genetic disorder, HD. The ascidians produce a wide variety of metabolites such as alkaloids, diterpenes, polyketides, peptides and polysaccharides with pronounced anticancer, anti-inflammatory, antioxidant and antiviral activities. Ascidians also have demonstrated commendable ameliorative and curative activates against neurological disorders. Though numerous ascidians have been explored for their biomedical activities, the existing pharmacopoeia warrants the exploitation of bioactive molecules with novel and unique structures from marine ascidians for the development of lead candidate compounds for HD, in future.

ACKNOWLEDGMENTS

The first author gratefully acknowledged to Council of Scientific & Industrial Research (CSIR) - New Delhi, India by for providing Senior Research Fellowship.

REFERENCES

[1] Roos RA. Huntington's Disease: A Clinical Review. *Orphanet Journal of Rare Diseases.* 2010 Dec;5(1):40.

[2] Djousse LM, Knowlton B, Cupples LA, Marder K, Shoulson I, Myers RH. Weight Loss in Early Stage of Huntington's Disease. *Neurology.* 2002 Nov 12;59(9):1325-30.

[3] Kingma EM, van Duijn E, Timman R, van der Mast RC, Roos RA. Behavioural Problems in Huntington's Disease using the Problem Behaviours Assessment. *General Hospital Psychiatry*. 2008 Mar 1;30(2):155-61.

[4] Kirkwood SC, Su JL, Conneally PM, Foroud T. Progression of Symptoms in the Early and Middle Stages of Huntington Disease. *Archives of Neurology*. 2001 Feb 1;58(2):273-8.

[5] Myers RH. Huntington's Disease Genetics. *NeuroRx*. 2004 Apr 1;1(2):255-62.

[6] Li SH, Li XJ. Huntingtin–Protein Interactions and the Pathogenesis of Huntington's Disease. *TRENDS in Genetics*. 2004 Mar 1;20(3):146-54.

[7] Schulte J, Littleton JT. The Biological Function of the Huntingtin Protein and Its Relevance to Huntington's Disease Pathology. *Current Trends in Neurology*. 2011 Jan 1;5:65.

[8] Ross CA, Tabrizi SJ. Huntington's Disease: From Molecular Pathogenesis to Clinical Treatment. *The Lancet Neurology*. 2011 Jan 1;10(1):83-98.

[9] Margolis RL, Ross CA. Diagnosis of Huntington Disease. *Clinical Chemistry*. 2003 Oct 1;49(10):1726-32.

[10] Hayden MR, Martin WR, Stoessl AJ, Clark C, Hollenberg S, Adam MJ, Ammann W, Harrop R, Rogers J, Ruth T, Sayre C. Positron Emission Tomography in the Early Diagnosis of Huntington's Disease. *Neurology*. 1986 Jul 1;36(7):888.

[11] Brandt J, Quaid KA, Folstein SE, Garber P, Maestri NE, Abbott MH, Slavney PR, Franz ML, Kasch L, Kazazian HH. Presymptomatic Diagnosis of Delayed-Onset Disease with Linked DNA Markers: The Experience in Huntington's Disease. *JAMA*. 1989 Jun 2;261(21): 3108-14.

[12] Jankovic J. Dopamine Depleters in the Treatment of Hyperkinetic Movement Disorders. *Expert Opinion on Pharmacotherapy*. 2016 Dec 11;17(18):2461-70.

[13] Bachoud-Lévi AC, Rémy P, Nǵuyen JP, Brugières P, Lefaucheur JP, Bourdet C, Baudic S, Gaura V, Maison P, Haddad B, Boissé MF.

Motor and Cognitive Improvements in Patients with Huntington's Disease after Neural Transplantation. *The Lancet.* 2000 Dec 9;356(9246):1975-9.

[14] Landles C, Bates GP. Huntingtin and the Molecular Pathogenesis of Huntington's Disease: Fourth in Molecular Medicine Review Series. *EMBO Reports.* 2004 Oct 1;5(10):958-63.

[15] Pringsheim T, Wiltshire K, Day L, Dykeman J, Steeves T, Jette N. The Incidence and Prevalence of Huntington's Disease: A Systematic Review and Meta-Analysis. *Movement Disorders.* 2012 Aug 1;27(9): 1083-91.

[16] Bossy-Wetzel E, Schwarzenbacher R, Lipton SA. Molecular Pathways to Neurodegeneration. *Nature Medicine.* 2004 Jul;10(7): S2.

[17] Ferrer I, Goutan E, Marın C, Rey MJ, Ribalta T. Brain-Derived Neurotrophic Factor in Huntington Disease. *Brain Research.* 2000 Jun 2;866(1-2):257-61.

[18] Zuccato C, Ciammola A, Rigamonti D, Leavitt BR, Goffredo D, Conti L, MacDonald ME, Friedlander RM, Silani V, Hayden MR, Timmusk T. Loss of Huntingtin-Mediated BDNF Gene Transcription in Huntington's Disease. *Science.* 2001 Jul 20;293(5529):493-8.

[19] Imarisio S, Carmichael J, Korolchuk V, Chen CW, Saiki S, Rose C, Krishna G, Davies JE, Ttofi E, Underwood BR, Rubinsztein DC. Huntington's Disease: From Pathology and Genetics to Potential Therapies. *Biochemical Journal.* 2008 Jun 1;412(2):191-209.

[20] Hobart W. W., Joseph J. B., & Thomas C. W. Molecular Aspects of Huntington's Disease. *Journal of Neuroscience Research.* 1998, 54, 301–308.

[21] Lin MT, Beal MF. Mitochondrial Dysfunction and Oxidative Stress in Neurodegenerative Diseases. *Nature.* 2006 Oct 18;443(7113):787.

[22] Cox SM, McKellin W. 'There's this Thing in Our Family': Predictive Testing and the Construction of Risk For Huntington Disease. *Sociology of Health & Illness.* 1999 Sep 1;21(5):622-46.

[23] Bonelli RM, Niederwieser G, Tribl GG, Költringer P. High-Dose Olanzapine in Huntington's Disease. *International clinical psychopharmacology.* 2002 Mar 1;17(2):91.

[24] Childs, E. (2010). Tetrabenazine. *Encyclopedia of Psychopharmacology.* Springer Berlin Heidelberg. 1306-1306.

[25] Paleacu D. Tetrabenazine in the Treatment of Huntington's Disease. *Neuropsychiatric Disease and Treatment.* 2007 Oct;3(5):545.

[26] Brotherton A, Campos L, Rowell A, Zoia V, Simpson SA, Rae D. Nutritional Management of Individuals with Huntington's Disease: Nutritional Guidelines. *Neurodegenerative Disease Management.* 2012 Feb;2(1):33-43.

[27] Chen CM, Lin YS, Wu YR, Chen P, Tsai FJ, Yang CL, Tsao YT, Chang W, Hsieh IS, Chern Y, Soong BW. High Protein Diet and Huntington's Disease. *PloS One.* 2015 May 19;10(5):e0127654.

[28] Coppen EM, Roos RA. Current Pharmacological Approaches to Reduce Chorea in Huntington's Disease. *Drugs.* 2017 Jan 1;77(1):29-46.

[29] White JK, Auerbach W, Duyao MP, Vonsattel JP, Gusella JF, Joyner AL, MacDonald ME. Huntingtin is Required For Neurogenesis and Is Not Impaired by the Huntington's Disease CAG Expansion. *Nature Genetics.* 1997 Dec;17(4):404.

[30] Andrews Thomasin C. & David J. Brooks. (1998). Advances in the Understanding of Early Huntington's Disease Using the Functional Imaging Techniques of PET and SPET." *Molecular medicine today* 4(12), 532-539.

[31] Jaspars M, De Pascale D, Andersen JH, Reyes F, Crawford AD, Ianora A. The Marine Biodiscovery Pipeline and Ocean Medicines of Tomorrow. *Journal of the Marine Biological Association of the United Kingdom.* 2016 Feb;96(1):151-8.

[32] Reen FJ, Gutiérrez-Barranquero JA, Dobson AD, Adams C, O'Gara F. Emerging Concepts Promising New Horizons For Marine Bio-Discovery and Synthetic Biology. *Marine drugs.* 2015 May 13;13 (5):2924-54.

[33] Leoutsakos V. *A short History of the Thyroid Gland.* Hormones-Athens-. 2004;3:268-71.

[34] Blunt JW, Copp B, Keyzers RA, Munro MH, Prinsep MR. *Marine Natural Products.*

[35] Gerwick WH, Moore BS. Lessons from the Past and Charting the Future of Marine Natural Products Drug Discovery and Chemical Biology. *Chemistry & Biology.* 2012 Jan 27;19(1):85-98.

[36] Mayer AM, Glaser KB, Cuevas C, Jacobs RS, Kem W, Little RD, McIntosh JM, Newman DJ, Potts BC, Shuster DE. The Odyssey of Marine Pharmaceuticals: A Current Pipeline Perspective. *Trends in Pharmacological Sciences.* 2010 Jun 1;31(6):255-65.

[37] Rocha-Martin J, Harrington C, Dobson AD, O'Gara F. Emerging Strategies and Integrated Systems Microbiology Technologies For Biodiscovery of Marine Bioactive Compounds. *Marine Drugs.* 2014 Jun 10;12(6):3516-59.

[38] Kumaran NS, Bragadeeswaran S, Balasubramanian T, Meenakshi VK. Bioactivity Potential of Extracts From Ascidian Lissoclinum Fragile. *African Journal of Pharmacy and Pharmacology.* 2012 Jul 8;6(25):1854-9.

[39] Koulman A, Pruijn LM, Sandstra TS, Woerdenbag HJ, Pras N. The Pharmaceutical Exploration of Cold Water Ascidians From the Netherlands: A Possible Source of New Cytotoxic Natural Products. *Journal of Biotechnology.* 1999 Apr 30;70(1-3):85-8.

[40] Jimenez PC, Fortier SC, Lotufo TM, Pessoa C, Moraes ME, de Moraes MO, Costa-Lotufo LV. Biological Activity in Extracts of Ascidians (*Tunicata, Ascidiacea*) from the Northeastern Brazilian Coast. *Journal of Experimental Marine Biology and Ecology.* 2003 Feb 26;287(1):93-101.

[41] Saravanan R. Isolation of Low-Molecular-Weight Heparin/Heparan Sulfate from Marine Sources. In *Advances in Food and Nutrition Research 2014* Jan 1 (Vol. 72, pp. 45-60). Academic Press.

[42] Subramani R, Aalbersberg W. Marine Actinomycetes: An Ongoing Source of Novel Bioactive Metabolites. *Microbiological Research.* 2012 Dec 20;167(10):571-80.

[43] Karthik R, Saravanan R. Marine Carbohydrate Based Therapeutics for Alzheimer Disease-Mini Review. *Journal of Neurology and Neuroscience.* 2015;6(5).
[44] Zhang C, Li X, Kim SK. Application of Marine Biomaterials for Nutraceuticals and Functional Foods. *Food Science and Biotechnology.* 2012 Jun 1;21(3):625-31.
[45] Pangestuti R, Kim SK. Neuroprotective Effects of Marine Algae. *Marine Drugs.* 2011 May 10;9(5):803-18.
[46] Lordan S, Ross RP, Stanton C. Marine Bioactives as Functional Food Ingredients: Potential to Reduce the Incidence of Chronic Diseases. *Marine Drugs.* 2011 Jun 14;9(6):1056-100.
[47] Senthilkumar K, Kim SK. Marine Invertebrate Natural Products for Anti-Inflammatory and Chronic Diseases. *Evidence-Based Complementary and Alternative Medicine.* 2013;2013.
[48] Sri Kumaran, N. & Bragadeeswaran, S. Nutritional Composition of the Colonial Ascidian *Eudistoma Viride* and *Didemnum Psammathodes. Biosciences Biotechnology Research Asia,* 2014, Vol. 11 Spl. Edn. 1, 331-338.
[49] Nanri K, Ogawa J, Nishikawa T. Tunic of a Pyurid Ascidian *Microcosmus Hartmeyeri* Oka is Eaten Locally in Japan. *Nanki Seibutu.* 1992;34(2):135.
[50] Davis AR. Over-Exploitation of *Pyura Chilensis* (Ascidiacea) in Southern Chile: The Urgent Need to Establish Marine Reserves. *Revista Chilena de Historia Natural.* 1995 Mar 1;68(1):7-1.
[51] Iyappan K, Ananthan G. Antibiotic Efficacy and Biochemical Composition of Ascidian, *Phallusia Nigra* (Savigny, 1816) from the Palk Bay, Southeast Coast of India.
[52] Bragadeeswaran S, Ganesan K, Prabhu K, Balasubramanian T, Venkateswarlu Y, Meenakshi VK. Pharmacological Properties of Biofouling Ascidian, *Polyclinum Madrasensis* Sebastian, 1952 from Tuticorin Coast of India. *Advances in Environmental Biology.* 2010 May 1:138-47.

[53] Packiam CS, Margret RJ, Meenakshi VK. Spectrophotometric Studies of a Simple Ascidian *Ascidia Sydneiensis*. *Acta Chimica Pharmaceutica Indica.* 2015;5(2):68-72.

[54] Kostetsky EY, Naumenko NV, Gerasimenko NI. Phospholipid-Composition of Tunicates. *Biologiya Morya-Marine Biology.* 1983 Jan 1(2):51-6.

[55] Kusaka H., Kaga Y., Saiki Y., Ohta S. (1985). Seasonal Changes in the Fatty Acid Composition of Ascidian Lipids. *Journal of Japan Oil Chemists' Society.* 20;34(4):262-70.

[56] Vysotskii M. V. n-3 Polyunsaturated Fatty Acids in Lipids of Ascidian *Halocynthia roretzi*. *International Information System for The Agricultural Science And Technology*, 1992, 58(5):953-8.

[57] Jeong BY, Ohshima T, Koizumi C. Hydrocarbon Chain Distribution of Ether Phospholipids of the Ascidian *Halocynthia Roretzi* and the Sea Urchin *Strongylocentrotus Intermedius. Lipids.* 1996 Jan 1;31(1 Part1):9-18.

[58] Mimura T, Okabe M, Satake M, Nakanishi T, Inada A, Fujimoto Y, Hata F, Matsumura Y, Ikekawa N. Fatty Acids and Sterols of the Tunicate, *Salpa Thompsoni*, From the Antarctic Ocean: Chemical Composition and Hemolytic Activity. *Chemical and Pharmaceutical Bulletin.* 1986 Nov 25;34(11):4562-8.

[59] Deibel D, Cavaletto JF, Riehl M, Gardner WS. Lipid and Lipid Class Content of the Pelagic Tunicate *Oikopleura Vanhoeffeni*. *Marine Ecology Progress Series.* 1992 Nov 12:297-302.

[60] Pond DW, Sargent JR. Lipid Composition of the Pelagic Tunicate *Dolioletta Gegenbauri* (Tunicata, Thaliacea). *Journal of Plankton Research.* 1998 Jan 1;20(1):169-74.

[61] Viracaoundin I, Barnathan G, Gaydou EM, Aknin M. Phospholipid FA from Indian Ocean Tunicates *Eudistoma Bituminis* and *Cystodytes Violatinctus. Lipids*. 2003 Jan 1;38(1):85-8.

[62] Meenakshi VK, Gomathy S, Senthamarai S, Paripooranaselvi M, Chamundeswari KP. Analysis of Vitamins by HPLC and Phenolic Compounds, Flavonoids by HPTLC in *Microcosmus Exasperatus*. *European Journal of Zoological Research.* 2012;1(4):105-10.

[63] Lee KH, Hong BI, Jung BC, Cho HS, Park CS, Jea YG. Seasonal Variations of Nutrients in Warty Sea Squirt (*Styela Clava*). *Journal of The Korean Society of Food and Nutrition* (Korea Republic). 1995.

[64] Lambert G, Karney RC, Rhee WY, Carman MR. Wild and Cultured Edible Tunicates: A Review. *Management of Biological Invasions*. 2016;7(1):59-66.

[65] Choi DL, Jee BY, Choi HJ, Hwang JY, Kim JW, Berthe FC. First Report on Histology and Ultrastructure of an Intrahemocytic Para-Myxean Parasite (IPP) from Tunicate *Halocynthia Roretzi* in Korea. *Diseases of Aquatic Organisms*. 2006;72(1):65-9.

[66] Cho ND, Zeng J, Choi BD, Ryu HS. Shelf Life of Bottled Sea Squirt *Halocynthia Roretzi* Meat Packed in Vegetable Oil (BSMO). *Fisheries and Aquatic Sciences*. 2014 Mar 31;17(1):37-46.

[67] Tamilselvi M, Sivakumar V, Abdul Jaffar Ali H, Thilaga RD. Preparation of Pickle from *Herdmania Pallida*, Simple Ascidian. *World Journal of Dairy & Food Sciences*. 2010;5(1):88-92.

[68] Kang CK, Choy EJ, Lee WC, Kim NJ, Park HJ, Choi KS. Physiological Energetics and Gross Biochemical Composition of the Ascidian *Styela Clava* Cultured in Suspension in a Temperate Bay of Korea. *Aquaculture*. 2011 Sep 1;319(1-2):168-77.

[69] Ananthan G, Karthikeyan MM, Selva PA, Raghunathan C. Studies on the Seasonal Variations in the Proximate Composition of Ascidians from the Palk Bay, Southeast Coast of India. *Asian Pacific Journal of Tropical Biomedicine*. 2012 Oct 1;2(10):793-7.

[70] Harant, H. Les Tuniciers comestibies Atti del 11 congresso Inter. *Nazionvale d' Igiene di Medicina Mediterranca Palermo*, 1951, 1-3.

[71] Lambert CC, Lambert G. Non-indigenous Ascidians in Southern California Harbors and Marinas. *Marine Biology*. 1998 Mar 1;130(4):675-88.

[72] Margalino G, Destefano M. Contributo Alla Conoscenza Della Digeribilita Delle Ascidie Eduli. *Thalassia Jonica*. 1960;3:69-78. [*Contribution to the Knowledge of the Edibility of Edible Ascidians*. Thalassia Jonica]

[73] Kim SM. Antioxidant and Anticancer Activities of Enzymatic Hydrolysates of Solitary Tunicate (*Styela Clava*). *Food Science and Biotechnology*. 2011 Aug 1;20(4):1075.

[74] Belmiro CL, Castelo-Branco MT, Melim LM, Schanaider A, Elia C, Madi K, Pavão MS, de Souza HS. Unfractionated Heparin and New Heparin Analogues from Ascidians (Chordate-Tunicate) Ameliorate Colitis in Rats. *Journal of Biological Chemistry*. 2009 Apr 24;284 (17):11267-78.

[75] Shanmuga Priya, D., Sankaravadivu, S. & Kohila Subathra Christy, H. (2016). Antioxidant Activity of a Colonial Ascidian *Eudistoma Viride* using DPPH Method. *Ejpmr* 3(8), 427-429.

[76] Chan ST, Pearce AN, Januario AH, Page MJ, Kaiser M, McLaughlin RJ, Harper JL, Webb VL, Barker D, Copp BR. Anti-Inflammatory and Antimalarial Meroterpenoids from the New Zealand Ascidian *Aplidium Scabellum*. *The Journal of Organic Chemistry*. 2011 Oct 3;76(21):9151-6.

[77] Shanmuga Priya, D., Christy Kohila Subathra, H. & Sankaravadivu, S, et al., (2015). Antioxidant Activity of the Simple Ascidian *Phallusia nigra* of Thoothukudi Coast. *International Journal of Pharmaceutical Chemistry*, vol 05 (12).

[78] Inanami O, Yamamori T, Shionoya H, Kuwabara M. Antioxidant Activity of Quinone-Derivatives from Freeze-dried Powder of the Ascidians. In *The Biology of Ascidians* 2001 (pp. 457-462). Springer, Tokyo.

[79] Aknin M, Dayan TL, Rudi A, Kashman Y, Gaydou EM. Hydroquinone Antioxidants from the Indian Ocean Tunicate *Aplidium Savignyi*. *Journal of Agricultural and Food Chemistry*. 1999 Oct 18;47(10):4175-7.

[80] Sato A, Shindo T, Kasanuki N, Hasegawa K. Antioxidant Metabolites from the Tunicate *Amaroucium multiplicatum*. *Journal of Natural Products*. 1989 Sep;52(5):975-81.

[81] Appleton DR, Chuen CS, Berridge MV, Webb VL, Copp BR. Rossinones A and B, Biologically Active Meroterpenoids from the

Antarctic Ascidian, Aplidium Species. *The Journal of Organic Chemistry.* 2009 Oct 29;74(23):9195-8.

[82] Pearce AN, Chia EW, Berridge MV, Maas EW, Page MJ, Harper JL, Webb VL, Copp BR. Orthidines A–E, Tubastrine, 3, 4-Dimethoxyphenethyl-B-Guanidine, and 1, 14-Sperminedihom-Ovanillamide: Potential Anti-Inflammatory Alkaloids Isolated from the New Zealand Ascidian *Aplidium Orthium* That Act as Inhibitors of Neutrophil Respiratory Burst. *Tetrahedron.* 2008 Jun 9;64(24):5748-55.

[83] Gopalakrishnan S, Meenakshi VK, Shanmugapriya D. Anti-Inflammatory Activity of Simple Ascidian, *Phallusia nigra* Savigny. *International Journal of Pharmaceutical Sciences Review and Research.* 2013;22(2):162-7.

[84] Krishnaiah P, Reddy VN, Venkataramana G, Ravinder K, Srinivasulu M, Raju TV, Ravikumar K, Chandrasekar D, Ramakrishna S, Venkateswarlu Y. New Lamellarin Alkaloids from the Indian Ascidian *Didemnumobscurum* and Their Antioxidant Properties. *Journal of Natural Products.* 2004 Jul 23;67(7):1168-71.

[85] Pearce AN, Chia EW, Berridge MV, Clark GR, Harper JL, Larsen L, Maas EW, Page MJ, Perry NB, Webb VL, Copp BR. Anti-Inflammatory Thiazine Alkaloids Isolated from the New Zealand Ascidian *Aplidium* sp.: Inhibitors of the Neutrophil Respiratory Burst in a Model of Gouty Arthritis. *Journal of Natural Products.* 2007 Jun 22;70(6):936-40.

[86] Pearce AN, Chia EW, Berridge MV, Maas EW, Page MJ, Webb VL, Harper JL, Copp BR. E/Z-Rubrolide O, an Anti-Inflammatory Halogenated Furanone from the New Zealand Ascidian *Synoicum n.* sp. *Journal of Natural Products.* 2007 Jan 26;70(1):111-3.

[87] Rajesh RP, Murugan A. Central Nervous System Depressant, Anti-Inflammatory Analgesic and Antipyretic Activity of the Ascidian *Eudistoma virde*. *Pharmacol.* 2013;65:69.

[88] Appleton DR, Page MJ, Lambert G, Berridge MV, Copp BR. Kottamides A‾ D: Novel Bioactive Imidazolone-Containing Alkaloids from the New Zealand Ascidian *Pycnoclavella kottae*. *The Journal of Organic Chemistry*. 2002 Jul 26;67(15):5402-4.

[89] Meenakshi VK, Paripooranaselvi M, Sankaravadivoo S, Gomathy S, Chamundeeswari KP. Immunomodulatory Activity of *Phallusia Nigra* Savigny, 1816 against S-180. *Int J Curr Microbiol Appl Sci.* 2013;2(8):286-95.

[90] Meenakshi, V. K., Paripooranaselvi, M. & Senthamarai, S., et al., (2013). Immunomodulatory Activity of Ethanol Extract of *Phallusia nigra* Savigny 1816, against Dalton's Lymphoma Ascites. *European Journal of Applied Engineering and Scientific Research*, 2 (1), 20-24.

[91] Ananthan G, Iyappan K (2014). Immunomodulatory Activity of Ethanol Extract of the Ascidian *Didemnum Albidum*. *World Journal of Pharmacy and Pharmaceutical Sciences*, 3(12), 745-755.

[92] Azumi K, Yokosawa H, Ishii S. Halocyamines: Novel Antimicrobial Tetrapeptide-Like Substances Isolated from the Hemocytes of the Solitary Ascidian *Halocynthia Roretzi*. *Biochemistry*. 1990 Jan 1;29(1):159-65.

[93] Azumi K, Yokosawa H, Ishii S. Presence of 3, 4-Dihydro-Xyphenylalanine-Containing Peptides in Hemocytes of the Ascidian, *Halocynthia roretzi*. *Experientia*. 1990 Oct 1;46(10):1020-3.

[94] Azumi K, Yoshimizu M, Suzuki S, Ezura Y, Yokosawa H. Inhibitory Effect Of Halocyamine, an Antimicrobial Substance from Ascidian Hemocytes, on the Growth of Fish Viruses and Marine Bacteria. *Experientia*. 1990 Oct 1;46(10):1066-8.

[95] In IH, Zhao C, Nguyen T, Menzel L, Waring AJ, Lehrer RI, Sherman MA. Clavaspirin, an Antibacterial and Haemolytic Peptide from *Styela Clava*. *Chemical Biology & Drug Design*. 2001 Dec 1;58(6):445-56.

[96] Jang WS, Kim KN, Lee YS, Nam MH, Lee IH. Halocidin: A New Antimicrobial Peptide from Hemocytes of the Solitary Tunicate, *Halocynthia Aurantium*. *FEBS Letters*. 2002 Jun 19;521(1-3):81-6.

[97] Galinier R, Roger E, Sautiere PE, Aumelas A, Banaigs B, Mitta G. Halocyntin and Papillosin, Two New Antimicrobial Peptides Isolated from Hemocytes of the Solitary Tunicate, *Halocynthia Papillosa*. *Journal of Peptide Science*. 2009 Jan 1;15(1):48-55.

[98] Wyche TP, Hou Y, Vazquez-Rivera E, Braun D, Bugni TS. Peptidolipins B–F, Antibacterial Lipopeptides from an Ascidian-Derived *Nocardia* sp. *Journal of Natural Products*. 2012 Apr 6;75(4):735-40.

[99] Hirsch S, Miroz A, McCarthy P, Kashman Y. Etzionin, a New Antifungal Metabolite from a Red Sea Tunicate. *Tetrahedron Letters*. 1989 Jan 1;30(32):4291-4.

[100] Lee IH, Zhao C, Cho Y, Harwig SS, Cooper EL, Lehrer RI. Clavanins, α-Helical Antimicrobial Peptides from Tunicate Hemocytes. *Febs Letters*. 1997 Jan 3;400(2):158-62.

[101] In IH, Zhao C, Nguyen T, Menzel L, Waring AJ, Lehrer RI, Sherman MA. Clavaspirin, an Antibacterial and Haemolytic Peptide from *Styela Clava*. *Chemical Biology & Drug Design*. 2001 Dec 1;58(6):445-56.

[102] Sugumaran M, Robinson WE. Bioactive Dehydrotyrosyl and Dehydrodopyl Compounds of Marine Origin. *Marine Drugs*. 2010 Dec 6;8(12):2906-35.

[103] Sugumaran M, Robinson WE. Structure, Biosynthesis and Possible Function of Tunichromes and Related Compounds. *Comparative Biochemistry and Physiology Part B: Biochemistry and Molecular Biology*. 2012 Sep 1;163(1):1-25.

[104] Wang W, Kim H, Nam SJ, Rho BJ, Kang H. Antibacterial Butenolides from the Korean Tunicate *Pseudodistoma Antinboja*. *Journal of Natural Products*. 2012 Nov 12;75(12):2049-54.

[105] Tadesse M, Svenson J, Jaspars M, Strøm MB, Abdelrahman MH, Andersen JH, Hansen E, Kristiansen PE, Stensvåg K, Haug T. Synoxazolidinone C; a Bicyclic Member of the Synoxazolidinone

Family with Antibacterial and Anticancer Activities. *Tetrahedron Letters*. 2011 Apr 13;52(15):1804-6.

[106] Reyes F, Fernandez R, Rodríguez A, Francesch A, Taboada S, Avila C, Cuevas C. Aplicyanins A–F, New Cytotoxic Bromoindole Derivatives from the Marine Tunicate *Aplidium Cyaneum*. *Tetrahedron*. 2008 May 26;64(22):5119-23.

[107] Miyata Y, Diyabalanage T, Amsler CD, McClintock JB, Valeriote FA, Baker BJ. Ecdysteroids from the Antarctic Tunicate *Synoicum Adareanum*. *Journal of Natural Products*. 2007 Nov 27;70(12):1859-64.

[108] Carroll AR, Nash BD, Duffy S, Avery VM. Albopunctatone, an Antiplasmodial Anthrone-Anthraquinone from the Australian Ascidian *Didemnum Albopunctatum*. *Journal of Natural Products*. 2012 Jun 8;75(6):1206-9.

[109] Donia MS, Wang B, Dunbar DC, Desai PV, Patny A, Avery M, Hamann MT. Mollamides B and C, Cyclic Hexapeptides from the Indonesian Tunicate *Didemnum Molle*. *Journal of Natural Products*. 2008 Jun 11;71(6):941-5.

[110] Schmitz FJ, Bowden BF, Toth SI. Antitumor and Cytotoxic Compounds From Marine Organisms. In *Pharmaceutical and Bioactive Natural Products* 1993 (pp. 197-308). Springer, Boston, MA.

[111] Degnan BM, Hawkins CJ, Lavin MF, McCaffrey EJ, Parry DL, Van den Brenk AL, Watters DJ. New Cyclic Peptides with Cytotoxic Activity from the Ascidian *Lissoclinum Patella*. *Journal of Medicinal Chemistry*. 1989 Jun;32(6):1349-54.

[112] Edler MC, Fernandez AM, Lassota P, Ireland CM, Barrows LR. Inhibition of Tubulin Polymerization by Vitilevuamide, A Bicyclic Marine Peptide, at a Site Distinct From Colchicine, the Vinca Alkaloids, and Dolastatin 10. *Biochemical Pharmacology*. 2002 Feb 15; 63(4):707-15.

[113] Ireland CM, Fernandez A, inventors; University of Utah Research Foundation (UURF), assignee. Cyclic Peptide Antitumor Agent from an Ascidian. *United States Patent US 5,830,996*. 1998 Nov 3.

[114] Rinehart Jr KL, Gloer JB, Cook Jr JC, Mizsak SA, Scahill TA. Structures of the Didemnins, Antiviral and Cytotoxic Depsipeptides from a Caribbean Tunicate. *Journal of the American Chemical Society.* 1981 Apr;103(7):1857-9.

[115] Aiello A, Carbonelli S, Esposito G, Fattorusso E, Iuvone T, Menna M. Turbinamide, a New Selective Cytotoxic Agent from the Mediterranean Tunicate *Sidnyum turbinatum. Organic letters.* 2001 Sep 20;3(19):2941-4.

In: Food for Huntington's Disease
Editors: M. Mohamed Essa et al.
ISBN: 978-1-53613-854-2
© 2018 Nova Science Publishers, Inc.

Chapter 9

TERPENOIDS AND HUNTINGTON'S DISEASE

R. Balakrishnan[1], K. Tamilselvam[1],
T. Manivasagam[2], A. Justin Thenmozhi[2],
M. Mohamed Essa[3,4,5] and N. Elangovan[1,*]

[1]Department of Biotechnology, School of Biosciences,
Periyar University, Salem, Tamil Nadu, India
[2]Department of Biochemistry and Biotechnology,
Annamalai University, Annamalainagar, Tamil Nadu, India
[3]Dept of Food Science and Nutrition,
College of Agriculture and Marine Sciences,
Sultan Qaboos University, Oman
[4]Ageing and Dementia Research Group,
Sultan Qaboos University, Oman
[5]Food and Brain Research Foundation, Chennai,
Tamil Nadu, India

---

* Corresponding Author Email: elangovannn@gmail.com.

ABSTRACT

According to the report published by the WHO, the morbidity due to neurodegenerative diseases (NDDs) is projected to be second highest cause of the death in 2040. Huntington's disease (HD) is a genetic NDD characterized by the progressive cognitive decline, motor dysfunction and psychiatric disturbance. These pathological abnormalities are mainly due to abnormal gene transcription and the deregulation of various biochemical and molecular processes. Oxidative stress is reported to be an important hallmark of in HD, so treatment with antioxidants along with other therapeutic agents, is gaining more significance in the pharmacotherapy of HD. Terpenoids and terpenes are the naturally occurring organic compounds ubiquitously present in plant resins and essential oils. Numerous experiments have indicated that the herbal oils extracted from medicinal plants exhibit a variety of biological functions and can be utilized as remedy for various diseases. Here we discuss the possible beneficial effect of terpenoids on HD.

INTRODUCTION

Huntington's disease (HD) is a brain disease, in which neuronal loss occurs progressively like other NDDs. In the final phase of HD, patients lose the control of basic movements needed for facial expression, communication and personal freedom. In 1993 the Huntington's Disease Collaborative Research Group that indicated the mutation in the Huntingtin gene leads to HD. The lack of promising therapeutic agents or any prospects for curing this disturbing loss of muscular control during the final stages of this diseases progression is threatening (Mac Donald et al., 1993).

Clinical Description

The main symptoms of HD include motor dysfunction, cognitive impairment and psychiatric disturbances. Additional symptoms with low prevalence are disturbances in sleep-and circadian rhythms, unintended weight loss and autonomic nervous system dysfunction. In the final stage of the disease the patient fully depends on others for day to day activities ultimately ending in death. The most common cause of death in HD patients is pneumonia, followed by suicide (Sturrock and Leavitt, 2010).

Juvenile Huntington's Disease

In the Juvenile Huntington's disease (JHD), symptoms and signs of HD occur prior to the age of 20 years. Behavioral impairment and problems with learning are the first signs. Hypokinetic and bradykinetic behavior with dystonic components are the motor symptom of HD. Chorea does not appears in the first decade but is mostly found only in the second decade. Epileptic fits occurs frequently. In most cases of JHD the CAG repeat length is more than 55. In 75% of the juveniles the father is the affected by HD (Ross and Margolis, 2002).

Motor Symptoms

The movement difficulties occur with both involuntary and voluntary movements. The involuntary movements are initially hyperkinetic followed by bradykinesia resulting in hypokinesia and a rigid-akinetic state. Another abnormal involuntary movement is the Chorea, orchoreoathetosis, which is an irregular and continuous jerky or writhing motion (Kumar et al., 2010).

Non-Motor Symptoms

Patients suffering from HD have meticulous and distinctive cognitive impairments with sub cortical dementia. Common cognitive features include bradyphrenia, defective recall, deterioration of complex intellectual functions, difficulty in executing functions, and personality changes. Apart from various cognitive abnormalities, various other psychiatric disturbances such as depression, anxiety, irritability, aggression, impulsivity, and a tendency towards suicide are also the key features of HD (Kumar et al., 2010).

PATHOLOGICAL FEATURES OF HD

Oxidative Stress in Huntington's Disease

Oxidative stress is a general term used to describe a serious imbalance between the production of reactive oxygen species (ROS) on one hand and the antioxidant defenses on the other. Susceptible neurons in the brain of HD patients do not tolerate the increase in ROS production (Stack et al., 2008). Enhanced ROS levels may trigger various intracellular cascades of oxidative stress by oxidizing DNA and proteins leading to lipid peroxidation processes in cellular membranes (Bogdanov et al., 2001). Initial post-mortem studies the brains of HD patients failed to detect any changes in the oxidative damage to DNA, lipids in the caudate nucleus, putamen and frontal cortex (Alam et al., 2000). Recent experiments have indicated an increment in the levels of oxidative indices in brain of HD patients. Various markers including cytoplasmic lipofuscin, accumulation of oxidative markers in DNA bases, DNA strand breaks and other cellular macromolecules associated with lipid peroxidation and protein nitration were also enhanced in HD patients (Lee et al., 2011). The main source of ROS in neurons is the mitochondria and mitochondrial dysfunction in HD is directly linked with oxidative stress (Tabrizi et al., 2000). Significantly diminished activities of mitochondrial complexes II/III and IV have been reported in the striatum of HD patients (Brennan et al., 1985). Both the oxidative stress and mitochondrial dysfunction are related to each other and are reported to exacerbate the other by positive feedback mechanisms, ultimately leading to the degeneration of susceptible neuronal groups including the striatal medium-sized spiny neurons in the HD brain (Polidori et al., 1999).

Mitochondrial Dysfunction and Huntington's Disease

Various studies have shown evidence of the involvement of mitochondrial dysfunction during HD (Brennan et al., 1985). Nuclear magnetic resonance spectroscopy explores the enhanced lactate levels in the basal ganglia and cortex. Biochemical experiments showed the diminished activities of complexes II and III of the ETC in the brain of HD patients (Browne et al., 1997). The striatal cells of mHTT-knock-in mouse embryos showed the impairments in mitochondrial respiration and ATP production (Chen, 2011). Both 3-nitropropionic acid and malonate, mitochondrial toxins, selectively inhibits succinate dehydrogenase and complex II and exhibit clinical and pathological symptoms that closely resemble HD (Tabrizi et al., 2000).

Neuroinflammation

There are abundant studies on the biology of microglia and their response to neuroinflammation (Hanisch and Kettenmann, 2007). Microglia is the resident immune cells present in the CNS. They structurally and functionally resemble peripheral tissue macrophages and are the main mediators of inflammation in brain (Ransohoff and Perry, 2009). Microglia are reported to be involved in numerous acute and chronic neurological diseases (Sugama et al., 2009). They are present as the 'resting' or 'surveilling' stage in the healthy adult brain and are characterized by a small cell body with minimal expression of surface antigens. Upon a CNS injury, they are rapidly activated, converted to less ramified cells and play an important role in the pathogenesis of NDDs. Neuroinflammation is triggered by pro-inflammatory indices like prostaglandins, cytokines and nitric oxide (Alexi et al., 2000). The postmortem human HD brain showed an enhanced profile of inflammatory mediators (Silvestroni et al., 2009). Some inflammatory mediators such as IL-1β and TNF-α were enhanced in the striatum only, whereas IL-6, IL-8 and MMP-9 increased in the cortex and cerebellum (Przedborski, 2007). The inflammatory mediators found in the striatum reflect the pathology, where as deregulated factors (IL-6, IL-8 and MMP-9) indicate the effect of HTTexp (Bjorkqvist et al., 2008). Therefore, neuroinflammation in HD seems to be triggered by the interactions of microglia, neurons, and macroglia.

Apoptosis

Traditionally, neuronal cell death occurs through two mechanisms: apoptosis or necrosis. Apoptotic cells display distinct morphological changes including membrane blebbing, cytoplasmic shrinking, chromatin condensation and reversed orientation of phosphatidiylserine in the mitochondrial membrane, ultimately leading to the cells being phagocytized by a neighboring cell (Ferrer, 1999). In necrosis, cells swell and rupture, inducing an inflammatory response. DNA get fragmented and used as a marker of apoptosis. Nuclear shrinkage and random DNA cleavage are found in necrotic tissue. Apoptotic cell death can commence through many factors including excitotoxicity, metabolic stress and oxidative, withdrawal of neurotrophic factors and environmental toxins (Sastry and Rao, 2000). Caspases are the cysteine aspartic acid proteases which are closely linked with cell death in apoptosis. Two main types of caspases are initiator caspases (caspase8) and the effectors caspases (caspase3). Trimerisations of death receptors induce the activation of initiator caspases (8 and 10) leadings to the activation of effectors caspases (Chen, 2011). Release of cytochrome c from the mitochondrial so activates the initiator caspases (9) (Chan and Mattson, 1999).

Current Therapeutic Approaches for HD

Many agents and surgical procedures have been evaluated in HD for their efficacy in suppressing dopamine agonists, chorea, dopamine antagonists, glutamate antagonists, including dopamine-depleting agents, acetylcholinesterase inhibitors, benzodiazepines, antiseizure medications, cannabinoids, lithium, fetal cell transplantation and deep brain stimulation (Pidgeon and Rickards, 2013). Additional side effects include: orthostatic hypotension, nausea and vomiting, tremor, memory problems, confusion, insomnia, dizziness, diarrhea, balance and gait difficulties, headaches, nervousness/anxiety, panic attacks, blurred vision and paranoia (Jancovic and Beach 1997). The present approaches do not extensively mitigate the symptoms of HD and also fail to slow down the progression of HD. Hence, alternate approaches are being exploited to improve the existing pharmacotherapy for HD.

Terpenoids

Terpenoids are a group of naturally occurring compounds, which are mainly found in plants, while others are obtained from other sources. They are volatile substances that give fragrance to plants and flowers. They are also present in the leaves and fruits of conifers, higher plants, citrus and eucalyptus. Terpenoids contribute to the flavors of spices like clove, cinnamon and ginger, as well as the scent of eucalyptus, the yellow color in sunflowers, and the red color in tomatoes (New man et al., 2000). Well-known terpenoids include camphor, salvinorin, menthol, citral A in the plant *Salvia divinorum*, the cannabinoids found in *cannabis* bilobalide and ginkgolide and found in Ginkgobiloba, as well as the curcuminoids found in turmeric and mustard seed (Luttgen et al., 2000).

Terpenoids include monoterpenes (D-limonene, geraniol, perillyl alcohol and carvone) and sesquiterpenes (farnesol) which are the main constituents of essential oils while diterpenes (trans-retinoic acid and retinol), Sesterterpenes (lupeol and ursolic acid) triterpenes (betulinic acid and oleanic acid), tetraterpenes (lycopene, lutein, α-carotene and β-carotene) and other terpenes are constituents of resins, rubber, balsams, and waxes (Eisenreich et al., 1998). Many terpenes have biological activities (against malaria, cancer, inflammation, NDDs and a variety of infectious viral and bacterial diseases that are used for the treatment of human diseases. The worldwide sales of terpene-based pharmaceuticals in 2002 were approximately US $12 billion (Rohdich et al., 2000).

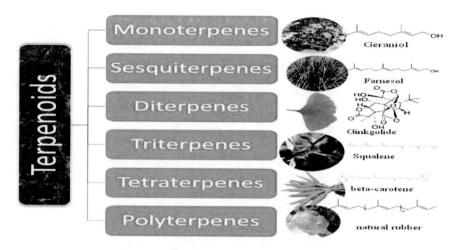

Figure 1. Classification of Terpenoids.

Table 1. Types of Terpenoids

S. No.	Class	Value of n	Number of carbon atoms
1.	Hemiterpenoids	1	5
2.	Monoterpenoids	2	10
3.	Sesquiterpenoinds	3	15
4.	Diterpenoids	4	20
5.	Sesterpenoids	5	25
6.	Troterpenoids	6	30
7.	Tetraterpenoids	8	40
8.	Polyterpenoids	>8	>40

Monoterpenoids

Monoterpenoids consist of a ten carbon backbone (2 isoprene units) structure and can be separated in to three subclasses: monocyclic, bicyclic and acyclic. Inside each group, the monoterpenoids may be simple unsaturated hydrocarbons or have functional groups such as ketones, alcohols and aldehydes. Common aliphatic examples include citral, geraniol, lavandulol, linalool and myrcene (Wagner et al., 2003). The important representatives of monocyclic monoterpenoids are eucalyptol, limonene, thymol, perillaldehyde, carvone, α-terpineol, geraniol and menthol (Singh, 2007).

Sesquiterpenoids

Sesquiterpenoids are derived from three isoprene units and exist in several forms, including monocyclic tricyclic longifolene, (zingiberene), linea (farnesol), copaene as well as the alcohol patchoulol and bicyclic (Caryophyllene) frame works (Davis et al., 2000).They are the most diverse group of terpenoids (Wang et al., 2013).

Diterpenoids

Diterpenoids are secondary metabolites containing twenty carbon atoms that derive from the condensation of 4 isoprenyl units. As other terpenoids, they are widespread in the plant kingdom, Most terpenoids biologically derive from geranylgeranyl diphosphate, which forms acyclic (phytanes), bicyclic (clerodanes, halimanes and labdanes), tricyclic (rosanes, cassanes, vouacapanes, abietanes, podocarpanes, pimaranes), tetracyclic (kauranes, aphidicolanes, stemaranes, atisanes, stemodanes, gibberellanes and trachylobanes), and macrocyclic diterpenes (ingenanes, tiglianes, daphnanes, cembranes and taxanes) according to the cyclization that occurs (Lonzotti, 2013).

Table 2. The Most Common Plants Containing Terpenoids

Plant		Terpenoid compounds	Activity
Coriandrum sativum L. (Apiaceae)	Fruits	Camphor, Linalool, geranylacetate	Carminative, spasmolytic
Boswellia Serrate Roxb ex Colebr. (Burseraceae)	Gum-resin dried	Boswellic acids	Anti-inflammatory, Analgesic
Cinnamomum verum J. S. Presl. (5*Cinnamomum zeylanicum* Nees) (Lauraceae)	Bark	β-caryophyllene, cinnamylacetate, Cinnamaldehyde, 1,8-cineole, eugenol, linalool,	Antimicrobial, anti-inflammatory, Antispasmodic
Artemisia absinthium L. (Asteraceae)	Herbs	(Z)-epoxyocimene, β-curcumen, trans-sabinyl acetate and α-Thujone, chrysanthenyl acetate, spathulenol and α-bisabolol	Antimicrobial, Digestive, apetizer, spasmolytic
Eucalyptus globules Labill. (Myrtaceae)	Leaves	β-pinene, 1, 8-Cineole, p-cymene, pinocarveol, α-terpineol, myrtenol, α-pinene	Antiseptic, carminative, expectorant
Euphrasia officinalis L. *Euphrasia rostkoviana* Hayne (Scrophulariaceae)	Herbs	Aucubin	Anti-inflammatory, Antiphlogistic
Foeniculum vulgare Miller subsp	Fruits	Anethole, estragole, fenchone	Secretolytic, antitumor, antioxidant, Spasmolytic, carminative, antimiocrbial, estrogenic, Expectorant

Plant		Terpenoid compounds	Activity
Gentiana lutea L. (Gentianaceae)	Roots	Secoiridoid glycosides (sweroside, swertiamarin, gentiopicroside)	Digestive, hepatoprotective, analgesic, and wound-healing
Ginkgo biloba L. (Ginkgoaceae)	Leaves	Ginkgolides A, B, C, J, bilobalide	Antioxidant, improving cognition, and memory
Hyssopus officinalis L. (Lamiaceae)	Herb	Marrubiin, oleanolic acid, pinocamphone, isopinocamphone, β-pinene, limonene	Expectorant, antiseptic
Inula helenium L. (Asteraceae)	Roots	Eudesmane, guaiane, germacrane types of sesquiterpenoids lactones	Antitumor, anti-inflammatory
Juniperus communis L. (Cupresaceae)	Pseudofruits	α-Pinene, limonene, myrcene, sabinen, terpinen-4-ol	Diuretic, antiseptic, anti-inflammatory
Kigelia africana (Lam.) Benth. (Bignoniaceae)	Root bark	Verminoside	Anti-inflammatory, antiphlogistic
Lavandula angustifolia Miller (Lamiaceae)	Flowers	Linalool, linalylacetate, cis-ocimen, terpinen-4-ol, limonene, 1,8-cineole, camphor, lavandulyl acetate, lavandulol	Sedative, analgetic, antiinflammatory, antibacterial
Melaleuca alternifolia (Maiden and Betch)	Leaves	α-terpinene, terpinen-4-ol, 1,8-Cineole, γ-terpinene	Anibacterial, Immunostimulant, antiseptic, anti-inflammatory
Melissa officinalis L. (Lamiaceae)	Leaves	β-caryophyllene, Citral, neral, germacrene D, citronellal, oleanolic acids and ursolic	Antimicrobial, sedative, antiviral, antispasmodic

Table 2. (Continued)

Plant		Terpenoid compounds	Activity
Myristica fragrans Houtt. (Myristicaceae)	Seeds	Limonene, pinene, α-pinene, β-sabinene	Carminative, Digestive
Pelargonium graveolens (Geraniaceae)	Leaves	β-phellandrene, limonene, geraniol, terpinen-4-ol, 1,8-cineole, linalyl acetate, citronellylformate, linalool, isomenthone, citronellol	Analgesic
Pimpinella anisum L. (Apiaceae)	Fruits	α-terpineol, anisaldehyde, estragole, linalool, anethole	Antimiocrbial, antitumor, carminative, expectorant, antisecretolytic, antispasmodic and antioxidant
Mentha x piperita L. (Lamiaceae)	Leaves	Limonene, menthol, Viridiflorol, 1,8-cineole, menthone, isomenthone, menthyl acetate, menthofuran	Choleretic, carminative, antimicrobial, spasmolytic, digestive
Pinus silvestris L. (Pinaceae)	Resin obtained from live trees	α-pinene and β-pinene, turpentine, terpinolene, camphene, dipentene, turpentine, mainly the monoterpenes Δ3-carene,	Antiseptic, expectorant, anti-inflammatory, analgesic
Plantago lanceaolata L. (Plantaginaceae)	Leaves	Asperuloside, catalpol, aucubin	Antibacterial, expectorant, antioxidant, immunostimulant, anti-inflammatory

Plant		Terpenoid compounds	Activity
Rosmarinus officinalis L. (Lamiaceae)	Leaves	Carnosol, α-pinene, 1,8-cineole, camphor	Antioxidant, spasmolytic, anticancer, Carminative, antiviral
Salvia officinalis L. (Lamiaceae)	Leaves	Oleanolic acid, α- and β-pinene, carvacrol, thujone, camphor, borneol, ursolic, geraniol and 1,8-cineole	Antimicrobial, crminative, estrogenic, antiChE, antihidrotic, Anti-inflammatory
Stevia rebaudiana (Bert.) Bertoni (Asteraceae)	Leaves	Steviol, dulcoside A, stevioside, steviolbioside, rebaudioside AF	Antihyperglycemic, glucagonostatic, insulinotropic and anticancer
Syzygium aromaticum (L.) Merill et L. M. Perry (Myrtaceae)	Flowers	β-caryophyllenee, acetyl eugenol, eugenol	Antiviral, antifungal, analgesic, antimicrobial
Thymus vulgaris L., *Thymus zygis* L. (Lamiaceae)	Herb	β-myrcene, oleanolic acids, p-cymene, γ-terpinene, ursolic, thymol, terpinen-4-ol, linalool and carvacrol	Antibacterial, expectorant, spasmolytic, secretomotoric, anti-inflammatory
Zingiber officinale Roscoe (Zingiberaceae)	Rhizome	Camphene, β-phellandrene, α-Zingiberene, β-bisabolene, geraniol, α-farnesene, zingiberol, β-sesquiphellandrene, 1,8-cineole, ar-curcumene	Digestive, carminative, anti-inflammatory, antiemetic
Tripterygiumwil fordii Hook. f. (Celastraceae)		Triptolide (structurally unique diterpenetriepoxide)	Antiproliferative, anticancer, immune modulation, anti-inflammatory and proapoptotic activity

Triterpenoids

Terpenoids form a large group of natural products which includes steroids and consequently sterols, derived from precursors. Nearly two hundred different triterpene skeletons exist from natural sources and represent structurally cyclization products of Squalene, which is the immediate biological precursor of all triterpenoids. Some biologically active triterpenoids include (β-amyrin, cycloartenol, cyclopuxin, cephalosporin, linosterol, cedrelon and friedelin) (Horborne, 1998).

Protective Effects of Herbs and Secondary Metabolites in HD

Many of the thousands of plant species growing throughout the world have a direct pharmaceutical action on the body. Natural compounds with the effects of calcium antagonization, anti-inflammation, anti-oxidant, neurofunctional and anti-apoptosis regulation exhibit preventive or therapeutic effects on various neurodegerative diseases. A number of the plants containing terpenoids have shown efficacy against HD, are discussed below:

Bacopa Monnieri

Bacopa monnieri and *Bacopa monniera* (BM) is are creeping perennials with small oblong leaves and purple flowers, they are found in warm wetlands and are native to India and Australia. Generally found as a weed in rice fields, BM grows throughout East Asia and the United States. The entire plant is used medicinally (Barrett and Strother, 1978). The major chemical constituents present in the plant are the dammarane type of tri-terpenoid saponins as well as Bacosides A and B. Among various constituents, Bacoside A has shown to improve memory. A variety of clinical trials have also shown beneficial effects of Brahmi in improving memory. They widely used neurotoxin 3-Nitropropionicacid (3-NP), utilized to induce an experimental model of HD, inactivate the mitochondrial enzyme succinate dehydrogenase (SDH) complex II and complex III of the electron transport chain. It also increases the levels of ROS, MDA, and free fatty acids, suggesting the vital role in oxidative stress for the manifestation of neurotoxicity (Andreassen et al., 2000; Coles et al., 1979). The dietary intake of BM leaf powder significantly decreased the basal levels of several oxidative markers, enhanced thiol-related antioxidant molecules enhanced and activities of antioxidant enzymes suggesting its antioxidant potential (Calabrese et al., 2008). One study has show that dietary BM supplements leads to significant protection against a neurotoxicant-induced oxidative damage in the brain (Shinomol and Muralidhara, 2011). The study further suggests that due to a strong antioxidant effect and a protective effect against stress-mediated neuronal dysfunctions, BM can be useful in HD treatment.

Ginkgo Biloba

Ginkgo biloba, normally known as ginkgo tree or the maiden hair tree is the only living species in the division *Ginkgophyta*, all others being extinct. It is found in fossils dating back 270 million years. Native to China the tree is widely cultivated, has been throughout human history. It has various uses in traditional medicine and as a source of food. The main terpenoid constituents present in the leaf are the trilactonic diterpenes: Ginkgolide J-M, Ginkgolide A-C and a trilactonic sesquiterpene: Bilobalide. Ginkgo leaf extract has exhibited protective effects against neurodegenerative diseases like cancer, cardiovascular diseases, tinnitus, stress, dementia (Alzheimer's disease), geriatric complaints like vertigo, psychiatric disorders and age-related macular degeneration likes schizophrenia (Ramassamy et al., 2007). The *G.biloba* extract (100 mg/kg, i.p. for 15 days) improved the 3-NP induced neurobehavioral deficits and also decreased the level of striatal MDA (Smith and Luo, 2004). Standardized *G.biloba* extract (EGb 761) also caused down-and up-regulation of striatal glyceraldehydes-3-phosphate dehydrogenase and *Bcl-xl* expression levels, respectively. These biochemical results, supported by the histopathological studies suggested neuroprotective role of EGb 761 in HD (Mahdy et al., 2011).

Curcuma Longa

Curcuma Longa (CL) also known as Cúrcuma is a small perennial herb native to India. It bears numerous rhizomes on its root system which are the source of its culinary spice known as Turmeric (Cúrcuma-rizoma secco in polvere) and its medicinal extract called Curcumin (Cúrcuma extracto refinado). CL contains yellow coloring matter, different essential oil, starch, curcuminiods and sesquiterpenes. Chronic administration of curcumin consistently improved body weight, reversed motor deficits, and increase SDH activity in 3-NP treated rats (Chainani, 2003). The improved 3-NP-induced motor and cognitive impairment along with a strong antioxidant property indicates that curcumin could be useful as well as act as a lead molecule in the treatment of HD (Kumar et al., 2007).

Ginsenosides

Ginsenosides or panaxosides are a class of naturally produced steroid glycosides and triterpene saponins. Compounds in this family are found almost exclusively in the plant genus *Panax* (ginseng), which has a long history of use in traditional medicine that has led to the study of the pharmacological effects of ginseng compounds. Ginsenosides can be isolated from various parts of the plant, though typically from the roots, it has been most widely studied due to its use in traditional Chinese medicine. Ginseng contains a series of tetracyclic dammarane triterpenoid saponin glycosides called, ginsenosides, which are the active constituents (Liu and Xiao, 1992) Ginsenosides, depending on their structural differences, are classified in to three categories: the panaxadiols (Rc,Rd,Rg3,Rh2,Rs1 and Rb1-Rb3), panaxatriols (Rf, Re, Rh1 and Rg1-2) and oleanolic acid derivatives (Ro) (Rausch et al., 2006). Ginsenosides Rd, Rb1 and Rb3 have exhibited a neuroprotective effect against 3-NP-induced striatal neuronal damage (Kim et al., 2005; Lian et al., 2005). Ginsenoside Rc, Rg5 and Rb1 have shown to protect medium spiny neurons from glutamate-induced apoptosis in genetically modified rodents (Radad et al., 2006). It has been hypothesized that the neuroprotective effect of these ginsenosides could be due to their ability to inhibit glutamate-induced Ca2+ responses in cultured spinal neuronal cultures (Keum et al., 2000).

Such reports strongly support that potential of ginseng and ginsenosides can be exploited to develop new therapeutics for the treatment of HD and other neurodegenerative disorders.

Centella Asiatica

Centella asiatica, (CA), commonly known as centella, Asiatic pennywort or Gotu kola, is an herbaceous, frost-tender perennial plant in the family Apiaceae. It is native to the wetlands in Asia and is used as a culinary vegetable as well as a medicinal herb. The most important chemical constituents from CA are triterpenoid saponins including madecassic acid, madecassoside, asiaticoside and Asiatic acid. Other saponins present in minor quantities are brahmoside and brahminoside. Various triterpene acids such as brahmic, betullic, acid and isobrahmic acid can be derived from the plant. The essential oil from the leaves of the plant contains monoterpenes, including β-pinene, γ-pinene, α-pinene and bornyl acetat. A part from these constituents lipids, flavones and sterols have also been reported from CA (Soumy anath et al., 2005). CA attenuated the 3-NP-induced depletion of GSH levels, total thiols, and endogenous antioxidants in the striatum and other brain regions (Shinomol and Muralidhara, 2008). It also exhibited protection against the 3-NP-induced mitochondrial dysfunctions viz., the reduction in the activity of SDH, electron transport chain enzymes, and decreased mitochondrial viability (Shinomol and Muralidhara, 2008). The results of this study clearly indicate that the protective effect of CA against neuronal damage induced by OS and mitochondrial dysfunctions along with its memory enhancing activity can be helpful in controlling HD-related impairments.

Cannabis Sativa

The unique smell of cannabis does not arise from cannabinoids, but from over hundred terpenoid compounds (Turner et al., 1980). Terpenoids derive from repeating units of isoprene, such as sesquiterpenoids (C15), monoterpenoids (with C10 skeletons), diterpenoids (C20), and triterpenoids (C30). The final structure of the terpenoids ranges from simple linear chains to complex poly cyclic molecules, and they may include aldehyde, ether, alcohol, ketone, or ester functional groups.

CONCLUSION

The above data clearly indicates that the oxidative stress plays a significant role in the pathophysiology of HD. Further, the plants rich in terpenoids having well established antioxidant and neuroprotective effects have shown beneficial effects against the symptoms of HD. Still ample work is required to fully elucidate the mechanism of these plants and phytochemicals against HD. Furthermore, lot of other plants containing terpenoid with significant antioxidant and neuroprotective potential can be explored for their protective effect against HD.

REFERENCES

Alam ZI, Halliwell B, Jenner P. No Evidence for Increased Oxidative Damage to Lipids, Proteins, or DNA in Huntington's Disease. *J Neurochem* 2000; 75:840-6.

Alexi T, Borlongan CV, Faull RL, Williams CE, Clark RG, Gluckman PD. Neuroprotective Strategies for Basal Ganglia Degeneration: Parkinson's and Huntington's Diseases. *Prog Neurobiol* 2000; 60:409-70.

Andreassen OA, Ferrante RJ, Hughes DB, Klivenyi P, Dedeoglu A, Ona VO. Malonate and 3-Nitropropionic Acid Neurotoxicity are Reduced in Transgenic Mice Expressing a Caspase-1 Dominant-Negative Mutant. *J Neurochem* 2000; 75:847-52.

Barrett SC. Strother JL. Taxonomy and Natural History of Bacopain California. *Syst Bot* 1978; 5:408-419.

Bjorkqvist M. A Novel Pathogenic Pathway of Immune Activation Detectable Before Clinical Onset in Huntington's Disease. *J Exp Med* 2008; 205:1869-1877.

Bogdanov MB, Andreassen OA, Dedeoglu A, Ferrante RJ, Beal MF. Increased Oxidative Damage to DNA in a Transgenic Mouse Model of Huntington's Disease. *J Neuro chem* 2001; 79:1246-9.

Bordelon YM, Mackenzie L, Chesselet MF. Morphology and Compartmental Location of Cells Exhibiting DNA Damage After Quinolinic Acid Injections into Rat Striatum. *J. Comp. Neurol* 1999; 412:38-50.

Brennan WAJr, Bird ED, Aprille JR. Regional Mitochondrial Respiratory Activity in Huntington's Disease Brain. *J Neurochem* 1985; 44:1948-50.

Browne SE, Bowling AC, MacGarvey U, Baik MJ, Berger SC, Muqit MM. Oxidative Damage and Metabolic Dysfunction in Huntington's Disease: Selective Vulnerability of the Basal Ganglia. *Ann Neurol* 1997; 41:646-53.

Calabrese C, Gregory WL, Leo M, Kraemer D, Bone K, Oken B. Effects of a Standardized *Bacopa Monnieri* Extract on Cognitive Performance, Anxiety, and Depression in the Elderly: A Randomized, Double-Blind, Placebo-Controlled Trial. *J Altern Complement Med* 2008; 14:707-13.

Chainani-Wu N. Safety and Anti-Inflammatory Activity of Curcumin: A Component of Turmeric (*Curcuma longa*). *J Altern Complement Med* 2003; 9:161-8.

Chan SL, and Mattson MP. Caspases and Calpain Substrates: Roles in Synaptic Plasticity and Cell Death. *J. Neurosci. Res* 1999; 58:67-190.

Chen CM. Mitochondrial Dysfunction, Metabolic Deficits, and Increased Oxidative Stress in Huntington's Disease. *Chang Gung Med J* 2011; 34:135-52.

Coles CJ, Edmondson DE, Singer TP. Inactivation of Succinate Dehydrogenase by 3-Nitropropionate. *J Biol Chem* 1979; 254:5161-7.

Consroe P. 1998. Brain Cannabinoid Systems as Targets for the Therapy of Neurological Disorders. *Neuro boil Dis* 5:534-51.

Davis EM, Croteau R. Cyclization Enzymes in the Biosynthesis of Monoterpenes, Sesquiterpenes, and Diterpenes. *Biosynth Arom Polyket Isopren Alkal* 2000; 209:53-95.

Eisenreich W, Schwarz M, Cartayrade A, Arigoni D, Zenk MH, Bacher A. The Deoxyxylulose Phosphate Pathway of Terpenoid Biosynthesis in Plants and Microorganisms. *Chem Biol* 1998; 5(9):R221-R233.

Ferrer I. Role of Caspases in Ionizing Radiation Induced Apoptosis in the Developing Cerebellum. *Dev. Neurobiol* 1999; 41:549-558.

Hanisch UK, Kettenmann H. Microglia: Active Sensor and Versatile Effect or Cells in the Normal and Pathologic Brain. *Nat Neurosci* 2007; 10:1387-1394.

Harborne JB. Phytochemical Methods. A Guide to Modern Techniques of Plant Analysis. 3rd.ed. London, UK: *Thompson Science* 1998;1317.

Jankovic J, Beach J. Long-Term Effects of Tetrabenazine in Hyperkinetic Movement Disorders. *Neurology* 1997;48:358-62.

Keum YS, Park KK, Lee JM, Chun KS, Park JH, Lee SK. Antioxidant and Anti-Tumor Promoting Activities of the Methanol Extract of Heat-Processed Ginseng. *Cancer Lett*. 2000; 13:41-8.

Kim JH, Kim S, Yoon IS, Lee JH, Jang BJ, Jeong SM. Protective Effects of Ginseng Saponins on 3-Nitropropionic Acid-Induced Striatal Degeneration in Rats. *Neuropharmacology* 2005;48:743-56.

Kumar P, Kalonia H, Kumar A. Huntington's Disease: Pathogenesis to Animal Models. *Pharmacol Rep* 2010; 62:1-14.

Kumar P, Padi SS, Naidu PS, Kumar A. Possible Neuroprotective Mechanisms of Curcumin in Attenuating 3-Nitropropionic Acid-Induced Neurotoxicity. *Methods Find Exp Clin Pharmacol* 2007; 29:19-25.

Lanzotti V. Diterpenes for Therapeutic Use. In: *Natural Products: Phytochemistry, Botany and Metabolism of Alkaloids, Phenolics and Terpenes*. Berlin Heidel berg: Springer-Verlag 2013; 317191.

Lee J, Kosaras B, DelSignore SJ. Modulation of Lipid Peroxidation and Mitochondrial Function Improves Neuropathology in Huntington's Disease Mice. *Acta Neuropathol* 2011; 121:487-98.

Lian XY, Zhang Z, Stringer JL. Protective Effects of Ginseng Components in a Rodent Model of Neurodegeneration. *Ann Neurol* 2005; 57:642-8.

Liu CX, Xiao PG. Recent Advances on Ginseng Research in China. *J Ethnopharmacol* 1992; 36:27-38.

Luttgen H, Rohdich F, Herz S, Wungsintaweeku IJ, Hecht S, Schuhr CA, Fellermeier M, Sagner S, Zenk MH, Bacher A, Eisenreich W. Biosynthesis of Terpenoids: YchB Protein of *Escherichia Coli* Phosphorylates the 2-Hydroxy Group of 4-Diphosphocytidyl-2 C methyl-D-Erythritol. *Proc Natl Acad Sci* 2000; 97:1062-1067.

Mac Donald ME, Ambrose, CM, Duyao MP, Myers R H, Lin C, Srinidhi L, Barnes G, Taylor SA, James M, Groot N, Mac Farlane H: Anovel Genes Containing a Trinucleotide Repeat that is Expanded and Unstable on Huntington's Disease Chromosomes. *Cell* 1993; 72:971-983.

Mahdy HM, Tadros MG, Mohamed MR, Karim AM, Khalifa AE. The Effect of *Ginkgo Biloba* Extract on 3-Nitropropionic Acid-Induced Neurotoxicity in Rats. *Neurochem Int* 2011; 59:770-8.

Newman DJ, Cragg GM, Snader KM. The Influence of Natural Products Upon Drug Discovery. *Nat Prod Rep* 2000; 17(3):215-234.

Pidgeon C, Rickards H. The Pathophysiology and Pharmacological Treatment of Huntington's Disease. *Behav Neurol* 2013; 26:245-253.

Polidori MC, Mecocci P, Browne SE, Senin U, Beal MF. Oxidative Damage to Mitochondrial DNA in Huntington's Disease Parietal Cortex. *Neurosci Lett* 1999; 272:53-6.

Przedborski S. Neuroinflammation and Parkinson's Disease. *Hand B Clin Neurol* 2007; 83:535-551.

Radad K, Gille G, Liu L, Rausch WD. Use of Ginseng in Medicine with Emphasis on Neurodegenerative Disorders. *J Pharmacol Sci* 2006; 100:175-86.

Ramassamy C, Longpre F, Christen Y. *Ginkgo biloba* Extract (EGb761) in Alzheimer's Disease: Is There Any Evidence? *Curr Alzheimer Res* 2007; 4:253-62.

Ransohoff RM, Perry VH. Microglial Physiology: Uniquestimuli, Specialized Responses. *Annu Rev Immunol* 2009; 27:119-145.

Rausch WD, Liu S, Gille G, Radad K. Neuroprotective Effects of Ginsenosides. *Acta Neuro boil Exp* (Wars) 2006; 66:369-75.

Rohdich F, Wungsintaweeku IJ, Luttgen H, Fischer M, Eisenreich W, Schuhr CA, Fellermeier M, Schramek N, Zenk MH, Bacher A. Biosynthesis of Terpenoids: 4-Diphosphocytidyl-2-C-Methyl-D-Erythritol Kinase from Tomato. *Proc Natl Acad Sci* 2000; 97: 8251-8256.

Ross CA, Margolis RL. Huntington Disease. *American College of Neuropsycho Pharmacol* 2002.

Sastry PS, and Rao KS. Apoptosis and the Nervous System. *J Neurochem* 2000; 7 4:1-20.

Shinomol GK, Muralidhara. *Bacopa monnieri* Modulates Endogenous Cytoplasmic and Mitochondrial Oxidative Markers in Prepubertal Mice Brain. *Phytomedicine* 2011; 18:317-26.

Shinomol GK, Muralidhara. Prophylactic Neuroprotective Property of Centella Asiatica Against 3-Nitropropionic Acid Induced Oxidative Stress and Mitochondrial Dysfunctions in Brain Regions of Prepubertal Mice. *Neurotoxicology* 2008; 29:948-57.

Silvestroni A, Faull RL, Strand AD, Moller T. Distinct Neuroinflammatory Profile in Post-Mortem Human Huntington's Disease. *Neuroreport* 2009; 20:1098-1103.

Singh G. *Chemistry of Terpenoids and Carotenoids*. New Dehli: Discovery Publisher Pvt. Ltd; 2007;1286.

Smith JV, Luo Y. Studies on Molecular Mechanisms of *Ginkgo Biloba* Extract. *Appl Microbiol Biotechnol* 2004; 64:465-72.

Soumyanath A, Zhong YP, Gold SA, Yu X, Koop DR, Bourdette D. *Centella Asiatica* Accelerates Nerve Regeneration Upon Oral Administration and Contains Multiple Active Fractions Increasing Neurite Elongation *In Vitro*. *J Pharm Pharmacol* 2005; 57:1221-9.

Stack EC, Matson WR, Ferrante RJ. Evidence of Oxidant Damage in Huntington's Disease: Translational Strategies Using Antioxidants. *Ann N Y Acad Sci* 2008; 1147:79-92.

Sturrock A, Leavitt BR. The Clinical and Genetic Features of Huntington Disease. *J Geriatr Psychiatry Neurol* 2010; 23:243-59.

Sugama S, Takenouchi T, Cho BP, Joh TH, Hashimoto M, Kitani H. Possible Roles of Microglial Cells For Neurotoxicity in Clinical Neurodegenerative Diseases and Experimental Animal Models. *Inflamm Allergy Drug Targets* 2009; 8:277-284.

Tabrizi SJ, Workman J, Hart PE, Mangiarini L, Mahal A, Bates G: Mitochondrial Dysfunction and Freeradical Damage in the Huntington R6/2 Transgenic Mouse. *Ann Neurol* 2000; 47:80-6.

Tabrizi SJ, Workman J, Hart PE. Mitochondrial Dysfunction and Freeradical Damage in the Huntington R6/2 Transgenic Mouse. *Ann Neurol* 2000; 47:80-6.

Thompson CB. Apoptosis in the Pathogenesis and Treatment of Disease. *Science* 1995; 267:1456-1462.

Turner CE, Elsohly MA. Boeren EG. Constituents of *Cannabis Sativa* L. XVII. A Review of the Natural Constituents. *J.NatProd* 1980; 43:169-234.

Wagner KH, Elmadfa I: Biological Relevance of Terpenoids-Overview Focusing on Mono-, Di and Tetraterpenes. *Ann Nutr Metab* 2003; 47:95-106.

Wang L, Yang B, Lin XP, Zhou XF, Liu Y. Sesterterpenoids. *Nat Prod Rep* 2013; 30:45573.

In: Food for Huntington's Disease ISBN: 978-1-53613-854-2
Editors: M. Mohamed Essa et al. © 2018 Nova Science Publishers, Inc.

Chapter 10

THERAPEUTIC OPTIONS FOR HUNTINGTON'S DISEASE: AYURVEDIC MEDICINAL PLANTS

J. Nataraj[1,2], T. Manivasagam[1,*], A. Justin Thenmozhi[1], C. Saravana Babu[3] and M. Mohamed Essa[4,5,6]

[1]Department of Biochemistry and Biotechnology,
Annamalai University, Tamil Nadu, India
[2]Department of Biochemistry,
Vinayaka Mission Research Foundation, Salem, India
[3] Department of Pharmacology, JSS College of Pharmacy,
JSS Academy of Higher Education and Research,
SS Nagar, Mysore, Karnataka, India
[4]Department of Food Science and Nutrition,
Sultan Qaboos University, Oman
[5]Ageing and Dementia Research Group,
Sultan Qaboos University, Muscat, Oman
[6]Food and Brain Research Foundation, Chennai, Tamil Nadu, India

---

[*]Corresponding Author Email: mani_pdresearchlab@rediffmail.com.

ABSTRACT

Ayurveda is an ancient medical system, one of the world's oldest, originating from India. It is considered as the most recognized and widely practiced alternative medicine. Throughout history, medicinal herbs were used for treating diseases in India. Most of the current pharmacotherapies, mainly targeting the neurotransmitters, yield symptomatic intervention that focus on the motor aspects of Huntington's disease (HD). Ayurvedic herbs and products offer relief without side effects, even with prolonged administration. Neurodegenerative diseases (NDs) are currently considered a major cause of mortality and disability in older people, thus enhancing their life span is a major task in the field of medical research. The symptoms of NDs are described in Ayurvedic texts alongside with the therapeutic potential of numerous plants. In this chapter, the role of the Ayurvedic medicinal plant, *Withania somnifera* (ashwagandha), on neurodegenerative diseases such as Huntington's disease treatment is discussed.

Keywords: Huntington's disease, neurodegenerative diseases, Ayurvedic medicinal plants

INTRODUCTION

In 1872, George Huntington published the description of a disease, which would bear his name (Huntington 1872). His two publications were case studies that were based on patients who were under the care of his father who was also a physician. This neurodegenerative disease (ND) is inherited from one generation to another and is characterized by excessive motor movements and psychological problems. Although earlier descriptions about this ND were available (Harper 2002; Lund 1860), George Huntington's publication is considered to contain first complete description of HD.

Huntington's disease (HD) is a progressive neurodegenerative disease that has no effective cure. HD patients are treated symptomatically with drugs, but none modify the progress, onset, or ultimate fatality of HD. A key step in understanding the mechanism and drug development processes of HD occurred in 1993 after the cloning of the HD gene (Willard, 1993).

It leads to the creation of the cell-based and transgenic models that express the mutant HD gene, a great outcome for the drug discovery processes. They are invaluable tools for discovering targets, small therapeutic molecules, and characterizing pathogenic mechanisms by the mutant Huntingtin protein (mHTT) expression.

Epidemiology

HD is a very rare neuropsychiatric disease occurring with a prevalence of 5-10 per 100,000 in Caucasian populations (Roos, 2010). In Japan, is reported that the prevalence of HD is about 1/10 of the total population (Bates et al., 2002). Due to the advancement in the science and medical fields and the intake of herbal-based food and medicines, populations have increased in countries like India and China. This has led to an enhanced prevalence of HD.

Symptoms

The main hallmark of the HD is the uncontrolled movement of the legs, arms, face, head, and upper body. This disease also causes a diminished reasoning and thinking skills, including concentration, memory, judgment, as well as a reduced ability to plan and organize. In addition, HD induces changes in mood, especially anxiety, depression, uncharacteristic irritability, and anger. Obsessive-compulsive behavior is also found inducing a person to repeat the same question or activity multiple times (Fernandez-Alvarez, 2001).

Clinical Description

The symptoms and signs of HD include motor, psychiatric, and cognitive disturbances. Other less well-known, but prevalent and often devastating symptoms of HD include sudden weight loss and disturbances in the circadian rhythm, sleep-wake cycle, and autonomic nervous system. The mean age for the onset of HD is between 30 and 50 years, with occurrence ranging from 2 to 85 years. The mean duration of the disease is 17 to 20 years. The progression of HD leads to dependency in day-to-day activities and ultimately death. The main cause of death in HD is pneumonia, followed by suicide (Thorpy, 2012).

Causes and Risk Factors

The defective gene codes a protein that was named "Huntingtin" after linking it to HD. The Huntingtin protein (HTT) gene carries its blueprints in repetitions of simple nucleotides codes. This gene defect involves repeats of specific nucleotides in a small part of chromosome 7. The normal Huntingtin gene contains about 17 to 20 repetitions of this sequence among its total of more than 3,100. The HD defect causes the HTTto synthesize 40 or more repeats. By using genetic tests, the number of repeats present in an individual Huntingtin protein gene can be determined for HD (Moncke Buchner et al., 2001).

PATHOPHYSIOLOGY OF HUNTINGTON DISEASE

Gene mutation and repeat expansion play a key role in the pathophysiology of HD. This underlying defect of HD is caused by an abnormal CAG expansion of the Huntingtin gene (HTT), leading to an enhanced polyglutamine (polyQ) track in the HTT protein. Disease-causing mutations induce a CAG repeat 40 or more times. HTT is a 348-kD protein that is found ubiquitously in neurons. It is primarily cytoplasmic, but it is also present in the nucleus and other organelles, with enhanced levels present in the brain and testis. The poly Q expansion in the HTT protein leads to protein aggregation and cell toxicity. However, the mechanisms by which the mutant HTT protein induced HD have not yet been fully elucidated.

Pharmacological Treatment Options

Many agents and surgical procedures such as dopamine antagonists, dopamine-depleting agents, acetylcholinesterase inhibitors, glutamate antagonists, benzodiazepines, cannabinoids, lithium, dopamine agonists, fetal cell transplantation, and deep brain stimulation are considered as to be therapeutic treatments for HD (Armstrong and Miyasaki, 2012; Pidgeon and Rickards, 2013; Bagchi, 1983; Adam and Jankovic, 2008). These agents typically improve the hyperkinetic movement disorders of HD including chorea, ballism, dystonia, myoclonus, and tics. While choosing a pharmacological invention, Physicians should consider the possibility of negative or positive effects on the psychiatric issues also associated with HD, such as irritability, mania, anxiety, apathy, obsessive disorder, depression, and cognitive decline. Adjunctive therapies, behavioral plans, alternative and complementary therapies, and cognitive interventions also play key roles in addressing the HD symptoms.

Ayurvedic Way of Treating Neurodegenerative Diseases

Eight branches are practiced in Ayurveda: Kayachikitsa (internal medicine), Shalakya (ophthalmology and ENT), Shalya (surgery), Aagada (toxicology), Kaumarbhritya (pediatrics), Rasayana (rejuvenation), Bhuta Vidya (psychology), and Bajikarana (sexology). Among various disciplines, Rasayanatantra improves memory and longevity helping to attain a youthful appearance as well as maintain normal brain function and physical strength (Singh et al. 2008).

The Ayurvedic treatment of HD is aimed at managing the symptoms and enrouting the basic pathology of the disease. Medicines like Kutaj (*Holarrhina antidysentrica*), Kutki (*Picrorrhiza kurroa*), Patha

(*Cissampelo-spareira*), Saariva (*Hemidesmus indicus*), Patol (*Tricosan thedioica*), Guggulu (*Commipho ramukul*), Musta (*Cyperus rotundus*), Psyllium (*Planta goovata*), Amalaki (*Emblica officinalis*), Lashuna (*Allium sativum*), and Haritaki (*Terminalia chebula*) are utilized to regulate the cholesterol metabolism. Medicines such as Shankhpushpi (*Convolvulus pluricaulis*), Brahmi (*Bacopa monnieri*), Ashwagandha (*Withania somnifera*), Vacha (*Acorus calamus*), and Mandukparni (*Centella asiatica*) are used to alleviate or slow down the neurodegeneration and improve dementia, cognitive ability, and speech defects.

The common name of the Ashwagandha (*Withania somnifera*), belonging Solanaceae family, is "Indian Winter cherry" or "Ginseng". It is an important ayurvedic herb used as a Rasayana medicine for its board range of health effects. It can be described as an herbal substance, which expands happiness by promoting physical and mental health. It is taken by small children as a tonic to promote cognitive functions and by adults to enhance longevity. Among the ayurvedic medicine, Ashwagandha has plays major role, known as a "Sattvic Kapha Rasayana" Herb (Changhadi, 1938).

It is commonly used either as a finely ground and sieved powder or a churn along with water, honey, or ghee. It improves the function of the brain and enhances the memory. It also improves the function of the reproductive system and promotes a sexual and reproductive life. It is also considered to be adominant adaptogen, which increases the body's resistance to stress. It enhances the defense of the body by improving the T cell immunity and acts as an antioxidant protecting cells against free radical toxicity.

Recent studies showed that Ashwagandha administration slows, reverses, stops, or removes neuritic atrophy and synaptic loss in the brains of patients of other NDs like AD, PD and Creutzfeldt- Jakob disease. Glyco with anolides (withaferin- A) and sitoindosides VII–X of ashwagandha significantly reversed the ibotenic acid induced cognitive defects in AD (Bhattacharya et al., 1995). It has been described as a nervine tonic (Singh et al., 1988), which is appear to cure disease by inducing immunity (Singh et al., 1986) and longevity in the users. Its extract dose dependently improved the activities of the antioxidant enzyme, catecholamine levels, dopaminergic D2 receptor binding, and tyrosine hydroxylase (TH) expression induced by 6-hydroxydopamine (6-OHDA) in rats. Thus, these studies suggest that Ashwagandha may be effective in protecting the dopaminergic neuronal injury in Parkinson's disease (Nagashyana et al., 2000).

ORAL AYURVEDIC MEDICINES FOR HUNTINGTON'S DISEASE

Kashayam or Herbal Decoctions

- Maharasnadi kashayam to relieve dystonia and jerky movements and to treat the pain and swelling that the patient may suffer due to altered gait
- Prasarinyadi kashayam to relieve pain, swelling, and inflammation
- Drakshadi kashayam to balance both vata and pitta dosha to treat mental aspects of the disease
- Gandharvahastadi kashayam
- Sahacharadi Kashayam

Asava/Arishtamor Herbal Fermented Liquids

- Balarishtam to calm the nerves
- Saraswath arishtam to improve memory and concentration
- Ashwagandha arishtam to improve muscle strength and induce sleep
- Draksh arishtam to calm the mind and treat mania

Vati/Gulika or Tablets and Capsules

- Ogarajaguggulu to relieve pain and inflammation
- Brahmibati to improve memory and concentration

- Shallakito relieve dystonia
- Ksheerabala 101 capsule
- Rasayanam or Rejuvenators and Leham or Confections
- Ashwagand harasayanam to improve motors skills
- Ajashwagand harasayanam
- Ajamamsarasayanam
- Drakshadirasayanam or drakshadileham
- Kushmandarasayanam

CAN AYURVEDA CURE HUNTINGTON'S DISEASE?

Since this is a genetic disorder, a complete cure cannot be promised. But the mental aspects can be improved so as to enable the patient to get through daily life, at least in the early and middle stages. Physical symptoms are the hardest to cure. However, if the disease is diagnosed early, then motor skills can be maintained or even improved. Since it is a chronic disorder, treatment will be required on a continuous basis for a very long time. If the symptoms are severe and persist for 2–6 weeks, choose the panchakarma therapy.

CONCLUSION

It may be concluded that HD is neurodegenerative disorder characterized by midlife onset, cognitive decline, involuntary movements, and behavioral disturbances. It is an autosomal and inherited disorder of the central nervous system involving widespread degenerative changes of the cerebral cortex and basal ganglia and other brain regions. Currently, there is no way to predict this disease prior to its occurrence. While HD progression cannot be reversed or stopped, therapies can partially alleviate symptoms and improve the quality of life of sufferers. Various treatments including pharmacological drugs such as dopamine antagonists, antidepressants, presynaptic dopamine depleters, anxiolytic benzodiazepines, anticonvulsants, tranquilizers, and Antibiotics only provide symptomatic relief of mental health care, speed, swallowing, and physical therapies. Other medications such aside benone, baclofen, and vitamin E were studied in clinical trials with limited samples. Modern research aiming to develop therapeutic agents that alter the course of neurodegenerative disease like HD by preventing neuronal death or stimulating neuronal recovery is needed. The goal of current research is to develop treatments that can prevent, retard, or reverse neuronal cell death. More specific treatments for Huntington's disease should become feasible with advances in knowledge of their etiology.

REFERENCES

Armstrong, M. J. Miyasaki, J. M. (2012). Evidence-Based Guideline: Pharmacologic Treatment of Chorea in Huntington Disease: Report of the Guideline Development Subcommittee of the American Academy of Neurology. *Neurology* 79, 597–603.

Bagchi, S. P. (1983). Differential Interactions of Phencyclidine with Tetrabenazine and Reserpine Affecting Intraneuronal Dopamine. *Biochem Pharmacol* 32, 2851–2856.

Bates, G., Harper, P. Jones, L. (2002). *Huntington's Disease*. Oxford University Press, 3.

Bhattacharya, S. K., Kumar, A. Ghosal, S. (1995). Effects of Glycowithanolides from *Withania somnifera* on Animal Model of Alzheimer's Disease and Perturbed Central Cholinergic Markers of Cognition in Rats. *Phytother Res.* 9, 110–113.

Bruyn, G. W. (1968). Huntington's Chorea: Historical, Clinical and Laboratory Synopsis. In *Handbook of Clinical Neurology.* 6, Editors. Vinken, P. J., Bruyn, G. W. Elsevier Amsterdam; 298-378.

Sharma, C. G. (1938). *Ashwagand harishta - Rastantra Sar Evam Sidhyaprayog Sangrah - Krishna-Gopal Ayurveda Bhawan (Dharmarth Trust)* Nagpur: 743–744.

Ellerby, L. M. (2002). Hunting for Excitement: NMDA Receptors in Huntington's Disease. *Neuron.* 33, 841–842.

Fernandez-Alvarez, E. Aicardi, J. (2001). *Movement Disorders in Children* Cambridge University Press. 36.

Harper, P. (2002). Huntington's Disease: A Historical Background. In *Huntington's Disease* (editors. Bates G., Harper P.S., Jones L.), Oxford, Oxford University Press. 3–37

Huntington's Disease Collaborative Research Group (1993). A Novel Gene Containing a Trinucleotide Repeat That is Expanded and Unstable on Huntington's Disease Chromosomes. *Cell* 72, 971–983.

Huntington, G. (1872).On chorea. In *The Medical and Surgical Reporter: A Weekly Journal,* (ed. Butler, S.W.), 317–321.

Kumar, P. Kumar, A. (2009). Possible Neuroprotective Effect of *Withania somnifera* Root Extract Against 3-Nitropropionic Acid-Induced Behavioral, Biochemical, and Mitochondrial Dysfunction in an Animal Model of Huntington's Disease. *J Med Food.* 12, 591–600.

Kumar, P., Kalonia, H. Kumar, A. (2011). Role of LOX/COX Pathways in 3-Nitropropionic Acid-Induced Huntington's Disease-Like Symptoms in Rats: Protective Effect of Licofelone. *Br J Pharmacol.* 164, 644–654.

Nagashyana, N., Sankarankutty, P., Nampoothiri, M. R. V., Moahan, P. Mohan Kumar, P. (2000) Association of L- Dopa with Recovery Following Ayurvedic Medication in Parkinson's Disease. *J Neurol Sci.* 176, 1121–1127.

Öncke Buchner, E., Reich, S., Mücke, M., Reuter, M., Messer, W., Wanker, E. E. Krüger, D. H. (2002). Counting CAG Repeats in the Huntington's Disease Gene by Restriction Endonuclease Eco P15I Cleavage. *Nucleic acids research.* 30, e83-e83.

Paleacu, D. (2007). Tetrabenazine in the Treatment of Huntington's Disease. *Neuropsychiatr Dis Treat* 3, 545–551.

Pidgeon, C. Rickards, H. (2013). The Pathophysiology and Pharma-Cological Treatment of Huntington Disease. *Behav Neurol* 26, 245–253.

Roos, R. A. (2010). Huntington's Disease: A Clinical Review. *Orphanet Journal of Rare Diseases*. 5, 40.

Singh, N. (1986). A Pharmaco-Clinical Evaluation of Some Ayurvedic Crude Plant Drugs As Anti-Stress Agents and Their Usefulness in Some Stress Diseases of Man. *Ann Nat Acad Ind Med.* 2:14–26.

Singh N. (1988). Effect of *Withania somnifera* and *Panax Ginseng* on Dopaminergic Receptors in Rat Brain During Stress. *36th Annual Congress on Medicinal Plant Research* (Freiburg) p. 28.

Tasset, I., Sánchez-López, F., Agüera, E., Fernández-Bolaños, R., Sánchez, F.M., Cruz Guerrero, A., Gascón-Luna, F. Túnez, I. (2012). NGF and Nitrosative Stress in Patients with Huntington's Disease. *J Neurol Sci.* 315, 133–136.

Thorpy, M. J. (2012). Classification of Sleep Disorders. *Neurotherapeutics.* 9, pp. 687-701.

Willard, H. F. (1993). The Needle Found! Trinucleotide Repeat Expansion in the Huntington's Disease Gene. *Hum Mol Genet.* 2, 497–498.

Zadori, D., Geisz, A., Vamos, E., Vecsei, L. Klivenyi, P. (2009). Valproate Ameliorates the Survival and the Motor Performance in a Transgenic Mouse Model of Huntington's Disease. *Pharmacol Biochem Behav.* 94, 148–153.

In: Food for Huntington's Disease
Editors: M. Mohamed Essa et al.
ISBN: 978-1-53613-854-2
© 2018 Nova Science Publishers, Inc.

Chapter 11

BENEFICIAL ROLES OF CURCUMIN, THE CURRY SPICE, IN HUNTINGTON'S DISEASE

C. Saravana Babu[1,], A. Bhat[1],*
R. Bipul[1], N. Chethan[1], A. H. Tousif[1],
A. M. Mahalakshmi[1], T. Manivasagam[2],
A. Justin Thenmozhi[2] and M. Mohamed Essa[3,4]

[1]Department of Pharmacology, JSS College of Pharmacy,
JSS Academy of Higher Education and Research,
SS Nagar, Mysore, KA, India
[2]Department of Biochemistry and Biotechnology,
Annamalai University, Annamalainagar, TN, India
[3]Department of Food Science and Nutrition, CAMS,
Sultan Qaboos University, Muscat, Oman
[4]Ageing and Dementia Research Group,
Sultan Qaboos University, Muscat, Oman

---

[*] Corresponding Author. Saravana Babu Chidambaram, Associate Professor, Department of Pharmacology, JSS College of Pharmacy, JSS Academy of Higher Education and Research, SS Nagar, Mysore - 570015, KA, India. Tel: +91-9940434129; Email: csaravanababu@gmail.com.

Abstract

Curcumin a highly bioactive principle obtained from *Curcuma longa*. It possesses a wide range of activities like anti-inflammatory, antioxidant, anticancer, neuroprotection etc. Various studies in animals have reported that it is against a wide range of human diseases, including diabetes, obesity, neurological and psychiatric disorders and cancer, as well as chronic illnesses affecting the eyes, lungs, liver, kidneys and gastrointestinal and cardiovascular systems. It is shown neuroprotective action in Alzheimer's disease, tardive dyskinesia, major depression, epilepsy, and other related neurodegenerative and neuropsychiatric disorders. The mechanism by which it acts as a neuroprotective is not clear. However it has been stated that it acts by its anti-inflammatory and antioxidant property. It inhibits reactive microglial and glial cells over-activation and prevents the neuronal cell death. Curcumin enhances neurogenesis, in the frontal cortex and hippocampal regions of the brain. Curcumin also modulates various neurotransmitters in brain. Curcumin is a promising natural agent however the problems associated with its low bioavailability requires great consideration. Glutamate toxicity is one of the major detrimental neurochemical pathways that causes increased intracellular calcium over-load, triggers inflammation and oxidative stress. Curcumin is shown to alleviate glutamate toxicity and in turn neuronal death via inhibition of oxidative stress and apoptosis. Glutamate toxicity also known as excitotoxicity is one of the key perpetrator in induction of neurodegeneration in Huntington's disease. The present chapter summarizes the mechanism of neuroprotective effect of curcumin in Huntington's disease.

Introduction

Neurodegeneration reduces the number of functional neurons and changes the synaptic plasticity. It is due to the activation of the proinflammatory factor, the accumulation of protein aggregates, and the production of the reactive oxidative species (Cole et al., 2007). Curcumin is a yellow colored pigment obtained from the rhizomes of turmeric which is used as a spice in food preparations as well as in folk medicine in south and central Asia. Curcumin because of its anti-oxidant, anti-inflammatory, and antiprotein-aggregate activities is a target drug in the treatment of various neurodegenerative disease like Parkinson disease, Alzheimer's disease (AD), multiple sclerosis, and Huntington's disease (HD) (Wang et al., 2017). It acts as an antioxidant by modulating the nuclear factor (Nrf2) which in turn leads to the upregulation of catalase (CAT), superoxide dismutase (SOD), and glutathione peroxidase (GPx) (Sethi et al., 2009). Curcumin downregulates inflammatory transcription factors like the Nuclear factor-kB (NF-kB), inflammatory cytokines, interleukins, chemokines, and the tumor necrosis factor-a (TNF-a), as well as inflammatory enzymes such as cycloxygenase-2 (COX-2) and inducible NO synthase (iNOS factor) (Aggarwal and Sung, 2009). Curcumin because of its poor absorption and quick biotransformation has a low bioavailability, however it can cross blood brain barrier (Lee et al., 2013).

EXCITOTOXICITY IN HUNTINGTON DISEASE

Excitotoxicity plays a major part in the degeneration of neurons in Huntington's disease (Mehta et al., 2013). Polyglutamine increase causes the hyper activation of the N-methyl-D-aspartate receptor (NMDAR and kainite receptors) (Song et al., 2003), which stabilizes the postsynaptic membrane NMDA receptors (Roche et al., 2001). While glutamate is inhibited at the synapses, it also affects the inositol, (1,4,5)-triphosphate receptor type 1, present in the endoplasmic reticulum membrane (Tang et al., 2003). Mutant huntingtin protein (MHTT) also contributes to excitotoxicity by downregulating the main astroglial glutamate transporter (GLT-1) (Liévens et al., 2001), which is responsible for the decrease in the uptake of glutamate (Shin et al., 2005). Most of these changes are responsible for glutamate-induced excitotoxicity by increasing intracellular Ca^{2+}, which disturbs the calcium homeostatic mechanism (Chen et al., 2000) and leads to harmful effects. Alterations in the calcium homeostasis were noted in HD mice (Tang et al., 2003). Calcium homeostasis in HD is considered as a potential target in the treatment of HD (Bezprozvanny, 2009). Excitotoxicity and mHTT also regulate a number of pathways mediated by kinases and phosphatase. Changes in the proteins responsible for glutamate signaling have been found in HD (Luthi-Carter et al., 2003).

Excitotoxicity is responsible for the decrease in neurons in HD due to the potentiation of glutamate release. In the early stages no major alterations in the expression of proteins were noticed in HD animal models (Giralt et al., 2009). Localization and expression of NMDA receptors play a crucial role in extra synaptic NMDAR activation and reduce ERK, which in turn inhibits CREB activation and BDNF production, leading to cell demise; synaptic NMDAR stimulation activates ERK that leads to effects in the nuclear homeostasis, in turn activating the transcription factor CREB and the production of BDNF (Hardingham and Bading, 2010). Glutamate transporters, like vesicular glutamate transporter 1 (VGluT1), are also affected in HD; VGluT1is responsible for bringing modifications to glutamate in the neurons, causing cell dysfunction in HD (Giralt et al., 2009). The alteration of the glutamate transporters in glial cells has been thought to be a promising therapeutic target in HD (Danbolt, 2001).

EXCITOTOXICITY TRIGGERED CYTOKINE RELEASE

It is a well-known fact that the overstimulation of the ion channel glutamate receptors (NMDA), due to their high permeability to Ca^{2+}, leads to neuronal demise and thus affecting the CNS functions (Choi et al., 1992; Nowak et al., 1984). The stimulation of the NMDAR via Kianic acid induces an activation of the mRNA for cytokines like interleukin-1β (IL-1β), interleukin-6, tumor necrosis factor (TNF-α), and the leukemia inhibitory factor in rats (Minami et al., 1991). Cytokines are responsible for neurodegeneration and neuromodulation in the brain after excitotoxicity (Yabuuchi et al., 1993). Kianic acid helps in the production of the endogenous interleukin-1 receptor antagonist (IL-1ra) in the brain of rats (Chau and Tai, 1981). IL-1ra mRNA expression is linked with declining pathological alterations in the brains of rats (Eriksson et al., 1998). Activation of microglia by Kianic acid is also responsible for the expression of cytokines, which mediate cellular communication (Minami et al., 1991).

EXCITOTOXICITY TRIGGERED OXIDATIVE STRESS

Oxidative stress is partly responsible for the development of neurodegenerative diseases. It damages nucleic acids, proteins, and lipids as well as facilitates the opening of mitochondrial permeability transition pore, thereby enhancing in the production of ROS, the aggravate energy fiasco, and stimulates the release of the proapoptotic agents like cytochrome c in cytoplasm (Nicholls, 2004). The aggravation of ROS and the alteration in the protective antioxidant mechanism leads to the neuronal cell demise (Farooqui and Farooqui, 2009). Nitric oxide (NO) production proliferates neurodegeneration. NO regulates cerebral vasoactivity, its production is enhanced by the release of glutamate followed by inhibition of glutamate removal, which over activates NMDAR and leads to excessive Ca^{2+} influx (Law et al., 2001). The deleterious effects of NO are caused by its action on the downstream metabolite $ONOO^-$. $ONOO^-$ regulates excitotoxicity and promotes oxidative DNA damage (Brown and Bal-Price, 2003). NO leads to an overexpression of metalloproteinases, damaging the surrounding neuronal cells. The overexpression of metalloproteinases also leads to cell detachment, causing anoikis. Thus the existence of NO and ONOO- accelerates the neuronal cell demise in neurodegenerative diseases. Intracellular ROS induce damage through mitochondrial changes, which cause the release of cytochrome c by activating the JNK pathway and the nuclear factor-κB (NF-κB) transcription factors (Berman and Hastings, 1999). Thus, keeping ROS in control is essential in the treatment of neurodegenerative diseases because it damages the neuronal cells (Maalouf et al., 2007).

EXCITOTOXICITY INDUCED APOPTOSIS

Glutamate potentiates caspase activity, which is in turn, removes trophic factors thereby activating the signaling pathway leading to neuronal apoptosis (Deckwerth and Johnson, 1993; Tenneti et al., 1998). By using a peptide inhibitor or a caspase pseudoenzyme, which guards substrates from metabolism, NMDA receptor-potentiated neuronal apoptosis could be enhanced by inhibiting the breakdown of caspase substrates. There are many caspases that have been cloned, but it is yet clear which one mediates neuronal apoptosis; several could potentially be responsible like CPP32 (caspase 3) and Nedd2 (caspase 2), depending on the cell type and form of the insult. Endogenous modulators of caspase activity are currently being studied. One of the major pathways that regulates the caspases is comprised of S-nitrosylation, a non-cGMP enabled activity of the NO group. The S-nitrosylation (a transfer of the NO group to a critical cysteine sulfhydryl) of various ion channels, enzymes, transcription factors, and other cellular proteins seems to be a universal regulatory event, similar to phosphorylation (Stamler et al., 1997). S-nitrosylation of the NMDA receptor changes its physiological functions (Lipton and Stamler, 1994). Caspase action may be reduced by the S-nitrosylation of an important cysteine residue present on an active site of caspase enzymes (Tenneti et al., 1997). It has been suggested that the apoptosis by the NO group may be reduced by decreasing caspase activity, whereas under other conditions, NO will react with O_2- to form peroxynitrite and precipitate cell demise (either apoptotic or necrotic depending on the concentration of the initial insult) (Tenneti et al., 1997).

ROLE OF CURCUMIN IN EXCITOTOXICITY

Excitotoxicity is mediated by NDMA receptors, which play a crucial part in the survival of the cell as the hyperactivity of NMDA receptors kills neuronal cells. In excitotoxic cell demise, two different patterns, like necrosis and apoptosis, have been recognized (Choi, 1992). NMDA-induced apoptosis affect GABAergic neurons which are also affected by excitotoxicity (Duarte et al., 1998). Curcumin protects GABAergic neurons from the pro-apoptotic activity of the excitotoxicity of NMDA. A decrease in intracellular Ca^{2+} homeostasis is responsible for the cell demise by apoptosis and/or necrosis (Orrenius et al., 2003). Ca^{2+} is a key secondary messenger for NMDA receptor-mediated synaptic activity and excitotoxicity (Arundine and Tymianski, 2003). Curcumin decreased the

NMDA-mediated Ca^{2+} levels, confirming that neuroprotection is achieved by decreasing the NMDA potentiated Ca^{2+} influx (Chen et al., 2015). Reduced Ca^{2+} influx by curcumin can be achieved through its effect on Muller cells by improving their buffer capacity. Curcumin attenuates intracellular signaling, which in turn modulates NMDA receptor function (Matteucci et al., 2005). Curcumin inhibits both serine-threonine and tyrosine kinases, regulators NMDA receptors, like cAMP-dependent protein kinase, protein kinase C, phosphorylase K, and Src-kinase (Aggarwal et al., 2003).

Curcumin decreases the activity of the NMDA receptor by affecting its phosphorylation. The NMDA receptor is a heteromeric ligand-gated ion channel having a number of receptor sub-units (NR1, NR2A-B, and NR3A) (Cull-Candy et al., 2001). The NR1 subunit appears to be ubiquitous and essential for Ca^{2+}-permeable receptor (Chen et al., 2003). The NMDAR activity is regulated by the phosphorylation of different subunits that play a part in the excitotoxic cell damage, the initiation of protein kinases (Greengard et al., 1991), or the inhibition of protein phosphatases (Westphal et al., 1999) enhancing the neuronal reactions to glutamate receptor agonists. Curcumin modulates the NMDA receptor activity without affecting its physiological function or inhibiting its pathological stimulation and thus helps protect neurons from demise.

CURCUMIN IN NEUROMUSCULAR DISEASE

Neurodegenerative diseases lead to the accumulation of the protein aggregates, oxidative stress, and the activation of proinflammatory factors. Curcumin has the desired characteristic of working as a neuroprotective drug. Curcumin decreases oxidative damage, prevents glial activation, binds amyloid plaques, and inhibits amyloid aggregation. Curcumin interacts with a number of targets such as transcription factors, inflammatory cytokines, antioxidants as well as other enzymes, kinases, and growth factors. This ability of curcumin to control a number of molecular links is the mechanism for its neuroprotective property. Its neuroprotective effect comes from its ability to act on oxidative stress, proinflammatory substances, and protein aggregation, which are evident in most of the neurodegenerative diseases. Curcumin has been shown to be a neuroprotective agent in various neurodegenerative diseases, like AD, by disrupting the prevailing plaques and partly repairing distorted neurites (Lim et al., 2001). Curcumin also modulates multiple cell signaling pathways and thus averts the progression of several autoimmune neurological diseases including MS (Qureshi et al., 2018). Curcuminoids in Parkinson disease by enhancing SOD/GSH/NGF/Hsp70 expressions, improving neuro functions in the *Substantia nigra* neurons (Mythri and Bharath, 2012). Curcumin treatment prevents the fibrillization of a-synuclein and increases the dopamine levels in early Parkinson disease (Zbarsky et al., 2005), epilepsy (Sumanont et al., 2006), cerebral injury (Ghoneim et al., 2002), age-associated neurodegeneration (Calabrese et al., 2003), schizophrenia (Bishnoi et al., 2008), Spongiform encephalopathies (Creutzfeld-Jakob disease) (Hafner-Bratkovic et al., 2008), neuropathic pain (Sharma et al., 2006a), and depression (Xu et al., 2005).

CURCUMIN IN CYTOKINE RELEASE

Curcumin inhibits the release of various cytokines. Abe et al. (1999) reported that curcumin inhibits IL1β, IL8, TNFα, the monocyte chemoattractant protein-1 (MCP1), and the macrophage inflammatory protein-1α (MIP1α) release from monocytes and macrophages. Jain et al. (2009) reported that curcumin significantly decreases the release of IL6, IL8, TNFα, and MCP1 from monocytes, which were grown in a high glucose atmosphere. Curcumin significantly reduced the levels of IL6, TNFα, and MCP1 in streptozotocin-induced hyperglycemic rats (Jain et al., 2009). Curcumin inhibits the release of IL6 in the rheumatoid synovial fibroblasts, IL8 in the human esophageal epithelial cells and alveolar epithelial cells, and IL1 in bone marrow stromal cells, colonic epithelial cells, and human articular chondrocytes (Kloesch et al., 2013; Raflee et al., 2009, Biswas et al., 2005; Xu et al., 1998). Curcumin blocks the release of

IL2, IL12, interferon-γ, and many other key cytokines (Gao et al., 2004; Fahey et al., 2007; Bachmeier et al., 2008; Xu et al., 1997).

CURCUMIN IN OXIDATIVE STRESS

Curcumin improves the systemic signs of oxidative stress (Sahebkar et al., 2015). It is also evident that curcumin can potentiate the actions of antioxidant enzymes like superoxide dismutase (SOD) (Menon and Sudheer, 2007). Curcumin protects against oxidative stress through a number of mechanisms. It scavenges most of the free radicals generated in neurodegenerative diseases by controlling the action of the antioxidants which neutralize the generated free radicals (Menon and Sudheer, 2007; Sahebkar et al., 2015); also, curcumin inhibits ROS-producing enzymes like lipoxygenase/cyclooxygenase and xanthine hydrogenase/oxidase (Sahebkar et al., 2015). Because of its lipophilic nature cucurmin can easily go against the free radicals, thus like vitamin E, it is a chain breaking antioxidant (Menon and Sudheer, 2007).

CURCUMIN IN APOPTOSIS

Curcumin inhibits the development of a wide range of tumor cells in different animal models. The mechanisms of its apoptotic induction are mixed, this includes inhibiting Akt dephosphorylation and NF-κB stimulation, reducing the levels of Bcl-2 and Bcl-XL potentiating cytochrome c release, increasing the progression and DNA damage gene (GADD153), and the stimulation of p38 and caspase-3 (Pan et al., 2001; Woo et al., 2003). The signaling pathways responsible for apoptosis in mammals are multifaceted and the pro- as well as the anti-apoptotic variations control the cell existence alterations from cell to cell (Cory and Adams, 2002). The mechanism curcumin uses to induce apoptosis in HT-29 cells is not clear. Mitochondrial and demise receptor pathways are the main apoptosis signaling pathways. Changes in the mitochondrial membrane potential and the relocation of cytochrome c from the mitochondria to cytosol in apoptosis are the beginning phases in the apoptotic cascade (Kluck et al., 1997). This cytochrome c forms an "apoptosome" of Apaf-1, cytochrome c, and caspase-9, which successively cleaves the effector caspase-3 (Li et al., 1997). Curcumin potentiates the release of cytochrome c from the mitochondria in a number of cell lines (Rashmi et al., 2003; Sen et al., 2005; Cao et al., 2007). Thus suggesting that the mitochondria are associated with curcumin-caused apoptosis. Curcumin acts as an antiproliferative by inducing apoptosis in HT-29 cells through the mitochondrial cell demise pathway. Curcumin reduces Bcl-2/Bax and Bcl-xL/Bad ratios, which in turn initiates caspase-3, the release of cytochrome c, and the collapse of $\Delta\Psi m$ It also downregulates survivin, another important anti-apoptotic protein (Wang et al., 2009).

CURCUMIN IN HUNTINGTON DISEASE

Huntington's disease (HD) is a neurological disease triggered by an increase of polyglutamine (polyQ) repeats inside the Huntingtin (HTT) protein with limited treatment options. This mutant Huntingtin (mHTT) protein with an extended polyQ upon expression generates inclusion bodies (IBs), increased cellular toxicity, the development of motor disabilities, and reduced viability in HD. Subcellular actions like oxidative stress, mitochondrial dysfunction, inflammation, and transcriptional dysregulation contribute to the development of HD (Chongtham and Agrawal, 2016).

Turmeric, is a dietary spice used in Asian food as well as in folk medicine in the management of different pathological conditions. Curcumin, due to its lipophilic nature, can cross the blood brain barrier (Lee et al., 2013). Curcumin has strong antioxidant, anti-inflammatory, and anti-protein aggregation activities; as a result it is used in the therapy of numerous neurodegenerative diseases (Menon and Sudheer, 2007). Curcumin also improved the polyQ induced motor neuronal dysfunction. Apoptosis is responsible for the neuronal demise in polyQ diseases including HD (Mattson, 2000; Saudou et al., 1998). Curcumin has an ability to suppress polyQ-induced neurodegeneration, thus potentially treat the neurodegenerative diseases with a high safety index. It retards any further damage to the neuronal architecture. By inhibiting the production of the elongated polyQ protein as well as neuronal damage during the non-feeding pupal period, it can affect the degree of retrieval in eye morphology and motor function. Curcumin inhibits the generation of Abeta40 fibrils in vitro (Yang et al., 2005). It can cross cell membranes and enter nuclei (Kunwar et al., 2009). Treatment with curcumin may also directly inhibit, or slow aggregate formation, resulting in a reduced density. Curcumin improves polyQ-induced neuronal dysfunction, inhibits neurodegeneration and cytotoxicity, thus it is a possible treatment of polyQ disease patients (Chongtham and Agrawal, 2016).

REFERENCES

[1] Aggarwal, B. B., Kumar, A., Bharti, A. C., 2003. Anticancer Potential of Curcumin: Preclinical and Clinical Studies. *Anticancer Res.* 23, 363–398.

[2] Aggarwal, B. B., Sung, B., 2009. Pharmacological Basis for the Role of Curcumin in Chronic Diseases: An Age-Old Spice with Modern Targets. *Trends Pharmacol. Sci.* 30, 85–94. https://doi.org/10.1016/j.tips.2008.11.002.

[3] Arundine, M., Tymianski, M., 2003. Molecular Mechanisms of Calcium-Dependent Neurodegeneration in Excitotoxicity. *Cell Calcium* 34, 325–337.

[4] Berman, S. B., Hastings, T. G., 1999. Dopamine Oxidation Alters Mitochondrial Respiration and Induces Permeability Transition in Brain Mitochondria: Implications for Parkinson's Disease. *J. Neurochem.* 73, 1127–1137.

[5] Bezprozvanny, I., 2009. Calcium Signaling and Neurodegenerative Diseases. *Trends Mol Med* 15, 89–100. Https://doi.org/10.1016/j.molmed.2009.01.001.

[6] Brown, G. C., Bal-Price, A., 2003. Inflammatory Neurodegeneration Mediated by Nitric Oxide, Glutamate, and Mitochondria. *Mol. Neurobiol.* 27, 325–355. Https://doi.org/10.1385/MN:27:3:325.

[7] Chen, K., An, Y., Tie, L., Pan, Y., Li, X., 2015. Curcumin Protects Neurons from Glutamate-Induced Excitotoxicity by Membrane Anchored AKAP79-PKA Interaction Network. *Evid Based Complement Alternat Med* 2015. https://doi.org/10.1155/ 2015/ 706207.

[8] Chen, M., Ona, V. O., Li, M., Ferrante, R. J., Fink, K. B., Zhu, S., Bian, J., Guo, L., Farrell, L. A., Hersch, S. M., Hobbs, W., Vonsattel, J. P., Cha, J. H., Friedlander, R. M., 2000. Minocycline Inhibits Caspase-1 and Caspase-3 Expression and Delays Mortality in a Transgenic Mouse Model of Huntington Disease. *Nat. Med.* 6, 797–801. https://doi.org/10.1038/77528.

[9] Chen, R.-W., Qin, Z.-H., Ren, M., Kanai, H., Chalecka-Franaszek, E., Leeds, P., Chuang, D.-M., 2003. Regulation of c-Jun N-Terminal Kinase, P38 Kinase and AP-1 DNA Binding in Cultured Brain Neurons: Roles in Glutamate Excitotoxicity and Lithium Neuroprotection. *J. Neurochem.* 84, 566–575.

[10] Choi, D. W., 1992. Excitotoxic Cell Death. *J. Neurobiol.* 23, 1261–1276. Https://doi.org/10.1002/neu.480230915.

[11] Chongtham, A., Agrawal, N., 2016. Curcumin Modulates Cell Death and Is Protective in Huntington's Disease Model. *Scientific Reports* 6, 18736. Https://doi.org/10.1038/srep18736.

[12] Cole, G. M., Teter, B., Frautschy, S.A., 2007. Neuroprotective Effects of Curcumin. *Adv Exp Med Biol* 595, 197–212.

[13] Cory, S., Adams, J. M., 2002. The Bcl2 Family: Regulators of the Cellular Life-Or-Death Switch. *Nat. Rev. Cancer* 2, 647–656. Https://doi.org/10.1038/nrc883.

[14] Cull-Candy, S., Brickley, S., Farrant, M., 2001. NMDA Receptor Subunits: Diversity, Development and Disease. *Curr. Opin. Neurobiol.* 11, 327–335.

[15] Danbolt, N. C., 2001. Glutamate Uptake. *Prog. Neurobiol.* 65, 1–105.

[16] Deckwerth, T. L., Johnson, E. M., 1993. Neurotrophic Factor Deprivation-Induced Death. *Ann. N. Y. Acad. Sci.* 679, 121–131.

[17] Duarte, C. B., Ferreira, I. L., Santos, P. F., Carvalho, A. L., Agostinho, P. M., Carvalho, A. P., 1998. Glutamate in Life and Death of Retinal Amacrine Cells. *Gen. Pharmacol.* 30, 289–295.

[18] Farooqui, T., Farooqui, A. A., 2009. Aging: An Important Factor for the Pathogenesis of Neurodegenerative Diseases. *Mech. Ageing Dev.* 130, 203–215. Https://doi.org/10.1016/j.mad.2008.11.006.

[19] Giralt, A., Rodrigo, T., Martín, E. D., Gonzalez, J. R., Milà, M., Ceña, V., Dierssen, M., Canals, J. M., Alberch, J., 2009. Brain-Derived Neurotrophic Factor Modulates the Severity of Cognitive Alterations Induced by Mutant Huntingtin: Involvement of Phospholipase C Gamma Activity and Glutamate Receptor Expression. *Neuroscience* 158, 1234–1250. https://doi.org/10.1016/j.neuroscience. 2008. 11.024.

[20] Greengard, P., Jen, J., Nairn, A. C., Stevens, C. F., 1991. Enhancement of the Glutamate Response by cAMP-Dependent Protein Kinase in Hippocampal Neurons. *Science* 253, 1135–1138.

[21] Hardingham, G. E., Bading, H., 2010. Synaptic Versus Extrasynaptic NMDA Receptor Signalling: Implications for Neurodegenerative Disorders. *Nat. Rev. Neurosci.* 11, 682–696. Https://doi.org/10.1038/nrn2911

[22] Jain, S. K., Rains, J., Croad, J., Larson, B., Jones, K., 2009. Curcumin Supplementation Lowers TNF-α, IL-6, IL-8, and MCP-1 Secretion in High Glucose-Treated Cultured Monocytes and Blood Levels of TNF-α, IL-6, MCP-1, Glucose, and Glycosylated Hemoglobin in Diabetic Rats. *Antioxid Redox Signal* 11, 241–249. Https://doi.org/ 10.1089/ars.2008.2140.

[23] Kluck, R. M., Bossy-Wetzel, E., Green, D. R., Newmeyer, D. D., 1997. The release of Cytochrome C from Mitochondria: A Primary Site For Bcl-2 Regulation of Apoptosis. *Science* 275, 1132–1136.

[24] Kunwar, A., Sandur, S. K., Krishna, M., Priyadarsini, K. I., 2009. Curcumin Mediates Time and Concentration Dependent Regulation of Redox Homeostasis Leading to Cytotoxicity in Macrophage Cells.

Eur J Pharmacol 611, 8–16. https://doi.org/10.1016/j.ejphar.2009.03.060.

[25] Law, A., Gauthier, S., Quirion, R., 2001. Say NO to Alzheimer's Disease: The Putative Links Between Nitric Oxide and Dementia of the Alzheimer's Type. Brain Res. Brain Res. Rev. 35, 73–96.

[26] Lee, W.-H., Loo, C.-Y., Bebawy, M., Luk, F., Mason, R. S., Rohanizadeh, R., 2013. Curcumin and Its Derivatives: Their Application in Neuropharmacology and Neuroscience in the 21st Century. *Curr Neuropharmacol* 11, 338–378. https://doi.org/10.2174/1570159X11311040002.

[27] Liévens, J. C., Woodman, B., Mahal, A., Spasic-Boscovic, O., Samuel, D., Kerkerian-Le Goff, L., Bates, G. P., 2001. Impaired glutamate uptake in the R6 Huntington's disease transgenic mice. *Neurobiol. Dis.* 8, 807–821. https://doi.org/10.1006/nbdi.2001.0430.

[28] Lipton, S. A., Stamler, J. S., 1994. Actions of Redox-Related Congeners of Nitric Oxide at the NMDA Receptor. *Neuropharmacology* 33, 1229–1233.

[29] Luthi-Carter, R., Apostol, B. L., Dunah, A. W., DeJohn, M. M., Farrell, L. A., Bates, G. P., Young, A. B., Standaert, D. G., Thompson, L. M., Cha, J. H. J., 2003. Complex Alteration of NMDA Receptors in Transgenic Huntington's Disease Mouse Brain: Analysis of mRNA and Protein Expression, Plasma Membrane Association, Interacting Proteins, and Phosphorylation. *Neurobiol. Dis.* 14, 624–636.

[30] Maalouf, M., Sullivan, P. G., Davis, L., Kim, D. Y., Rho, J. M., 2007. Ketones Inhibit Mitochondrial Production of Reactive Oxygen Species Production Following Glutamate Excitotoxicity by Increasing NADH oxidation. *Neuroscience* 145, 256–264. https://doi.org/10.1016/j.neuroscience.2006.11.065.

[31] Matteucci, A., Frank, C., Domenici, M. R., Balduzzi, M., Paradisi, S., Carnovale-Scalzo, G., Scorcia, G., Malchiodi-Albedi, F., 2005. Curcumin Treatment Protects Rat Retinal Neurons Against Excitotoxicity: Effect on ND Aspartate-Induced Intracellular Ca^{2+}

Increase. *Exp Brain Res* 167, 641–648. https://doi.org/10.1007/s00221-005-0068-0.

[32] Mattson, M. P., 2000. Apoptosis in Neurodegenerative Disorders. *Nat. Rev. Mol. Cell Biol.* 1, 120–129. https://doi.org/10.1038/35040009.

[33] Mehta, A., Prabhakar, M., Kumar, P., Deshmukh, R., Sharma, P. L., 2013. Excitotoxicity: Bridge to Various Triggers in Neurodegenerative Disorders. *Eur. J. Pharmacol.* 698, 6–18. https://doi.org/10.1016/j.ejphar.2012.10.032.

[34] Menon, V. P., Sudheer, A. R., 2007. Antioxidant and Anti-Inflammatory Properties of Curcumin. *Adv. Exp. Med. Biol.* 595, 105–125. https://doi.org/10.1007/978-0-387-46401-5_3.

[35] Mythri, R. B., Bharath, M.M.S., 2012. Curcumin: A Potential Neuroprotective Agent in Parkinson's Disease. *Curr. Pharm. Des.* 18, 91–99.

[36] Nicholls, D. G., 2004. Mitochondrial Dysfunction and Glutamate Excitotoxicity Studied in Primary Neuronal Cultures. *Curr. Mol. Med.* 4, 149–177.

[37] Nowak, L., Bregestovski, P., Ascher, P., Herbet, A., Prochiantz, A., 1984. Magnesium Gates Glutamate-Activated Channels in Mouse Central Neurones. *Nature* 307, 462–465.

[38] Orrenius, S., Zhivotovsky, B., Nicotera, P., 2003. Regulation of Cell Death: The Calcium-Apoptosis Link. *Nat. Rev. Mol. Cell Biol.* 4, 552–565. Https://doi.org/10.1038/nrm1150.

[39] Pan, M. H., Chang, W. L., Lin-Shiau, S. Y., Ho, C. T., Lin, J. K., 2001. Induction of Apoptosis by Garcinol and Curcumin Through Cytochrome C Release and Activation of Caspases in Human Leukemia HL-60 Cells. *J. Agric. Food Chem.* 49, 1464–1474.

[40] Qureshi, M., Al-Suhaimi, E. A., Wahid, F., Shehzad, O., Shehzad, A., 2018. Therapeutic Potential of Curcumin for Multiple Sclerosis. *Neurol. Sci.* 39, 207–214. Https://doi.org/10.1007/s10072-017-3149-5.

[41] Roche, K. W., Standley, S., McCallum, J., Dune Ly, C., Ehlers, M. D., Wenthold, R. J., 2001. Molecular Determinants of NMDA

Receptor Internalization. *Nat. Neurosci.* 4, 794–802. https://doi.org/10.1038/90498.

[42] Sahebkar, A., Banach, M., Serban, M.-C., Ursoniu, S., 2015. Effect of Curcuminoids on Oxidative Stress: A Systematic Review and Meta-Analysis of Randomized Controlled Trials. *Journal of functional foods.*

[43] Saudou, F., Finkbeiner, S., Devys, D., Greenberg, M. E., 1998. Huntingtin Acts in the Nucleus to Induce Apoptosis But Death Does Not Correlate with the Formation of Intranuclear Inclusions. *Cell* 95, 55–66.

[44] Sethi, G., Sung, B., Aggarwal, B. B., 2009. *The Role of Curcumin in Modern Medicine, in: Herbal Drugs: Ethnomedicine to Modern Medicine.* Springer, Berlin, Heidelberg, pp. 97–113. https://doi.org/10.1007/978-3-540-79116-4_7.

[45] Shin, J.-Y., Fang, Z.-H., Yu, Z.-X., Wang, C.-E., Li, S.-H., Li, X.-J., 2005. Expression of Mutant Huntingtin in Glial Cells Contributes to Neuronal Excitotoxicity. *J. Cell Biol.* 171, 1001–1012. https://doi.org/10.1083/jcb.200508072.

[46] Song, C., Zhang, Y., Parsons, C. G., Liu, Y. F., 2003. Expression of Polyglutamine-Expanded Huntingtin Induces Tyrosine Phosphorylation of N-Methyl-D-Aspartate Receptors. *J. Biol. Chem.* 278, 33364–33369. https://doi.org/10.1074/jbc.M304240200.

[47] Stamler, J. S., Toone, E. J., Lipton, S. A., Sucher, N. J., 1997. (S)NO Signals: Translocation, Regulation, and a Consensus Motif. *Neuron* 18, 691–696.

[48] Tang, T.-S., Tu, H., Chan, E. Y. W., Maximov, A., Wang, Z., Wellington, C. L., Hayden, M. R., Bezprozvanny, I., 2003. Huntingtin and Huntingtin-Associated Protein 1 Influence Neuronal Calcium Signaling Mediated by Inositol-(1,4,5) Triphosphate Receptor Type 1. *Neuron* 39, 227–239.

[49] Tenneti, L., D'Emilia, D. M., Lipton, S.A., 1997. Suppression of Neuronal Apoptosis by S-Nitrosylation of Caspases. *Neurosci. Lett.* 236, 139–142.

[50] Wang, J., Qi, L., Zheng, S., Wu, T., 2009. Curcumin Induces Apoptosis Through the Mitochondria-Mediated Apoptotic Pathway in HT-29 Cells. *J Zhejiang Univ Sci B* 10, 93–102. https://doi.org/10.1631/jzus.B0820238.

[51] Wang, X.-S., Zhang, Z.-R., Zhang, M.-M., Sun, M.-X., Wang, W.-W., Xie, C.-L., 2017. Neuroprotective Properties of Curcumin in Toxin-Base Animal Models of Parkinson's Disease: A Systematic Experiment Literatures Review. *BMC Complement Altern Med* 17. https://doi.org/10.1186/s12906-017-1922-x.

[52] Westphal, R. S., Tavalin, S. J., Lin, J. W., Alto, N. M., Fraser, I. D., Langeberg, L. K., Sheng, M., Scott, J. D., 1999. Regulation of NMDA Receptors by An Associated Phosphatase-Kinase Signaling Complex. *Science* 285, 93–96.

[53] Woo, J.-H., Kim, Y.-H., Choi, Y.-J., Kim, D.-G., Lee, K.-S., Bae, J. H., Min, D. S., Chang, J.-S., Jeong, Y.-J., Lee, Y. H., Park, J.-W., Kwon, T. K., 2003. Molecular Mechanisms of Curcumin-Induced Cytotoxicity: Induction of Apoptosis Through Generation of Reactive Oxygen Species, Down-Regulation of Bcl-XL and IAP, the Release of Cytochrome C and Inhibition of Akt. *Carcinogenesis* 24, 1199–1208. https://doi.org/10.1093/carcin/bgg082.

[54] Yang, F., Lim, G. P., Begum, A. N., Ubeda, O. J., Simmons, M. R., Ambegaokar, S. S., Chen, P. P., Kayed, R., Glabe, C. G., Frautschy, S. A., Cole, G. M., 2005. Curcumin Inhibits Formation of Amyloid Beta Oligomers and Fibrils, Binds Plaques, and Reduces Amyloid *In Vivo*. *J. Biol. Chem.* 280, 5892–5901. https://doi.org/10.1074/jbc.M404 751200.

ABOUT THE EDITORS

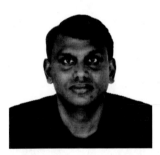

M. Mohamed Essa, PhD, is an Associate Professor of Nutrition at Sultan Qaboos University, Oman, and holding the visiting professor position in the neuropharmacology group, ASAM, at Macquarie University, Sydney, Australia. He is an editor-in-chief for the *International Journal of Nutrition, Pharmacology, Neurological Diseases* published by Wolters & Kluwer, US. He is also acting as associate editor for *BMC Complementary and Alternative Medicine*. Dr. Essa is involved as an editor/reviewer on the board of various well-known journals such as *Frontiers in Neurology, Frontiers in Bioscience, Biochemie, PloS One*, etc. Dr. Mohamed Essa is conducting research on the effect of dietary supplementation of natural products on neurodegenerative diseases. He is an expert in the field of nutritional neuroscience/neuropharmacology and has published one hundred and ten papers, forty one book chapters, and eight books. He has strong international collaborations with institutes in USA, Australia, Zurich and India. In 2015, Dr. Essa founded a new foundation named "Food and Brain Research Foundation" to support research in nutritional neuroscience. Dr. Essa is a recipient for many awards from local and international bodies. In 2015, his book, titled *Food and Brain Health*, was awarded as "Best Book in the World" by Gourmand Cookbook Awards and the same book was awarded "Best in the World of the Past Twenty Years" by Gourmand Cookbook Awards. In 2015 and 2016, Dr. Essa received the "National Research Award" under the health sector from The Research Council, Oman. In 2013 and 2017, he was awarded as a Distinguished Researcher, Sultan Qaboos University, Oman. One of his scientific images won the "Best of the Show," and "Best of Overall" in all categories in the "Science of Art- Photo Contest" at the ISN-ASN International meeting in Mexico, 2013. Furthermore, in 2010, Dr. Essa got the "Professional from Developing Country" award from IMFAR, USA. In 2009, he was awarded the ASN Young Investigator Educational Enhancement Award (ASN-YIEE-2009). In July of 2017, his book titled *Food and Parkinson's Disease* was awarded as best book in the world by Gourmand Cookbook Awards. He has over fifteen years of research experience and currently he has received many research grants from local and international agencies in the area of neuropharmacology and nutritional neurosciences (approximately 1.31 million USD).

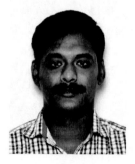

T. Manivasagam, PhD, is an Assistant Professor of Biochemistry at Annamalai University, India. He is working in the field of neuroscience and produced 10 pre-doctoral and 8 doctoral students. So far he published 89 papers and 12 book chapters. He received world best book award (3rd Place) for her book entitled *Food and Parkinson's Disease* by Gourmand Cook Book Awards in 2017. He has strong international collaborations with researchers in Oman, Australia and USA. He received "Young Scientist Award" from Annamalai University and Academy of Sciences, Chennai. He holds memberships in various international and national societies. He has received few awards and research grants from national and international agencies.

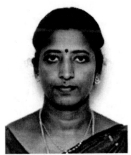

A. Justin Thenmozhi PhD, has been as an Assistant Professor in the Department of Biochemistry and Biotechnology, Annamalai University, India since 2007. She is working in the field of Neuroscience particularly in Alzheimer's disease and published 39 research papers in Peer reviewed journals, 6 book chapters and edited a book. She is serving as a reviewer in various well known journals such as Brain Research, Neurochemical Research, Chemico-Biological Interactions etc.,. She received world best book award (3rd Place) for her book entitled *Food and Parkinson's Disease* by Gourmand Cook Book Awards in 2017 under the category D9 Health and Nutrition Institutions. She has received the "Outstanding Women achiever Award in 2016" from Venus International Foundation. She has received research grants from UGC and DST, New Delhi, India. She has strong international collaborations with researchers in Oman, Australia and the United States of America.

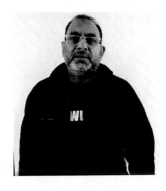

Qazi A. Hamid obtained his doctoral degree in biochemistry from one of the most prestigious universities of the world: Banaras Hindu University. He has accumulated over thirty years of experience in the field of cancer research, inflammation and recombinant immunology. Currently, he leads the operations of Rx Biosciences, Ltd as its Chief Executive Officer. For the last twelve years, the company has been involved in multidimensional research activities, particularly in the field of therapeutic antibodies. One of the main objectives of the company includes the discovery of new drug targets and therapeutic agents for diseases of great public significance such as prostate cancer and Alzheimer's disease. He is actively engaged in collaboration with leading pharmaceutical companies and federal government organizations within the United States such as the FDA, USDA and DOD. His current research focuses to develop therapeutic antibodies for neurodegenerative diseases including Alzheimer's and Huntington disease. Dr. Hamid has authored many peer reviewed scientific articles for international journals and has presented his findings at many national and international conferences. He has lead grant proposals awarded by National Cancer Institute, USA. Additionally, he has been on the reviewer's panel for National Institute of Health (NIH) along with some international scientific journals. Throughout most of his academic career, he has been ranked at the top, received prestigious honors and distinctions. He was awarded with a gold medal for ranking at the top in BS examination in the university. With all my academic achievements and professional expertise I feel very comfortable in writing about the book and would like to thank the authors for making a sincere effort to contribute in the wellbeing of mankind.

INDEX

A

acetylcholinesterase, 28, 102, 221, 243
acetylcholinesterase inhibitor, 28, 221, 243
acid, 5, 6, 12, 13, 14, 18, 19, 20, 23, 25, 29, 34, 36, 47, 50, 52, 54, 56, 60, 64, 65, 70, 71, 72, 73, 75, 76, 77, 78, 81, 82, 83, 84, 97, 100, 112, 114, 123, 125, 126, 128, 134, 136, 138, 142, 145, 148, 149, 150, 151, 155, 156, 157, 158, 190, 192, 199, 207, 219, 222, 225, 227, 230, 231, 232, 234, 235, 236, 244, 248, 254
adenosine, 65, 95
adrenal glands, 110
adrenocorticotropic hormone, 109
adverse effects, 51, 53, 142, 188
age, 2, 3, 10, 17, 19, 21, 29, 32, 33, 34, 64, 67, 89, 101, 108, 135, 154, 177, 182, 188, 217, 229, 242, 258, 261
aggregation, 2, 11, 34, 57, 58, 64, 79, 80, 118, 142, 146, 154, 242, 257, 260
alkaloids, ix, 12, 14, 67, 100, 190, 198, 199, 200, 201, 210, 213, 234
allergic reaction, 139
alpha-tocopherol, 145
alternative medicine, 240, 269
alters, 59, 68, 79, 131, 137, 172, 261
aluminium, 5, 23, 36, 67
amino acid, ix, 13, 22, 67, 68, 81, 95, 190, 192, 193, 196
amyloid beta, 31, 36, 38, 267
amyotrophic lateral sclerosis, 118, 135, 149, 158
analgesic, 99, 210, 225, 226, 227
antibiotic, 108, 113, 116, 123, 139, 190
anti-cancer, 94
anticoagulant, 69
anticonvulsant, 95, 98
antidepressant, 95, 247
anti-inflammatory agents, 188, 199
anti-inflammatory drugs, 10
antioxidant, 3, 7, 9, 11, 12, 13, 16, 18, 20, 24, 27, 28, 33, 34, 36, 37, 51, 56, 57, 58, 59, 67, 69, 75, 78, 94, 95, 118, 128, 144, 145, 146, 149, 150, 152, 156, 158, 197, 198, 199, 201, 218, 224, 226, 229, 230, 232, 245, 252, 253, 255, 259, 260
antitumor, 213, 224, 226
antitumor agent, 213
anxiety, 36, 42, 50, 111, 112, 113, 122, 128, 133, 137, 143, 218, 221, 233, 241, 243
apathy, 42, 143, 243

apoptosis, 7, 16, 37, 47, 49, 54, 73, 76, 82, 84, 88, 94, 153, 155, 158, 220, 228, 230, 234, 236, 237, 252, 255, 256, 259, 260, 263, 265, 266, 267
ascidians, 182, 190, 191, 192, 193, 195, 196, 197, 201, 205, 208, 209
ascorbic acid, 16, 19, 30, 35, 198
Asia, 33, 97, 182, 183, 206, 231, 252
Asian countries, x, 21, 183
aspartate, 23, 29, 253, 264, 266
aspartic acid, 5, 220
asthma, 18, 97, 98
astringent, 14, 67, 167, 174
astrocytes, 10, 17, 48
astrogliosis, 47, 49
atrophy, 43, 44, 184, 244
autism, 109, 111, 113, 115, 116, 134
autism spectrum disorder, 115, 130, 134
autoimmune diseases, 113
autonomic nervous system, 110, 216, 242
autonomic neuropathy, 18
autosomal dominant, 64, 161, 182
ayurveda, 25, 28, 98, 99, 240, 243, 246, 247
ayurvedic medicinal plants, 240

B

bacteria, 107, 108, 111, 112, 114, 116, 117, 119, 120, 122, 124, 126, 128, 132, 136, 196, 211
bacterial infection, 116
bacterial strains, 126
basal ganglia, 47, 49, 64, 89, 90, 146, 182, 184, 219, 232, 233, 246
behavior therapy, 50
behavioral disorder, 113
behavioral problems, 91
beneficial effect, 17, 20, 50, 56, 92, 124, 125, 146, 148, 149, 153, 156, 216, 228, 232
benthic invertebrates, 192

bioavailability, 8, 55, 56, 58, 148, 154, 252, 253
biochemistry, 81, 137
biodiversity, 189
biological activities, 67, 69, 97, 99, 222
biomedical applications, 201
biosynthesis, 136, 212, 234
biotechnology, 205
black tea, 4, 6, 29, 56, 59, 152
blood, 17, 21, 27, 28, 38, 53, 57, 65, 93, 96, 97, 112, 117, 125, 154, 182, 197, 253, 260
blood circulation, 97
blood flow, 38, 96
blood pressure, 21, 27, 94
body mass index, 185
body weight, 23, 56, 70, 71, 73, 74, 75, 77, 78, 230
bone marrow, 258
bowel, 122, 123, 132
brain, ix, x, 2, 3, 6, 10, 13, 16, 20, 24, 26, 34, 37, 38, 39, 43, 44, 45, 47, 48, 49, 53, 55, 57, 59, 63, 64, 65, 68, 70, 74, 81, 82, 83, 84, 87, 88, 102, 106, 109, 110, 111, 112, 113, 114, 115, 116, 117, 118, 119, 123, 124, 128, 129, 130, 131, 132, 133, 134, 135, 136, 137, 138, 142, 144, 146, 151, 154, 155, 156, 157, 162, 163, 167, 171, 178, 182, 183, 184, 185, 203, 215, 216, 218, 219, 221, 229, 231, 233, 234, 236, 239, 242, 243, 244, 246, 249, 252, 253, 254, 260, 261, 262, 263, 264, 265, 270, 272
brain activity, 123
brain damage, 38, 63
brain functions, 111
brain-derived neurotrophic factor, 83, 162, 203, 263

C

Ca^{2+}, 46, 47, 49, 65, 73, 152, 230, 253, 254, 256, 257
caffeine, 5, 26, 67, 82, 83, 84
CAG repeats, 44, 64, 66, 89, 143, 163, 178, 183, 187, 248
Cajal, 110
calcium, 19, 45, 76, 101, 127, 139, 178, 192, 228, 253, 261, 265, 266
cancer, 9, 18, 26, 30, 32, 33, 51, 58, 61, 94, 97, 109, 122, 126, 130, 149, 197, 222, 229, 252, 272
cannabinoids, 221, 231, 243
cannabis, 221, 231
carbohydrates, 5, 14, 192
carbon, 124, 127, 138, 222, 223
cardiovascular disease, 26, 58, 94, 103, 229
cardiovascular system, 182, 252
carotene, 19, 93, 101, 222
carotenoids, 19, 21, 26, 69, 198, 236
caspases, 220, 234, 256, 265, 266
catecholamines, 68, 75, 114
Caucasian population, 241
cell death, 8, 31, 54, 76, 148, 155, 183, 184, 185, 187, 220, 233, 247, 252, 262, 265
cell differentiation, 126
cell fate, 49
cell line, 16, 36, 66, 75, 76, 94, 118, 198, 200, 260
cell membranes, 10, 261
cell signaling, 258
central nervous system, 28, 129, 132, 136, 137, 160, 183, 184, 246
cerebellum, 24, 44, 50, 220, 234
cerebral amyloidosis, 8
cerebral cortex, 45, 50, 54, 68, 88, 143, 146, 183, 184, 185, 246
cerebrospinal fluid, 46
chemical, 67, 68, 88, 189, 190, 191, 195, 199, 205, 207, 228, 231

chemokines, 10, 119, 253
chemoprevention, 30
chemotaxis, 10, 28
childhood, 115, 183
children, 89, 102, 113, 115, 116, 134, 186, 244
Chinese medicine, 125, 230
cholesterol, 18, 20, 30, 94, 127, 192, 244
chorea, 40, 41, 43, 60, 64, 65, 88, 90, 91, 92, 102, 127, 143, 161, 168, 171, 182, 187, 188, 204, 221, 243, 247, 248
chromosome, 44, 182, 183, 242
chronic diseases, 123, 144, 154, 197, 206, 261
chronic fatigue, 122, 123
chronic fatigue syndrome, 123
chronic illness, 252
clinical symptoms, 43, 89, 177
clinical trials, 40, 121, 144, 151, 153, 163, 188, 228, 247
CNS, 13, 19, 32, 35, 48, 53, 99, 100, 109, 110, 111, 112, 113, 114, 117, 219, 254
coenzyme, 142, 144, 156, 163
coenzyme Q10, 19, 142, 144, 145, 147, 155, 156, 158, 163
cognitive deficit, 8, 12, 16, 22, 28, 50, 157, 164
cognitive dysfunction, 24, 42, 43, 82, 178
cognitive flexibility, 162
cognitive function, 7, 12, 25, 33, 36, 40, 91, 171, 244
cognitive impairment, 40, 50, 64, 68, 84, 88, 119, 149, 162, 216, 217, 230
cognitive performance, 32, 233
colitis, 123, 198, 209
composition, 36, 67, 81, 108, 111, 117, 124, 135, 160, 177, 192, 193, 206, 207, 208
compounds, ix, 5, 6, 12, 16, 21, 24, 25, 51, 63, 67, 78, 80, 95, 101, 125, 142, 144, 151, 152, 153, 182, 188, 190, 197, 199, 201, 205, 212, 213, 221, 224, 225, 226, 227, 228, 230, 231

Index

compulsive behavior, 168, 241
condensation, 49, 76, 220, 223
constipation, 17, 96, 100, 112, 174
consumption, 4, 7, 10, 25, 30, 33, 56, 59, 68, 81, 97, 115, 120, 174
coordination, 2, 56, 65, 75, 118, 143, 148, 161
cortex, 44, 45, 54, 70, 72, 162, 219, 220
cortical neurons, 25, 64, 89
cortisol, 83, 110, 113, 122
crocetin, 21, 23, 24, 25
cultivation, 14, 33, 68
curcumin, vii, 9, 10, 11, 25, 26, 28, 30, 31, 34, 35, 37, 38, 53, 55, 56, 60, 69, 74, 77, 80, 82, 83, 94, 96, 142, 144, 146, 147, 148, 153, 154, 155, 156, 157, 158, 230, 233, 234, 251, 252, 256, 257, 258, 259, 260, 261, 262, 263, 264, 265, 266, 267
cure, 3, 63, 65, 88, 92, 122, 163, 240, 244, 246
cyclooxygenase, 10, 74, 259
cysteine, 74, 95, 220, 256
cytochrome, 49, 56, 73, 220, 255, 259, 263, 265, 267
cytochrome c, 73, 220, 255, 259
cytokines, 10, 49, 71, 109, 110, 114, 116, 119, 122, 220, 253, 254, 257, 258
cytosine-adenine- guanine (CAG) repeat, 44, 64, 66, 89, 143, 162, 163, 178, 182, 183, 187, 217, 242, 248
cytotoxicity, 12, 54, 60, 148, 149, 261, 263, 267

D

deep brain stimulation, 221, 243
defects, 46, 147, 156, 244
defence, 16, 70, 150
defense mechanisms, 3
deficit, 56, 72, 134, 148

dementia, 2, 8, 34, 41, 51, 119, 127, 161, 182, 183, 186, 217, 229, 244, 264
dendritic cell, 30
depression, 42, 50, 92, 111, 112, 122, 128, 137, 143, 170, 171, 182, 183, 188, 218, 233, 241, 243, 258
derivatives, 10, 18, 33, 52, 53, 190, 197, 209, 213, 230, 264
diabetes, 13, 18, 51, 53, 99, 109, 112, 132, 150, 197, 252
diabetic neuropathy, 151
diagnosis, 43, 116, 163, 166, 183, 186, 202
diagnostic markers, 163
diarrhea, 93, 100, 112, 116, 122, 123, 124, 134, 139, 221
diet, ix, 3, 20, 51, 52, 100, 106, 108, 126, 148, 166, 175, 204
dietary habits, 166
dietary intake, 20, 186, 229
dietary spice, 260
dietary supplementation, 17, 269
digestion, 93, 96, 99, 108, 167
disease gene, 202, 248, 249
disease model, 59, 80, 154, 155, 262
disease progression, 12, 40, 43, 49, 89, 90, 162, 163
diseases, x, 1, 2, 10, 11, 13, 27, 51, 53, 55, 69, 82, 90, 93, 94, 96, 106, 109, 129, 141, 142, 144, 149, 160, 166, 168, 172, 174, 178, 191, 197, 201, 216, 222, 228, 232, 240, 249, 252, 255, 257, 260, 269, 273
disorder, ix, 40, 43, 64, 68, 83, 88, 115, 118, 128, 134, 137, 142, 143, 160, 182, 183, 186, 187, 188, 201, 243, 246
distribution, 61, 132, 207
diversity, 129, 189, 190, 191, 262
DNA, 7, 10, 17, 20, 49, 76, 143, 163, 177, 183, 202, 218, 220, 232, 233, 255, 259, 262
DNA damage, 7, 17, 20, 233, 255, 259
DNA strand breaks, 218

dopamine, 6, 11, 23, 29, 31, 34, 47, 55, 65, 75, 90, 146, 150, 158, 178, 187, 221, 243, 246, 247, 258
dopamine agonist, 221, 243
dopamine antagonists, 221, 243, 246
dopaminergic, 6, 23, 31, 35, 50, 54, 90, 91, 118, 128, 135, 146, 245, 249
drosophila, 17, 27, 54, 66, 148, 153
drug discovery, 34, 190, 191, 205, 235, 241
drugs, 1, 3, 50, 51, 63, 90, 91, 144, 160, 163, 176, 187, 189, 190, 191, 198, 204, 205, 206, 212, 240, 246, 249
dyspepsia, 13, 26, 96, 100
dystonia, 43, 102, 162, 183, 188, 243, 245, 246

ethnic groups, 143, 182
etiology, 89, 116, 247
Europe, x, 64, 67, 103, 145, 182, 183, 192
excitotoxicity, 45, 46, 47, 49, 64, 65, 76, 81, 128, 220, 252, 253, 254, 255, 256, 261, 262, 264, 265, 266
expectorant, 21, 93, 224, 226, 227
experimental autoimmune encephalomyelitis, 133
exploitation, 201, 206
exposure, 76, 116, 124, 149, 168
extraction, 14, 35, 36
extracts, ix, 6, 12, 13, 18, 21, 22, 24, 31, 51, 58, 79, 98, 198, 205

E

electron, 46, 54, 65, 72, 74, 145, 149, 163, 229, 231
encephalomyelitis, 113, 133
energy, 45, 46, 49, 64, 108, 124, 145, 150, 154, 156, 158, 171, 255
enterochromaffin cells, 110, 119
environmental change, 166
environmental factors, 128
environmental stimuli, 108
environmental stress, 109, 112
enzymes, 3, 11, 16, 27, 45, 53, 65, 70, 74, 113, 122, 125, 190, 228, 229, 231, 234, 245, 253, 256, 257, 259
epigallocatechin 3-gallate (EGCG), 2, 6, 7, 8, 33, 56, 57, 70, 75, 76, 77, 79, 80, 142, 145, 152, 153, 157
epigenetic modification, ix
epilepsy, 142, 252, 258
epithelial cells, 110, 115, 258
epithelium, 111, 117, 120
equilibrium, 3, 165, 172, 177
ester, 34, 36, 199, 232
ethanol, 99, 200, 211

F

facial expression, 162, 216
facial muscles, 41
families, 40, 42, 144
family history, 43, 163
family members, xi
fatty acids, 95, 98, 101, 135, 144, 190, 193, 229
fermentable carbohydrates, 114
fermentation, 56, 67, 125, 149
flatulence, 93, 96, 100, 170, 173, 174
flavonoids, v, 16, 19, 30, 31, 52, 56, 63, 66, 67, 70, 74, 78, 81, 83, 95, 152, 194, 199, 207
food, ix, x, xi, 9, 27, 30, 31, 36, 42, 65, 69, 80, 93, 99, 100, 102, 106, 115, 131, 142, 144, 145, 160, 167, 168, 174, 192, 193, 205, 209, 229, 241, 252, 260
food additive, 9
food intake, 42, 131
food products, 65
free radicals, 3, 10, 46, 145, 150, 259
fruits, 14, 16, 51, 53, 63, 80, 97, 98, 99, 123, 160, 221
functional food, 38, 140, 160, 177, 206, 266

G

gastrointestinal tract, 129, 135
gene expression, 28, 48, 67, 76, 162
gene silencing, 54
genes, 31, 77, 84, 107, 118, 125, 141, 235
genetic disorders, 186
genetic mutations, 142
ginger, 9, 88, 93, 98, 101, 221
ginseng, 230, 234, 235
glial cells, 3, 48, 184, 252, 254, 266
glucose, 3, 5, 18, 23, 45, 115, 130, 258
glucose tolerance, 115
glutamate, 23, 29, 45, 48, 49, 64, 68, 75, 85, 91, 178, 221, 230, 243, 252, 253, 254, 255, 257, 262, 263, 264, 265
glutamine, 20, 44, 54, 64, 79, 89, 162, 164, 184
glutathione, 3, 8, 20, 23, 35, 56, 70, 73, 74, 78, 82, 118, 147, 152, 253
grape-derived polyphenols, 58
growth, 9, 25, 28, 36, 49, 79, 118, 136, 161, 196, 200, 211, 257
growth factor, 49, 118, 257
gut brain axis, 109, 131

H

healing, ix, 93, 98, 225
health, 1, 4, 9, 20, 24, 33, 67, 88, 93, 94, 97, 106, 107, 119, 120, 127, 128, 137, 144, 166, 168, 176, 183, 244, 270
health effects, 127, 244
health promotion, 33
heart disease, 96, 197
heart failure, 185
herbal medicine, 40, 51
hippocampus, 8, 23, 44, 68, 70
histone, 117, 125, 128, 135, 149
histone deacetylase, 117, 128, 135, 149
history, 43, 51, 60, 93, 116, 143, 160, 191, 205, 229, 230, 232, 240
homeostasis, 3, 45, 47, 108, 253, 254, 256, 263
human, 2, 13, 28, 36, 51, 66, 89, 93, 101, 106, 107, 109, 110, 126, 129, 132, 138, 139, 144, 152, 164, 165, 184, 187, 190, 197, 198, 199, 200, 220, 222, 229, 236, 252, 258, 265
human body, 106, 107, 165
human brain, 13
human development, 184
human genome, 107
human health, 2, 152, 190
human neutrophils, 198, 199
huntingtin (HTT) protein, x, 45, 66, 143, 147, 162, 184, 202, 242, 253
Huntington's Disease, vi, 88, 102, 141, 142, 155, 179, 181, 182, 187, 202, 203, 236, 242, 247, 248, 253, 260, 262, 273

I

immune activation, 233
immune modulation, 227
immune regulation, 108
immune response, 110, 114, 120, 130
immune system, 107, 108, 110, 116, 120, 139
in vitro, 6, 7, 28, 33, 34, 102, 124, 138, 153, 199, 236, 261
in vivo, 7, 8, 28, 33, 38, 53, 138, 198, 267
India, 1, 10, 13, 37, 39, 63, 67, 69, 87, 88, 94, 95, 96, 98, 99, 101, 105, 106, 141, 159, 160, 181, 193, 198, 200, 201, 206, 208, 215, 228, 230, 239, 240, 241, 251, 270, 271
infection, 48, 96, 111, 114, 123, 138
inflammation, 8, 10, 24, 36, 48, 54, 81, 88, 90, 100, 113, 117, 118, 119, 124, 130,

135, 137, 146, 149, 158, 171, 176, 198, 219, 222, 228, 245, 252, 260, 272
inflammatory bowel disease, 109, 139
inflammatory disease, 122, 200
inflammatory mediators, 136, 220
inflammatory responses, 116, 136
ingestion, 57, 59, 120
ingredients, ix, 80, 84, 206
inherited disorder, 63, 246
injury, iv, 29, 34, 55, 64, 68, 85, 151, 163, 219, 245, 258
insomnia, 17, 92, 188, 221
intestine, 107, 108, 116, 127
intracellular calcium, 76, 252
irritable bowel syndrome, 131, 134, 140

K

kabam, 160, 165, 166, 168, 172
kidneys, 10, 252
kynurenine pathway, 65

L

lactate dehydrogenase, 73
lactate level, 45, 146, 219
lactic acid, 120, 122
large intestine, 127
lipid peroxidation, 6, 7, 13, 20, 24, 27, 28, 30, 72, 73, 74, 78, 102, 147, 218, 234
lipids, 20, 67, 192, 193, 207, 218, 231, 232, 255
liquid chromatography, 35
liver, 10, 20, 27, 91, 97, 147, 155, 198, 252
liver cells, 155
liver disease, 147
liver enzymes, 91
loss of appetite, 96, 169
low-grade inflammation, 117
lycopene, 21, 22, 70, 72, 82, 222

M

macrophage, , 3, 122, 125, 198, 200, 219, 258, 263
macrophage inflammatory protein, 258
macular degeneration, 19, 21, 32, 229
malnutrition, 172, 177
marine environment, 182, 189, 200
medical, ix, 26, 81, 93, 157, 160, 164, 177, 179, 180, 240, 241
medication, 90, 103, 248
medicine, 11, 13, 30, 51, 53, 69, 93, 94, 96, 98, 99, 120, 144, 146, 160, 165, 166, 176, 179, 203, 204, 229, 230, 235, 244, 252, 260
memory, 7, 8, 11, 12, 13, 15, 21, 24, 29, 70, 74, 78, 96, 102, 109, 113, 162, 167, 186, 221, 225, 228, 231, 241, 243, 244, 245
memory performance, 70, 78
mental health, 94, 244, 247
metabolism, 27, 47, 54, 55, 58, 106, 107, 108, 112, 118, 119, 122, 124, 129, 150, 156, 158, 179, 234, 244, 255
metabolites, 8, 28, 51, 54, 56, 75, 114, 127, 190, 191, 196, 199, 201, 205, 209, 223
mice, 6, 7, 8, 21, 23, 29, 32, 34, 35, 36, 38, 54, 66, 68, 84, 102, 111, 113, 118, 123, 124, 133, 137, 138, 139, 146, 147, 148, 150, 156, 178, 232, 234, 236, 253, 264
microbial communities, 107, 132
microbiome, 106, 107, 109, 110, 111, 112, 113, 114, 115, 116, 119, 120, 121, 124, 126, 128, 129, 130, 133
microbiota, 106, 107, 108, 110, 111, 112, 113, 114, 115, 116, 117, 118, 119, 122, 124, 129, 130, 131, 132, 134, 135, 136, 138, 139, 188
microorganisms, 106, 107, 108, 111, 120, 122, 127, 131, 234
mitochondria, 3, 45, 47, 49, 65, 73, 150, 157, 218, 260, 261, 262, 263, 267

mitochondrial damage, 128
mitochondrial DNA, 46, 47, 235
mitochondrial dysfunction, x, 2, 40, 45, 64, 84, 88, 145, 148, 151, 154, 157, 203, 218, 219, 231, 233, 236, 237, 248, 260, 265
mitochondrial toxins, 219
models of HD, 63, 65, 149, 151, 153
molecular biology, 107
molecular mimicry, 136
molecular weight, 196, 197
monocyte chemoattractant protein, 258
monocyte chemoattractant protein-1, 258
monoterpenoids, 223, 231
movement disorders, 127, 128, 161, 202, 234, 243

N

nerve, 11, 54, 63, 68, 72, 88, 98, 109, 114, 116, 182, 236
nerve growth factor, 68
nervous system, 2, 13, 55, 88, 93, 108, 109, 115, 116, 131, 132, 142, 210, 236
neurodegeneration, 2, 20, 44, 45, 47, 51, 64, 65, 81, 89, 112, 123, 132, 136, 139, 146, 147, 157, 163, 203, 235, 244, 252, 254, 255, 258, 261, 262
neurodegenerative diseases, ii, 2, 4, 19, 27, 33, 51, 53, 57, 106, 112, 119, 124, 126, 128, 130, 141, 142, 146, 158, 163, 183, 203, 216, 229, 237, 240, 243, 255, 258, 259, 260, 261, 263, 269, 273
neurodegenerative disorders, 1, 2, 20, 24, 35, 58, 88, 117, 141, 144, 153, 157, 178, 231, 235, 263, 265
neurogenesis, 33, 184, 204, 252
neuroinflammation, 2, 78, 119, 219
neurological disease, 47, 55, 96, 102, 112, 121, 147, 150, 160, 168, 171, 172, 173, 175, 182, 219, 258, 260, 269

neuromotor, 148
neuronal apoptosis, 82, 153, 155, 158, 255, 266
neuronal cells, 255, 256
neuronal density, 12
neurons, 2, 3, 7, 10, 13, 17, 20, 26, 36, 44, 45, 47, 48, 49, 60, 64, 89, 110, 118, 123, 128, 131, 135, 142, 149, 150, 153, 157, 161, 162, 183, 184, 218, 220, 230, 242, 252, 253, 254, 256, 257, 258, 262, 263, 264
neuropathic pain, 258
neuropathy, 76, 96
neuropharmacology, 264
neuroprotection, v, 1, 2, 3, 6, 7, 12, 15, 19, 22, 25, 31, 35, 40, 54, 60, 71, 72, 75, 85, 149, 156, 158, 252, 257, 262
neuroscience, 33, 130, 263, 264, 270, 271
neurosurgery, 102
neurotoxicity, 6, 12, 20, 23, 24, 25, 26, 36, 37, 60, 65, 70, 72, 82, 83, 84, 146, 148, 149, 156, 157, 158, 163, 229, 232, 234, 235, 237
neurotransmission, 84, 90, 91, 150
neurotransmitters, 11, 60, 68, 81, 113, 114, 134, 240, 252
neurotrophic factors, 118, 128, 220
New Zealand, 198, 199, 200, 209, 210, 211
nitric oxide, 2, 3, 7, 25, 27, 31, 46, 72, 74, 81, 82, 119, 200, 220, 262, 264
nitric oxide synthase, 7, 74
nitrite, 71, 72, 73, 74, 75, 78
NMDA receptors, 47, 65, 248, 253, 254, 256, 264, 267
N-methyl-D-aspartic acid, 187
non-steroidal anti-inflammatory drugs, 10
Nrf2, 7, 74, 78, 83, 152, 253
nuclei, 43, 44, 76, 261
nucleus, 44, 49, 53, 110, 116, 218, 242, 266
nutraceutical, 138, 154, 190
nutrients, 120, 172, 194, 208
nutrition, ix, 1, 30, 51, 111, 140, 190, 205

Index

nutritive value, 106, 182, 191, 192, 193

O

obesity, 18, 112, 252
oil, 8, 9, 55, 95, 97, 98, 230, 231
olanzapine, 50, 92, 204
oligomers, 38, 79, 267
oral ayurvedic medicines, 245
oral health, 38
organ, 55, 108, 142, 152
organelles, 3, 49, 242
orthostatic hypotension, 221
oxidation, 3, 10, 29, 56, 149, 155, 261, 264
oxidative damage, 23, 78, 118, 144, 198, 218, 229, 232, 233, 257
oxidative stress, x, 2, 3, 6, 7, 12, 16, 18, 19, 24, 25, 27, 29, 32, 33, 34, 35, 37, 40, 46, 49, 54, 56, 71, 74, 77, 78, 81, 88, 112, 117, 122, 123, 141, 144, 145, 148, 150, 151, 153, 157, 203, 216, 218, 229, 232, 233, 236, 252, 255, 257, 259, 260, 266

P

paanikamba vaatham, 169
pain, 96, 100, 109, 134, 171, 173, 174, 245
paneth cells, 110
Parkinson's Disease (PD), 2, 6, 10, 26, 116, 117, 118, 129, 138, 232, 244
pathogenesis, 10, 29, 66, 82, 102, 128, 144, 145, 156, 202, 203, 219, 237, 263
pathogens, 117, 120, 122, 125, 139
pathology, 10, 12, 28, 37, 44, 64, 81, 134, 135, 138, 161, 202, 203, 220, 243
pathophysiology, x, 139, 161, 232, 235, 242, 248
peptide, 7, 12, 28, 34, 37, 60, 110, 111, 112, 190, 196, 201, 211, 212, 213, 255
peripheral blood, 17, 199
peripheral blood mononuclear cell, 17

peripheral neuropathy, 18
pharmacological agents, 100, 144
pharmacological treatment, 235, 243, 248
pharmacotherapy, 202, 216, 221
phenolic compounds, 13, 100, 199, 207
phosphate, 46, 229, 234
phospholipids, 10, 43, 95, 193, 207
phosphorus, 127, 139, 192
phosphorylation, 8, 48, 152, 256, 257, 264, 266
phylum, 108, 192
physiology, 107, 110, 112, 235
pitham, 160, 165, 166
plants, 31, 51, 53, 68, 80, 93, 101, 123, 216, 221, 228, 232, 234, 240
pneumonia, 217, 242
potassium, 19, 101, 192
prebiotics, vi, 105, 106, 120, 124, 125, 126, 127, 136, 137, 138, 139, 140
probiotic, vi, 105, 106, 120, 121, 122, 123, 124, 126, 127, 128, 130, 133, 136, 137, 139, 140
progenitor cell, 138
progressive neurodegenerative disorder, 127
pro-inflammatory, 71, 74, 75, 109, 116, 117, 119, 122, 219
proliferation, 10, 25, 79, 123, 126, 138
prostaglandins, 10, 95, 220
prostate cancer, 94, 273
protection, 25, 34, 51, 54, 73, 113, 126, 142, 145, 148, 150, 151, 229, 231
protective mechanisms, 28
protein kinase C, 31, 257
protein kinases, 257
proteins, 2, 7, 44, 47, 49, 58, 77, 79, 113, 118, 141, 153, 190, 192, 194, 218, 232, 253, 254, 255, 256, 264
psychiatric disorder, 40, 68, 161, 229, 252
psychiatric illness, 131
psychiatric symptoms, 42, 186
psychological problems, 161, 240
psychological stress, 133

psychopharmacology, 204
psychotic symptoms, 50

Q

quinolinic acid, 77, 78, 81, 82, 83, 148, 233
quinone, 74, 145, 197

R

radical formation, 67
radicals, 3, 122, 259
reactive oxygen, 3, 13, 46, 49, 65, 218, 264, 267
red wine, 149
relief, 40, 50, 94, 144, 176, 240
researchers, 1, 108, 115, 126, 160, 182, 189, 191, 271, 272
respiration, 77, 82, 83, 219, 261
response, 28, 47, 72, 83, 92, 98, 113, 115, 119, 133, 148, 219, 220, 263
responsiveness, 112, 115
restoration, 142, 154
resveratrol, 53, 54, 58, 59, 60, 142, 145, 148, 149, 150, 151, 153, 155, 156, 157, 158
ribonucleotide reductase, 31
risk, 2, 10, 18, 47, 94, 102, 144, 163, 178, 183, 186, 203
risk factors, 242

S

schizophrenia, 12, 68, 83, 189, 229
science, 30, 93, 102, 165, 241, 271
scientific understanding, 58
secondary symptoms, 42
seed, 15, 58, 94, 101, 221
sensory symptoms, 186
serotonin, 11, 31, 75, 111, 113, 114, 132

sexual behavior, 185, 186
Siddha System of Medicine, vi, 164, 165, 166
Siddhars, 164
side effects, 3, 50, 91, 92, 94, 144, 163, 176, 187, 188, 221, 240
signal transduction, 131
signaling pathway, 16, 25, 47, 53, 59, 110, 114, 155, 158, 255, 259
skeletal muscle, 46, 89, 182
skin, 14, 94, 96, 149, 166, 169
sleep disorders, 50, 249
sleep disturbance, 171, 178
smooth muscle cells, 110
sodium, 91, 103, 117, 192
species, 3, 13, 49, 65, 66, 67, 99, 107, 108, 113, 117, 124, 128, 133, 138, 148, 189, 190, 192, 199, 210, 218, 228, 229, 252, 264, 267
speech, 90, 162, 167, 170, 186, 187, 244
spices, v, ix, 33, 87, 88, 92, 93, 94, 98, 99, 101, 221
spinal cord, 2, 89, 109, 117, 142
spinal cord injury, 109
starch polysaccharides, 124
sterols, 12, 190, 207, 228, 231
stomach, 93, 98, 100, 171
stress, 2, 16, 20, 24, 25, 27, 29, 32, 46, 47, 60, 68, 74, 84, 94, 110, 112, 113, 122, 131, 133, 146, 149, 151, 153, 216, 218, 220, 229, 244, 249, 252, 255, 258, 259
stress response, 113, 133
stressors, 109
striatum, 29, 44, 45, 54, 64, 70, 71, 73, 77, 84, 89, 147, 162, 184, 218, 220, 231, 233
stroke, 20, 23, 29, 37, 68, 96, 109, 197
survival, 20, 31, 33, 60, 76, 126, 142, 151, 153, 155, 158, 162, 249, 256
survival rate, 151
swelling, 49, 72, 167, 245
swollen glands, 94
symptomatic treatment, 92

symptoms, 10, 11, 26, 40, 41, 42, 43, 50, 51, 54, 65, 75, 78, 82, 89, 90, 106, 118, 121, 123, 137, 143, 144, 148, 149, 161, 164, 168, 171, 177, 183, 184, 185, 186, 187, 202, 216, 217, 219, 221, 232, 240, 241, 243, 246, 248
synaptic plasticity, 47, 233, 252
synaptic transmission, 150, 162
synbiotics, vi, 105, 106, 120, 126, 127, 137, 138, 139, 140
syndrome, 42, 115, 116, 122, 123, 188
synthesis, 3, 6, 45, 46, 49, 68, 108, 113

T

tannins, 13, 14, 16, 52, 53, 199
tardive dyskinesia, 43, 252
therapeutic agents, 96, 153, 189, 216, 247, 273
therapeutic benefits, 92, 154
therapeutic effect, 55, 95, 140, 144, 146, 153, 228
therapeutics, 34, 59, 81, 88, 177, 231
therapy, 30, 37, 50, 68, 83, 91, 92, 93, 102, 137, 144, 164, 177, 187, 233, 246, 260
tissue, 6, 48, 61, 77, 146, 219, 220
tissue homeostasis, 48
tonic, 11, 93, 99, 244
toxic effect, 54, 149, 172, 184
toxic metals, 151
toxicity, 12, 20, 25, 31, 46, 55, 59, 60, 71, 75, 79, 80, 135, 150, 155, 158, 184, 242, 244, 252, 260
toxicology, 243
toxin, 65, 122, 137, 145, 267
transcription, 10, 28, 34, 48, 125, 135, 162, 184, 203, 216, 253, 254, 255, 256, 257
transcription factors, 125, 253, 255, 256, 257
transplantation, 203, 221, 243

transport, 54, 113, 145, 146, 149, 163, 229, 231
treatment, 1, 3, 8, 11, 13, 20, 23, 24, 26, 29, 35, 50, 51, 54, 70, 71, 72, 73, 74, 75, 76, 77, 78, 79, 90, 91, 92, 93, 94, 96, 97, 100, 102, 113, 120, 122, 123, 124, 127, 133, 134, 139, 143, 145, 146, 148, 149, 150, 151, 153, 155, 158, 160, 163, 164, 165, 176, 179, 182, 187, 188, 200, 202, 204, 216, 222, 229, 230, 231, 235, 237, 240, 243, 246, 247, 248, 252, 253, 255, 258, 260, 261, 264
trial, 26, 90, 91, 92, 102, 140, 144, 145, 179, 233
tumor, 54, 55, 138, 139, 200, 234, 253, 254, 259
tumor cells, 259
tumor growth, 200
tumor necrosis factor, 200, 253, 254
tumor progression, 138
turmeric, 9, 24, 26, 28, 37, 55, 63, 65, 69, 80, 88, 93, 94, 96, 101, 146, 221, 230, 233, 252, 260
tyrosine, 7, 23, 245, 257, 266
tyrosine hydroxylase, 23, 245

U

ubiquitin, 2, 45, 116, 144
ubiquitin-proteasome system, 2, 45

V

vaatham, 160, 165, 166, 167, 168, 169, 170, 171, 172, 173, 174, 175
vagus nerve, 117, 137
vegetables, 20, 51, 67, 80, 123, 160, 175
vitamin A, 19
vitamin B2, 21
vitamin C, 13, 14, 18, 29, 30, 67, 101
vitamin E, 19, 50, 150, 247, 259

vitamin K, 108
vitamins, ix, 26, 67, 95, 122, 192, 194, 207

worldwide, 10, 56, 64, 96, 99, 100, 178, 183, 222

W

water, 11, 22, 53, 56, 70, 152, 160, 165, 167, 174, 175, 194, 205, 244
weight gain, 92
weight loss, 42, 143, 182, 183, 186, 216, 242
wetlands, 228, 231

Y

yeast, 57, 79, 196

α

α-lipoic acid, 18, 20, 25, 142, 145, 151